Essentials of MRI Safety

T0201247

Essentials of MRI Safety

Donald W. McRobbie, PhD

Associate Professor, Discipline of Medical Physics
School of Physical Sciences
University of Adelaide
Adelaide, Australia

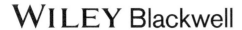

Registered Office(s)
John Wiley & Sons, Inc., 111 River Street, Hoboken, NJ 07030, USA
John Wiley & Sons Ltd, The Atrium, Southern Gate, Chichester, West Sussex, PO19 8SQ, UK

Editorial Office
9600 Garsington Road, Oxford, OX4 2DQ, UK

For details of our global editorial offices, customer services, and more information about Wiley products visit us at www.wiley.com.

Wiley also publishes its books in a variety of electronic formats and by print-on-demand. Some content that appears in standard print versions of this book may not be available in other formats.

Library of Congress Cataloging-in-Publication Data

Names: McRobbie, Donald W., 1958– author.
Title: Essentials of MRI safety / Donald W. McRobbie, PhD, Associate
    Professor, Discipline of Medical Physics, School of Physical Sciences,
    University of Adelaide, Adelaide, South Australia, Australia.
Description: First edition. I Hoboken : Wiley-Blackwell, 2020. I Includes
    bibliographical references and index.
Identifiers: LCCN 2020003790 (print) I LCCN 2020003791 (ebook) I ISBN
    9781119557173 (paperback) I ISBN 9781119557166 (adobe pdf) I ISBN
    9781119557159 (epub)
Subjects: LCSH: Magnetic resonance imaging–Health aspects. I Magnetic
    resonance imaging–Safety measures. I Magnetic resonance
    imaging–Standards.
Classification: LCC RC78.7.N83 M38 2020 (print) I LCC RC78.7.N83 (ebook)
    I DDC 616.07/548–dc23
LC record available at https://lccn.loc.gov/2020003790
LC ebook record available at https://lccn.loc.gov/2020003791

Cover Design: Wiley
Cover Images: (clockwise) Courtesy of Donald McRobbie, © Elsevier,
© yojunior24/Shutterstock, © metamorworks/Shutterstock

Set in 10/12pt TradeGothic by SPi Global, Pondicherry, India

SKY10070022_041124

Contents

Contents

Foreword: essentials

In recent years MRI safety has received increased media attention amidst growing public concern. From controversies over the use and side-effects of gadolinium to projectile accidents, a serious adverse MRI event always makes news. It doesn't have to. It is possible to practice completely without incident, as long as you understand the *essence* of MRI safety.

I started my career at the University of Aberdeen investigating the biological effects of magnetic fields because, even back in 1981, the safety of MRI was already on the scientific agenda. Since then there have been innumerable technical and clinical advances, but some of our MRI safety practice has not developed at the same rate. Often departmental practices and individual beliefs (I can't say "knowledge") are based more upon historical custom and hearsay than upon science. This book aims to place MRI safety practice firmly on a scientific basis, equipping you to recognize and assess potential risk and also its absence.

What about all the maths? Surely we don't need it? We do. It is essential because MRI safety without a solid theoretical and numerical foundation is just guesswork, folklore or worse. If you are allergic to maths, then you may be relieved to learn that all the difficult material is contained in Chapter 2 and the appendices. The other chapters contain the minimum of theory necessary to attain an understanding of each topic, and much of the maths is restricted to illustrative numerical examples. I have avoided complex electromagnetic (EM) modeling and complex algebra. All the examples can be solved approximately using simple "back of an envelope" calculations. Whilst this lacks the rigor or accuracy of EM modeling or solving Maxwell's equations, it provides insight into how physical parameters relate to safety issues. Examples are purely illustrative, but should be sufficient for readers to identify and make estimates of risk.

This book is also written in the context of the MRI safety roles: MR Medical Director (MRMD), MR Safety Officer (MRSO), and MR Safety Expert (MRSE). In order to develop the required knowledge for these roles, each chapter contains revision questions for self-assessment, one hundred in total. Beware: some of the questions have multiple correct answers. For the aspiring MRSE every chapter, including the appendices, is essential. For the other roles and for the general readership of MR practitioners more selective reading is possible. Use of the Further reading and resources at the end of each chapter is highly recommended and, in some instances, essential as they contain authoritative sources, reviews, guidance, and standards.

Finally, a word of caution and a disclaimer. This book does not provide definitive guidance on the scanning of individual patients with specific implants. For that you must adhere to the most current implant information and observe the MRI conditions, conducting benefit versus risk analyses if required, and with appropriate clinical authorization. Neither does the book endorse any specific practice over and above adhering to MRI implant conditions, pharmaceutical labeling, available professional body guidance, standards, and exposure limits.

Acknowledgments

I would like to thank colleagues and friends who have helped me on this MRI safety journey, with the kind provision of materials, or with the production of this book. These include Gregory Brown, Anastasia Papadaki, Frank Shellock, Marc Agzarian, Jeff Hand, Stephen Keevil, Denise Newsom, Adam Waldman, Catriona Todd, Amrish Mehta, Frank de Vocht, Kristel Schaap, Nick Ferris, Emanuel Kanal, Titti Owman, Miles Capstick, Niels Kuster, Kjell Hansson-Mild, John Powell, Thomas Vaughan, Wellesley Were, Kelly Parker, Daniel Zappia, David Price, Marc Rea, Rebecca Quest, Irving Weinberg, Gary Liney, Anneke Cox, Dawn Phillips-Jarrett, Julian Byrne, Jessica Driscoll, Celine Duraffourd, Eike Davis, Antoine Daridon, Helen Estall, Colin Robertson, Nicola Baker, Dan Krainak, Simon Grant, Zoltan Nagy, Eugenio Mattei, Kawin Setsompop, Stephen Wastling. My thanks also go to James Watson, Tom Marriott, Baskar Anandraj and Sonali Melwani at Wiley, Mary Malin at Transtype for copy-editing, and to the team at Wiley for bringing the book to production. Finally I am indebted to my original University of Aberdeen supervisors from whom I learned so much and who set me on this journey: Meg Foster and the late Jim Hutchison in whose memory the book is dedicated. As ever my gratitude to Kathryn, Laura, and Andrew for encouragement and support.

In memoria James Hutchison 1940–2018

1

Systems and safety: MR hardware and fields

INTRODUCTION

Magnetic resonance imaging (MRI) has grown, from its initial development in the late 1970s to early 1980s, to become one of the most utilized diagnostic imaging modalities. In 2015 there were 103 million MR examinations performed in hospitals from a population of 1.1 billion people in 29 developed countries. A total of 33 000 scanners were in use in 36 countries serving a combined population of 1.7 billion [1].

The two greatest advantages of MRI are its superior soft tissue discrimination compared to X-rays or CT, and a lack of exposure to ionizing radiation. MRI uses a combination of magnetic fields of varying frequencies: radiofrequency in the megahertz (MHz) region; audio or "very low frequencies" (VLF) up to tens of kilohertz (kHz); and a static field (zero hertz). None of these possesses sufficiently localized concentrations of electromagnetic (EM) energy to damage atoms, molecules, or cells (Figure 1.1). The risk of cancer induction from magnetic field exposures encountered in MRI is quite possibly zero – unlike X-rays, CT, mammography, or the radioactive tracers used in nuclear medicine. This makes MRI very attractive for serial examinations, for scans of children whose tissues are more sensitive to the ionizing radiation used in alternative modalities, or for research studies on groups of healthy volunteers.

So, is MRI safe?

Obviously not, or there would be no need for this book. Whilst later chapters will show that MRI is relatively benign from a biological point of view, the *practice* of MRI may involve significant risk to the patient and to others present during the examination. The MRI examination room is potentially the most hazardous environment within the radiology department because of the possibility of catastrophic and fatal accidents where practice is poor or where safety protocols are not fully observed or understood.

Nowhere is this better illustrated than in the tragic case of a six-year old boy who in 2001 was struck by an oxygen tank which had flown into the scanner, later dying from his injuries. This prompted a root and branches review of MR safety practice within the USA by the American College of Radiology [2] leading to a series of recommendations. It is concerning, that even today, not all these recommendations are routinely followed in every institution. In a 10-year review of MRI-related incidents reported to the US Food and Drug Administration (FDA) 59% were thermal (excessive heating, burns), 11% mechanical (cuts, fractures, slips, falls, crush and lifting injuries), 9% from projectiles, and 6% acoustic (hearing loss) [3] (Figure 1.2).

Essentials of MRI Safety, First Edition. Donald W. McRobbie.
© 2020 John Wiley & Sons Ltd. Published 2020 by John Wiley & Sons Ltd.

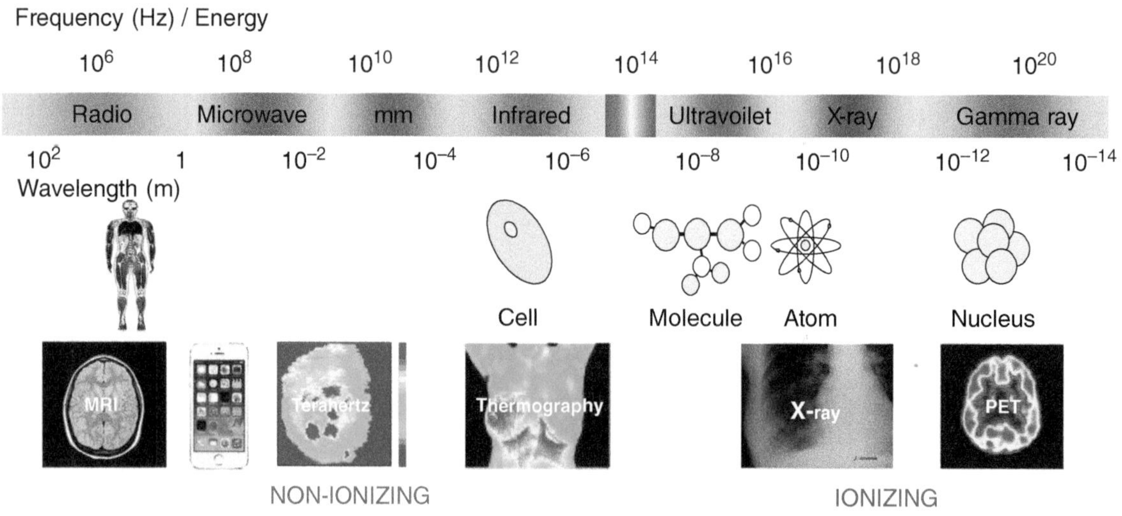

Frequency (Hz) / Energy

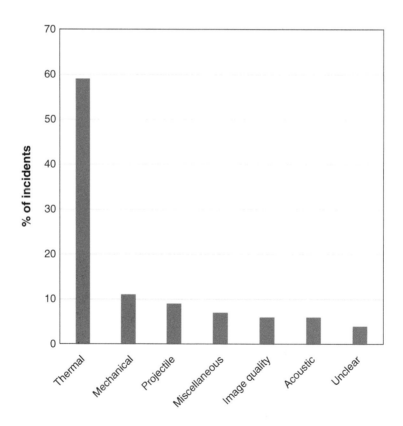

Figure 1.1   The electromagnetic spectrum showing frequency and wavelength of radiations, relative scale, and applications.

Figure 1.2   MRI adverse events reported to the FDA. Data from [3].

   A significant source of risk from MRI arises when patients have implants, particularly active implanted medical devices (AIMDs), such as cardiac pacemakers or neuro-stimulators. However, whereas a decade ago, custom might have been pre-cautionary – not to scan these patients, modern practice is moving towards finding ways to scan whenever there may be significant benefit to the patient. This requires that all MR practitioners have a deeper understanding of the possible interactions between the device, human tissues, and the scanner, and of MR safety in general. That is the purpose of this book, to ensure all MR practitioners have sufficient knowledge to practise safely for the benefit of their patients.

OVERVIEW OF MRI OPERATION

MRI relies upon the properties of nuclear magnetism. The nucleus of an atom consists of subatomic particles: electrically neutral neutrons and positively charged protons. In an atom the electrical charge of the protons is usually balanced by the negative charge of the surrounding electron cloud. MRI concerns the nucleus of hydrogen, mainly as it occurs in water and fat molecules.

Nuclear magnetic resonance

Hydrogen is the simplest element in the universe with the atomic number of one, meaning its nucleus possesses a single proton. The proton is said to exhibit a property known as *spin*. The consequences of spin only become observable in an externally applied magnetic field (denoted B_0) in which the proton spins *precess*, like spinning tops or gyroscopes, around the direction of B_0. In the external field the proton spins must adhere to specific energy levels or quantum basis states (Figure 1.3a). A slight imbalance between the populations of these results in a net magnetization, M_0 (Figure 1.3b). M_0 can be manipulated by applying the appropriate frequency (or energy) of electromagnetic radiation. This is the *Larmor* or *resonance frequency*:

$$f_0 = \gamma B_0 \tag{1.1}$$

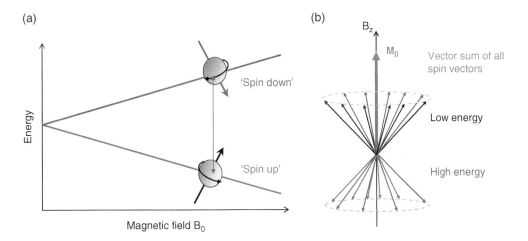

Figure 1.3   Nuclear magnetism: (a) basis state energy differences; (b) formation of macroscopic magnetization M_0 from the sum of basis state spin vectors.

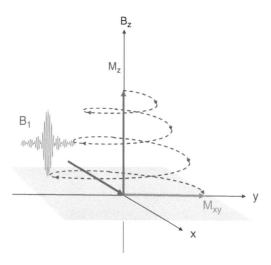

Figure 1.4   Excitation of the macroscopic magnetization **M** by the B_1 RF field.

where the subscript "0" means "at resonance". $\bar{\gamma}$ ("gamma bar") is the *gyromagnetic* ratio of the hydrogen nucleus. When frequency f is expressed in MHz and B_0 in tesla, $\bar{\gamma}$ has a value of approximately 42.58 MHz T^{-1}. This simple relationship underpins all of MRI.

The radiofrequency energy is applied as a magnetic field B_1 orthogonal to the direction of B_0 (Figure 1.4). Whilst B_1 is present the magnetization precesses around both B_0 and B_1 directions, tipping away from the z-axis (usually head–foot) of the scanner. B_1 is applied in a short burst as a RF pulse. The angle of deflection away from the z-axis is known as the flip angle α. For a simple rectangular shaped RF pulse this is

$$\alpha = \gamma B_1 t_p \qquad (1.2)$$

where t_p is the duration of the pulse (in seconds), B_1 is the amplitude of the "excitation" pulse (in tesla), and $\gamma = 2\pi \times \bar{\gamma}$ (2.68×10^8 radians s^{-1}).

Example 1.1 B_1 amplitude

What B_1 amplitude is required for a 1 ms rectangular shaped RF pulse to produce a flip angle of 90°?

Express α in radians ($= \frac{\pi}{2}$). From Equation 1.2

$$B_1 = \frac{\alpha}{\gamma t_p} = \frac{0.5 \times \pi}{2.68 \times 10^8 \times 0.001} = 5.9\,\mu T$$

Once excited, the magnetization recovers towards its initial equilibrium value M_0 by two independent relaxation processes: T_1 *relaxation* restores the longitudinal or z-component of magnetization towards M_0; T_2 *relaxation* causes the transverse component, the *signal*, to decay to zero. T_1 and T_2 *relaxation times* vary by tissue type and exhibit changes due to pathology, often increasing where disease or injury is present.

Image formation

Image formation is achieved by varying the value of magnetic field in the z- or B_0 direction. The field variation is applied by passing electrical pulses through one or more sets of *gradient coils*, forming the gradient pulses. The gradients, known as G_x, G_y, G_z, are designed to produce linear variations in the z-component of the magnetic field with respect to the x, y, and z axes (Figure 1.5). In terms of their function in image formation they are known as slice-select (G_{SS}), phase-encode (G_{PE}), or frequency-encode (G_{FE}).

Slice selection

By applying a narrow bandwidth B_1 pulse, shaped to include a limited range of frequencies, simultaneously with the slice select gradient G_{SS}, the excitation region is restricted to a narrow slice of the patient's anatomy with a width or thickness:

$$sw = \frac{\Delta f}{\gamma G_{SS}} \qquad (1.3)$$

The slice thickness can be controlled by changing the amplitude of the slice-select gradient or by changing the bandwidth of the RF pulse. The slice orientation can be selected by using different gradient coils (or a combination of coils for oblique views). By changing the RF frequency images may be acquired as a series of 2D multiple slices at different locations (Figure 1.6).

In-plane localization

The localization of the MR signal within a slice is usually achieved by two processes: phase-encoding (PE) and frequency-encoding (FE), each using gradient pulses along orthogonal directions. These pulses encode the MR signal in terms of spatial frequencies. Image acquisition requires multiple repetitions of the basic block of a *pulse sequence* using a different amplitude

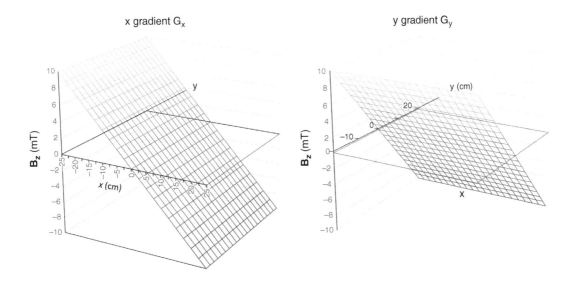

Figure 1.5 B_z from magnetic field gradients G_x and G_y.

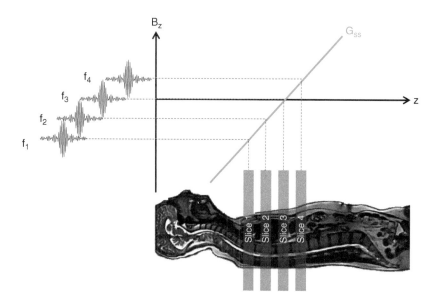

Figure 1.6 Multiple slice imaging. Changing the frequency of each RF pulse whilst a gradient G_{ss} is applied selects a different slice position.

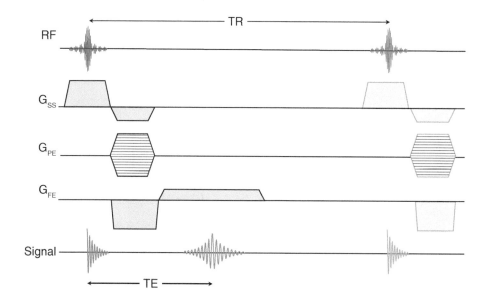

Figure 1.7 Simple 2D gradient echo (GRE) pulse sequence showing pulse amplitudes and timings of the components.

of PE pulse each time (Figure 1.7). TR is the time interval between successive repetitions. Image reconstruction is achieved by the mathematical operation of a two-dimensional (2D) Fourier transform.

The application of a second set of PE gradients in conjunction with the selection of a thicker slab of tissue makes three-dimensional (3D) imaging possible (Figure 1.8).

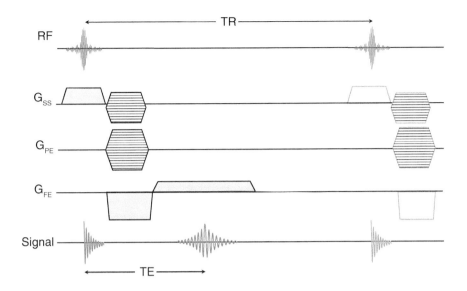

Figure 1.8 **3D imaging sequence with a second phase-encode gradient in the slab direction.**

Pulse sequences

A clinical scanner has many different pulse sequences available, broadly designated as either *gradient echo* (GRE) or *spin echo* (SE). In GRE (e.g. Figure 1.7) each signal collected arises from a low flip angle RF pulse, typically less than 40°. T_1-weighted images are generated using so-called spoiled gradient echo. Rewound GRE uses slightly higher flip angles (>40°), producing bright-fluid images, popular in cardiac MRI. GRE images are shown in Figure 1.9.

The SE sequence was initially developed for its ability to recover signal loss arising from B_0 inhomogeneities. These occur across the field-of-view (FOV) as dephasing, or "fanning out", of transverse components of the magnetization (Figure 1.10) following a 90° pulse. By applying a 180° pulse orthogonal to the 90° pulse (and also to B_0), the fan of magnetization vectors is twisted around in such a way that those with a phase lag advance in phase and vice-versa. At time TE, equal to twice the interval between the 90° and 180° pulses, the magnetization rephases, giving a strong echo whose magnitude depends upon the tissue T_2.

Spin echo can be further enhanced by using multiple 180° pulses to form a series or train of echoes, each of which can have different phase-encoding applied. In Turbo or Fast Spin Echo (TSE/FSE) the overall scan time is reduced by the echo train length (ETL) or Turbo-factor (TF). Typical ETL/TFs are in the range 3–20, although single shot acquisitions with 128–256 echoes are also possible.

The addition of a preparation 180° pulse prior to the 90° inverts the magnetization to lie along the -z axis. As each tissue recovers towards $+M_0$, there is a time at which its magnetization passes through zero. An image formed at this point, will not contain signal from that tissue. Short TI Inversion Recovery (STIR) removes fat from the image, whilst FLuid Attenuated Inversion Recovery (FLAIR) removes the cerebrospinal fluid (CSF). Typical SE images are shown in Figure 1.11.

Parallel imaging

In parallel imaging a multi-element RF receive array coil is used to provide additional spatial information, and to reduce the number of lines of signal required to form an image. Parallel imaging reduces the number of TR periods of an acquisition by an amount known as the reduction factor R, SENSE factor or iPAT factor. The use of parallel imaging reduces the patient's overall RF exposure.

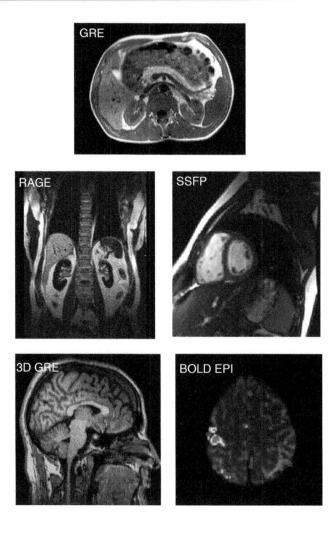

Figure 1.9   Gradient echo images: Gradient echo (GRE) abdomen; Rapid Acquired Gradient Echo (RAGE); 3-D Gradient Echo (3D GRE); Steady State Free Precession (SSFP) heart; BOLD-EPI with brain activation map overlay. Source: Flinders Medical Centre, Adelaide, Australia; Charing Cross Hospital, London, UK. Reproduced with permission.

Overview of MRI applications

Since its adoption in the late 1980s the scope of MRI's clinical applications has grown, and continues to grow. Brain, spine, and musculoskeletal imaging were the first major applications.

MRI's ability to differentiate between grey and white matter in the brain led to its deployment in neuroradiology, particularly for white matter disease and brain tumors. The development of diffusion-weighted imaging (DWI) gives MRI the ability to detect acute stroke and chronic infarct. Functional MRI (fMRI) is a popular tool in neuroscience research which utilizes the Blood Oxygenation Level Dependent (BOLD) effect to map neural activation. White matter connectivity can be investigated using diffusion tensor imaging (DTI) or high angular diffusion imaging (HARDI) and tractography. In musculoskeletal MRI soft tissue components, muscle, bone marrow, fat, and cartilage are all visible. Whilst tendon, ligament, and cortical bone are inferred by their absence of signal, edema resulting from injury is highly conspicuous.

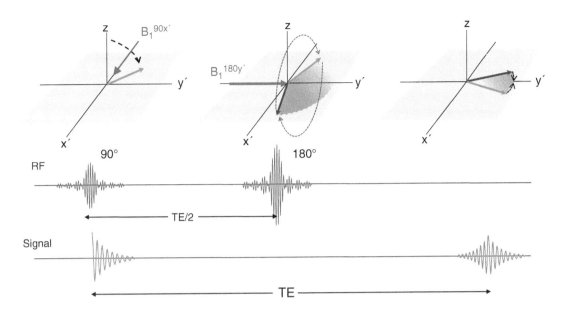

Figure 1.10   Spin echo formation: following a 90° pulse aligned with the x′ axis, magnetization in the x′y′ plane dephases; a 180° pulse aligned with the y′-axis inverts the phase of the magnetization to form a spin echo at time TE. The prime (′) indicates a frame of reference rotating at the Larmor frequency.

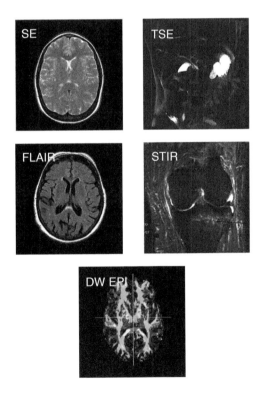

Figure 1.11   Spin echo images: (a) Spin echo (SE) T_2-weighted brain; single shot Turbo (fast) Spin Echo (TSE) MR cholangio-pancreatogram; Fluid Attenuated Inversion Recovery (FLAIR) brain; Short TI Inversion Recovery (STIR) knee; Diffusion EPI (Echo Planar Imaging) showing white matter directional anatomy. Source: Flinders Medical Centre, Adelaide, Australia. Reproduced with permission.

MRI has a major role in oncology through tumor imaging, often using DWI for diagnosis, staging, and treatment assessment. Applications include breast, bowel, prostate, liver, pancreas, female pelvis, in addition to brain and spine. MR *spectroscopy* (MRS) provides in-vivo bio-chemical information on tumor and tissue metabolism. Through sensitizing the MR signal to flow or by the injection of a gadolinium-based contrast agent (GBCA) angiographic images can be obtained to investigate vascular disease. The development of rapid GRE sequences has facilitated cardiac MR for heart morphology and function studies. GRE using the in-phase–out-of-phase technique is applied in liver and abdominal imaging of adenoma and cirrhosis, whilst TSE/FSE can indicate cysts, hepatocellular carcinoma and metastases. Single-shot TSE/FSE is used for MR cholangio–pancreatography (MRCP) in the biliary system. Some of these are illustrated in Figures 1.8 and 1.10.

MRI HARDWARE

The heart of the MRI system is the magnet, creating the static B_0 field that produces the tissue magnetization. The B_1 pulse that manipulates the magnetization is generated by a RF transmit coil (Tx) or coils fed by high-powered broadband RF amplifiers. The pulse shapes are generated digitally and converted to analog waveforms prior to amplification. The gradient coils provide the pulses used for spatial encoding of the signal. Finally, the MR signal is detected by receiver coils (Rx). These are usually positioned close to the anatomy of interest to maximize the signal received. Most receive coils are *array* or matrix coils formed from numerous minimally interacting smaller *elements*. The advantages of array coil technology include improved signal-to-noise ratio (SNR) and the ability to utilize parallel imaging techniques. Once detected, the MR signal is demodulated, i.e. the RF "carrier" component (at f_0) is removed, as the spatial information is stored in the VLF signal region. With "direct digital" systems, demodulation and digitization are applied directly to the amplified RF signal, close to or at the coil. The ensuing signals are transmitted digitally or optically and stored for reconstruction. Figure 1.12 shows a schematic of a typical MR system. The gradient and RF amplifier systems, control and signal processing systems, and cooling equipment are situated in the equipment or technical room, external to the MR examination or magnet room. The console and host computer are located in the control room (Figure 1.13).

Magnet system

The magnet is the largest single component of the system. Most systems use superconducting magnets. Superconductivity is a quantum mechanical property whereby, below a critical temperature T_c, an electrical conductor loses its electrical resistance, enabling large electrical currents to be sustained in perpetuity without a driving voltage from a power supply. As long as the windings are kept sufficiently cold, the current and hence the magnet's field persists indefinitely. Liquid helium with a boiling point of −269 °C (4.3 K or kelvin) is used for cooling. Safety consequences of this are considered in Chapter 12.

Superconductivity

Superconductivity was discovered by Dutch scientist Heike Kamerlingh Onnes in 1911, but it took until 1957 for Bardeen, Cooper, and Schrieffer to formulate a quantum mechanical theory (BCS theory) to account for the phenomenon. The electrical resistance of a non-superconducting metal, such as copper, depends upon its temperature, decreasing with lower temperatures, but possessing a finite resistance even at absolute zero (−273.15 °C). Below T_c the electrons in a

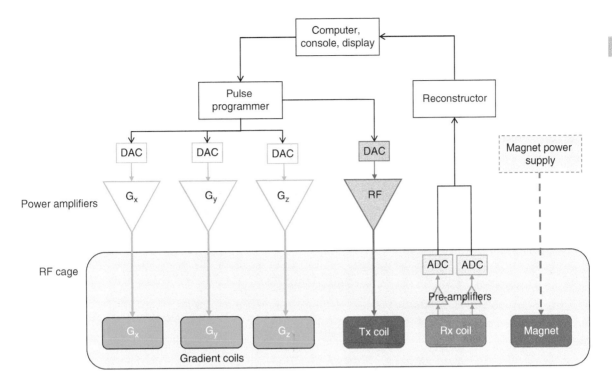

Figure 1.12 Schematic of principal MRI system components: DAC is digital-to-analog convertor; ADC is analog-to-digital convertor; Tx transmit; Rx receive; black lines denote digital signal; colored lines denote analog signal. The magnet power supply is only required for the initial ramp-up.

superconductor pair up into "Cooper pairs" acting as a superfluid resulting in zero resistance (Figure 1.14a).

Niobium titanium (Nb-Ti) alloy used in MR magnets is a type 2 superconductor.[1] It has a second, higher critical temperature at which some magnetic flux may exist within the material. Superconductivity behaves as a thermodynamic phase with a relationship between temperature, field, and current density (Figure 1.14b). There is a critical field B_c and current density J_c above which the superconductive state cannot exist. This puts an ultimate limit on the field strength that can be achieved. Nb-Ti has a T_c of 9.5 K and B_c of 15 T. Niobium-tin (Nb-Sn) alloy can sustain higher fields.

High temperature superconductors can have T_c above 90K and can be cooled using liquid nitrogen (N) with a boiling point of 77 K (−196 °C) or with cooled helium gas. These have been used to produce 0.5 T MRI magnets, but not operating in a persistent current mode. Research is ongoing with the prospect of simplifying the cooling system and reduced dependence upon helium. Helium is a by-product of natural gas extraction, a limited resource. Nitrogen can be produced from the atmosphere.

Superconducting MR magnets

Superconducting magnets are capable of generating magnetic flux densities, colloquially referred to as "magnetic field strength", up to 7 T (tesla) in currently available systems. 1.5 and 3 T

---

[1] In type 1 superconductors the magnetic field inside the material is zero due to the Meissner Effect.

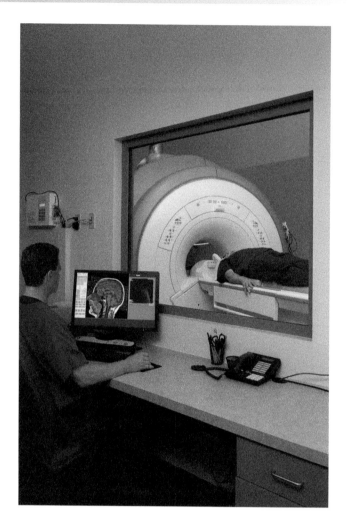

Figure 1.13   MRI operator's console in the control room with observation window into the magnet room. Source: James Steidl/iStockphoto.

systems are most common. B_0 is orientated horizontally along the scanner bore or patient aperture, by convention denoted as the z-axis.

Figure 1.15 shows a schematic of a modern MRI magnet in cross-section. There are two sets of windings: the field coils and the shield coils. The shield coils are wound in opposition to the field coils in order to reduce the extent of the *fringe field*. The windings are held in a large vessel or *cryostat* and bathed in liquid helium. Surrounding this is a vacuum to prevent conduction and convection heating, and layers of highly reflective sheeting to prevent radiative heating.

During operation some helium will evaporate or "boil off". In older magnets this was wasted as exhaust, but modern magnets have a refrigeration system, the *cold head* or *cryo-cooler* which re-condenses the gas as liquid. Such "zero boil-off" systems generally do not require helium replenishment. If electrical power is lost, the reliquification will not occur, but the magnet can stay cold for several days. This allows new systems to be transported cold.

To generate the field initially, a power supply is required. The process of energizing the magnet or "ramping up" involves a gradual increase of electrical current. A superconducting switch or shunt is maintained in a non-superconductive state by a small heater whilst the current grows. At the desired current the heater is turned off and the switch becomes superconducting, completing the electrical

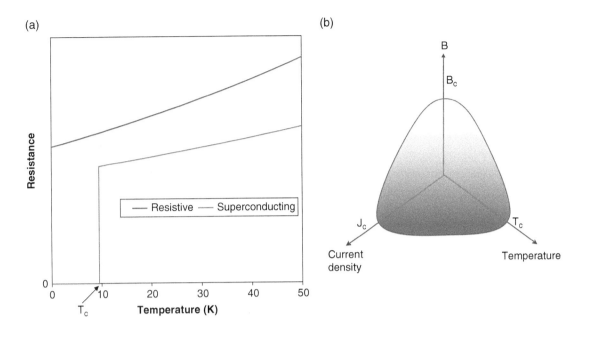

Figure 1.14   Superconductivity: (a) resistance v temperature for a superconductor and a non-superconductor; (b) Superconducting phase diagram: each of temperature, current density and magnetic field must be below a critical value T_c, J_c, B_c to maintain the superconductive state.

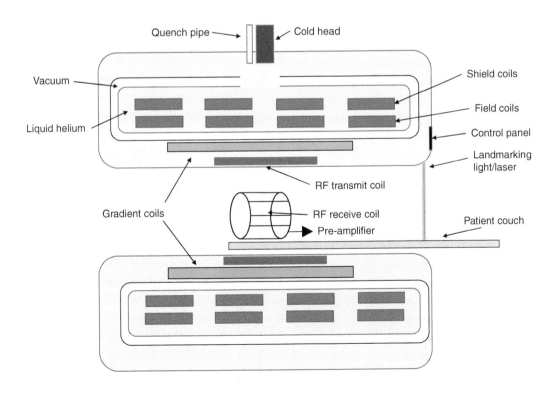

Figure 1.15   Schematic of a self-shielded superconducting MRI system.

circuit. The power supply can then be disconnected and removed from site. The reverse process, ramping down, can be used to reduce or remove the field when required, e.g. for a major hardware upgrade or after a non-injurious ferromagnetic incident to remove the offending object.

The Nb-Ti wires are 50–150 μm in diameter, embedded in a copper matrix. This provides additional mechanical strength – they are subject to significant magnetic forces – and provides a means for conducting excess heat and current in the event of a magnet failure or *quench* to prevent damage to the more delicate Nb-Ti filaments. In the superconducting state, the copper matrix acts like an insulator, providing isolation between the Nb-Ti strands.

Short larger-bore magnets

A recent industry trend has been to reduce the length of the magnet, typically to around 1.6 m and to increase the diameter of the bore from 60 to 70 cm to afford better patient comfort and to accommodate larger patients. This has implications for safety as it affects the fringe field (see Fringe field spatial gradient, page 19).

Other magnets

Other configurations of MRI systems are also available, although less common. Resistive magnets producing fields up to 0.4 T are sometimes configured as open or C-arm systems, affording better access to the patient and a less claustrophobic experience. Resistive magnets have one safety-related advantage: the field can be routinely switched off.

Permanent magnets are used in low field niche scanners for extremity imaging or in "upright systems". These employ various rare earth materials such as neodymium-iron-boron (Nd-Fe-B). Their magnetic field is always present.

Imaging gradients subsystem

Magnetic field gradients G_x, G_y, and G_z used to spatially select or encode the MR signal during acquisition are generated by three sets of gradient coils. The field generated is *always* along z. Gradient coils usually require water cooling as they have typically hundreds of amperes (A) of electricity pulsed through them. Specialist hybrid amplifiers and power supplies are used to generate these strong pulses. A consequence of gradient pulsing is the generation of acoustic noise (Chapter 7).

Gradient pulses usually have a trapezoidal waveform (Figure 1.16). The ability of the gradient system to switch rapidly, known as the *slew rate* (SR), is defined as the maximum amplitude divided by the *rise time* required to achieve that amplitude:

$$SR = \frac{\text{Maximum ampitude}}{\text{minimum time required}}$$ (1.4)

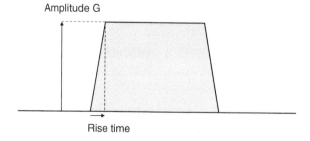

Amplitude G

Rise time

Figure 1.16   Trapezoidal gradient pulse.

Example 1.2   Gradient performance

What is the (theoretical) maximum field produced by a 40 mTm^{-1} gradient system with a slew rate of 200 T m^{-1}s^{-1}? What is the minimum rise time?

Assuming that the gradient is linear over a 50 cm FOV, the maximum amplitude at the edge, 25 cm from the iso-center is

$$G_{max} = 40 \times 0.25 = 10 \; mT.$$

The minimum rise time is

$$t_{min} = \frac{40 \times 10^{-3}}{200} = 0.2 \; ms.$$

Radiofrequency subsystem

The radiofrequency system comprises two subsystems: transmit and receive. RF transmit is more important for MR safety.

RF transmission

In most instances a body RF transmit coil is used (Figure 1.17). This typically has a "birdcage" design, operating in *quadrature* to produce a *circularly-polarized* magnetic field B_1. Some coils may operate in transmit and receive mode (T/R) denoted symbolically as in Figure 1.18. Examples are dedicated T/R head and knee coils. Tx coils usually have a cylindrical geometry, entirely encompassing the anatomical region to produce a uniform B_1 so that everything in the FOV experiences the same flip angle.

The coils operate in a resonant mode as tuned circuits, resulting in current amplification to achieve greater B_1 at the Larmor frequency. They are driven by powerful RF amplifiers, rated at tens of kilowatts (kW). An important aspect of RF generation is impedance matching, usually to 50 Ω (ohms), to ensure the maximum power transfer from the amplifier to the coil. B_1 is of the order of micro-tesla (μT) peak amplitude.

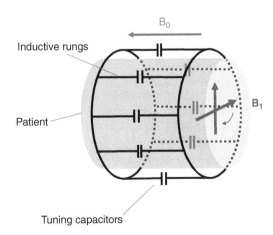

Figure 1.17   Transmit 8-rung 'birdcage' coil to produce a circularly polarized (rotating) B_{1+} field orthogonal to B_0.

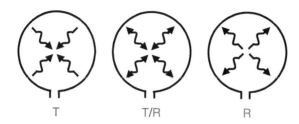

Figure 1.18   IEC 60601-2-33 [4] compliant coil labeling: left- transmit only; middle- transmit-receive; right- receive only.

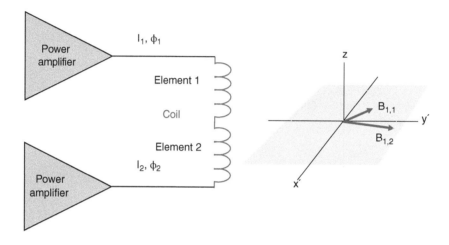

Figure 1.19   Parallel transmit: two (or more) independent RF power amplifiers drive elements of the transmit coil.

In 3 T systems, operating at 128 MHz, the B_1-field in tissue is often quite non-uniform. In this instance *parallel transmit* systems can help. These utilize multi-element Tx coils powered by independent amplifiers capable of changing both the amplitude and phase (relative direction) of the RF pulses (Figure 1.19).

RF reception

The purpose of the RF receiver coils is to detect the tiny (micro-volt) MR signals. A parallel tuned circuit is used (Figure 1.20) to magnify the voltage prior to pre-amplification and further processing. The receive coil requires protection circuitry to prevent the large transmit pulses from coupling into the coil. A simple means of achieving this is to use crossed diodes and a detuning capacitor. During the large Tx pulses the diodes conduct and so the total capacitance becomes the sum of both capacitors and the circuit is off-resonance. During signal detection the diodes do not conduct, and C_d is "invisible." A fault in this circuitry can lead to large induced currents in the coil and potential heating or burns for the patient.

ELECTROMAGNETIC FIELDS

The extent and magnitude of the fields involved in MRI are summarized in Table 1.1 and Figure 1.21.

(a)

(b)

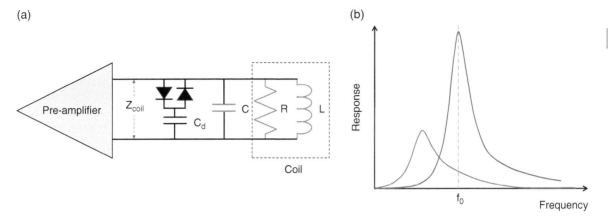

Figure 1.20 Receive coil and pre-amplifier: (a) the coil has inductance L and resistance R; C_d is a detuning capacitor; (b) response of the coil during signal reception (red line) and RF transmission (blue line).

Table 1.1 Magnetic fields in MRI.

Field	Amplitude	Frequency / Slew rate	Pulse duration
Static field B_0	0.2-7 T	0 Hz	Always present
Static fringe field spatial gradient dB/dz	0-25 T m^{-1}	0 Hz	Always present
Imaging gradients G_x, G_y, G_z	0-80 mT m^{-1}	0-10 kHz 0-200 T m^{-1} s^{-1}	0-10 ms
RF transmit field B_1	0-50 µT	8-300 MHz	0-10 ms

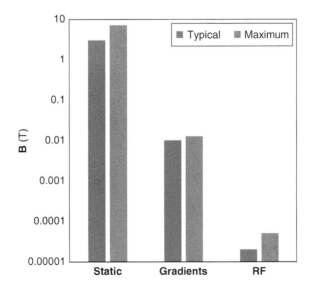

Figure 1.21 Relative magnitude of magnetic fields used in MRI.

Static field

Definition of magnetic flux density and the tesla

Whilst MR practitioners commonly refer to their magnets in terms of "magnetic field strength", this nomenclature is scientifically incorrect. The proper term is *magnetic flux density*, denoted as **B**. **B** is a vector field with components in each direction B_x, B_y and B_z. MRI is only sensitive to B_z and that is what we refer to colloquially as the "field." Magnetic flux density has the SI (International System) unit of the tesla (T). An older unit is the gauss (G). One tesla equals 10 000 G.

The scientific definition of the tesla is in terms of force. Referring to Figure 1.22, one tesla is the amount of magnetic flux density which exerts a force of one newton (N) on a charged particle of charge one coulomb (C) moving at right angles to the field direction with a velocity of one meter per second (m s^{-1}). It's not an easy definition, but the fact that it is defined in terms of force is highly apt for MR safety!

MYTHBUSTER:

The unit of "magnetic field strength" is not the tesla, but is amperes per meter. B is the *magnetic flux density*.

So, what is magnetic field strength in actuality? It is given the symbol **H** and has units of amperes per meter (A m^{-1}). It is defined in terms of a cylindrical electromagnet, just like our scanner – the current in the windings generates an **H**-field. In free space

$$B = \mu_0 H \tag{1.5}$$

μ_0 is the magnetic *permeability* in a vacuum, equal to $4\pi \times 10^{-7}$ henrys per meter (H m^{-1}).

One way of visualizing magnetic fields is through magnetic field lines. If you have ever done the experiment of introducing iron filings to the proximity of a simple bar magnet you may have observed the pattern shown in Figure 1.23a. These illustrate the magnetic "lines of force". A small compass needle positioned anywhere will align with these. We can think of the magnetic flux density as being the intensity of grouping of these lines: the more closely grouped together, the stronger the B-field.

B₀ fringe field

The most uniform and dense grouping of lines of force for an MR magnet (Figure 1.23b) occurs within the bore. As we move away from the bore the lines diverge and consequently the B-field decreases. We call this region the *fringe field*. Your scanner manufacturer provides field maps showing fringe field contours at 0.5, 1, 3, 5, 10, 20, 40, and 200 mT [4] (Figure 1.24). These are important for MRI suite design (Chapter 12). A modern MRI system utilizes self-shielding in order to reduce the spatial extent of the fringe field (Figure 1.25).

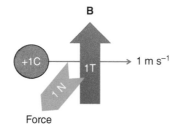

Figure 1.22   Definition of the SI unit tesla.

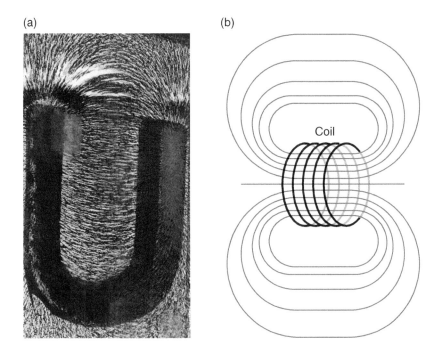

(a)   (b)

Coil

Figure 1.23   Magnetic field lines of force: (a) seen in the pattern of iron filings around a permanent magnet; (b) from an electromagnet.

Fringe field spatial gradient

As we move further from the bore of the magnet, the lines of force diverge, and the fringe field decreases (Figure 1.23b). The amount it decreases with distance is known as the *fringe field spatial gradient*, specified in T m^{-1}. The fringe field spatial gradient is responsible for the attractive force on ferromagnetic objects. Your manufacturer is required to provide you with information about the fringe field gradient. Figure 1.25 shows how the B_0 field and its spatial gradient dB/dz vary along the z-axis. The fringe field is compressed for the shielded magnet but produces a stronger spatial gradient close to the bore entrance. This is highly significant for projectile safety.

MYTHBUSTER:

The fringe spatial field gradient is always present as long as the main static B_0 field exists. It should not be confused with the imaging gradients.

The imaging gradients

Gradient amplitude is measured in mT m^{-1} (milli-tesla per meter). When a gradient pulse is applied, e.g. along the x-axis, the total B experienced at a point x is

$$B(x) = B_0 + x\,G_x \qquad (1.6)$$

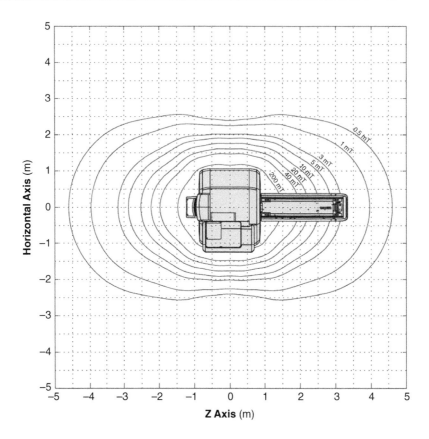

Figure 1.24 Fringe field contours at 0.5, 1, 3, 5, 10, 20, 40 and 200 mT for a 3 T MR magnet. Reproduced with permission of Siemens Healthineers.

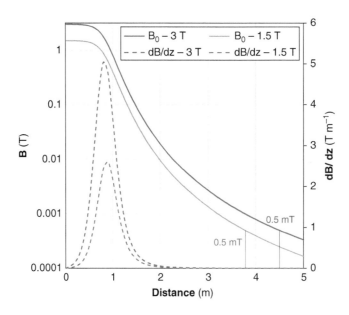

Figure 1.25 The magnitude of the B_0 fringe field (solid lines, logarithmic LH scale) and its spatial gradient dB/dz (dashed lines, linear RH scale) along the z-axis simulated for shielded 1.5 and 3 T MRI magnets. The vertical lines indicate the locations of the 0.5 mT contour. The iso-center is located at z=0, and the bore entrance at 0.8 m.

Example 1.3 B_z from a gradient

In a 1.5 T MRI system with a gradient amplitude of 10 mT m^{-1} what is the total magnetic field at a point $x = 10$ cm from the iso-center?

$$B_z(x) = 1.5 + 0.1 \times 10 \times 10^{-3} = 1.501\,T$$

At a point $x = -10$ cm, the resultant B-field is 1.499 T.

The contribution to the overall magnetic field of the gradients is small, but we could not image without them. The strength of the field produced by the gradients decreases rapidly outside the bore of the magnet, and is negligibly small away from the magnet.

As the gradients are switched, they produce *time-varying magnetic fields*. The *rate of change* of field is given by the derivative of B with respect to time, or dB/dt (measured in T s^{-1}). For a trapezoidal gradient waveform (Figure 1.16)

$$\frac{dB}{dt} = \frac{\Delta B}{\Delta t} \tag{1.7}$$

where ΔB is the change in B produced by the gradient and Δt is the time over which the change occurs. dB/dt is important when considering acute physiological effects, such as peripheral nerve stimulation (PNS). See Chapter 4.

Example 1.4   Gradient dB/dt

In the example of Figure 1.16 if the peak gradient amplitude is 10 mT and the rise time 0.1 ms, what is the dB/dt?

$$\frac{dB}{dt} = \frac{10\,mT}{0.1\,ms} = 100\,T\,s^{-1}$$

Radiofrequency field

Figure 1.26 shows simulations of the electric and magnetic fields generated around an eight-rung birdcage transmit coil [5]. The magnetic B_1-field is highly uniform, whilst the electric field (E) is concentrated around the rungs. In air B_1 decreases rapidly beyond the limits of the transmit coil.[2] B_1 is produced as a pulse consisting of a "carrier" frequency (at the Larmor frequency) multiplied by a shape or envelope (Figure 1.27). The simple rectangular pulses of Equation 1.2 are seldom used in practice and a more general expression for flip angle is

$$\alpha = \gamma \int_0^{t_p} B_1(t)\,dt \tag{1.8}$$

This is equal to the area under the curve of the pulse envelope. Three important points arise:

1. for the same pulse shape and duration, the B_1 amplitude is proportional to the flip angle;
2. for the same pulse shape and duration, the B_1 amplitude required to produce a given flip angle is independent of B_0;
3. the peak amplitude of B_1 alone is not sufficient to characterize the RF exposure.

---

[2] This is not true in tissue. See Chapter 2, page 54.

MYTHBUSTER:

The amplitude of the B_1 RF excitation pulse does not depend upon the static field strength B_0.

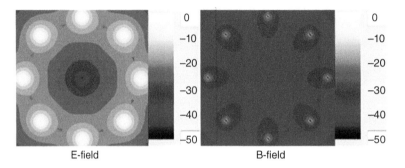

E-field   B-field

Figure 1.26   Simulated electric (L) and magnetic fields (R) from an eight-rung birdcage coil. Scale in dB. Source [5], licensee BioMed Central Ltd.

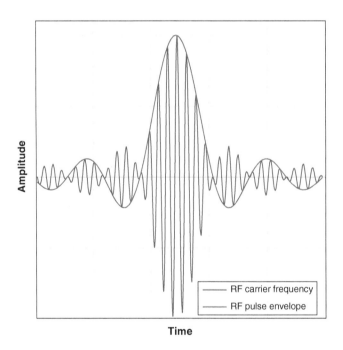

Time

Figure 1.27   RF pulse consisting of the carrier (Larmor) frequency multiplied by a shape function or pulse envelope. The example shown is a truncated sinc (sinx/x) function.

B_{1+} and B_{1+}RMS

The parameter B_{1+}RMS is used to characterize the average B_1 exposure. The "+" refers to the rotating component of B_1 responsible for excitation of the magnetization. An efficient coil should not generate a B_{1-}. RMS stands for root-mean-square and is a type of averaging used for time-varying

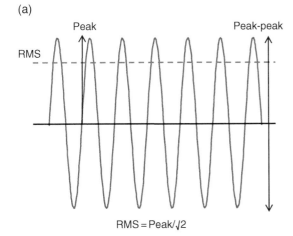

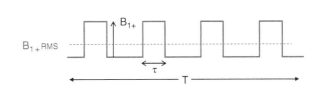

Figure 1.28   (a) the RMS value of a sinusoid is the peak amplitude divided by √2; (b) B_{1+}RMS for a train of N RF pulses of amplitude B_{1+}, duration τ within time T.

waveforms. For example, the RMS value for a sinusoidal waveform is $1/\sqrt{2}$ or approximately 0.71 of the peak amplitude (Figure 1.28a). B_{1+}RMS is defined as

$$B_{1+RMS} = \sqrt{\frac{\int_0^T \left(B_{1+}(t)\right)^2 dt}{T}} \qquad (1.9)$$

calculated over 10 second intervals (T=10 s). The easiest way to visualize this is to consider a regular train of N rectangular RF pulses (Figure 1.28b), each of amplitude B_{1+} and duration t_p. In this case

$$B_{1+RMS} = B_{1+}\sqrt{\frac{N\,t_p}{TR}} \qquad (1.10)$$

Consequently B_{1+}RMS depends upon the

- flip angle
- number of RF pulses (echoes, slices, etc.)
- RF pulse shape
- TR.

B_1 is also a time-varying magnetic field. We can calculate the magnitude of dB/dt for a circulating field $B_{1+}e^{-i\omega t}$ as[3]

$$\left|\frac{dB_1}{dt}\right| = \left|\frac{d}{dt}B_{1+}e^{-i\omega t}\right| = \omega B_{1+} = 2\pi f B_{1+} \qquad (1.11)$$

The rate of change is proportional both to the frequency and the amplitude. As B_{1+} is typically μT and f in MHz, RF dB/dt is of the order of a few tesla per second.

---

[3] Using complex notation where $i = \sqrt{-1}$, the operator $e^{i\omega t}$ signifies circular motion.

Scanning modes

The IEC standard 60601-2-33 [4] defines three modes for scanning:

- **Normal mode**: mode of operation of the MR equipment in which none of the outputs has a value that may cause physiological stress to patients.
- **First-level controlled mode**: mode of operation of the MR equipment in which one or more outputs reach a value that may cause physiological stress to patients which needs to be controlled by medical supervision.
  - Software allowing access to this mode must require specific acknowledgement by the operator that the first-level controlled mode has been entered.
- **Second-level controlled mode**: mode of operation of the MR equipment in which one or more outputs reach a value that may produce significant risk for patients, for which explicit ethical approval is required (i.e. a Human Studies protocol approved to local requirements).

"Outputs" refers to the magnitude of the magnetic fields. Clinical scanners are usually restricted to the Normal and First Level Modes.

OTHER MEDICAL DEVICES

Along with an understanding of MRI hardware and fields it is important to understand how these interact with other medical devices. A system to categorize the MRI safety (we used to say "compatibility") of other devices: implants, accessories, medical equipment, tools, fire extinguishers, gas tanks, etc. uses three labels [6]:

- *MR Safe* means that the device poses no risk to the patient in the MR environment. Image quality may be affected.
- *MR Conditional* means that the device poses no additional risk to the patient when introduced to the MR environment under specified conditions.
- *MR Unsafe* means that the device may not be introduced into the MR environment as it poses significant risk to the patient and/or staff.

The approved signs are shown in Figure 1.29. The "MR environment" generally means the MR examination room, or areas with a fringe field exceeding 0.5 mT, rather than just the scanner itself. The safety of implants is considered in Chapters 9–11.

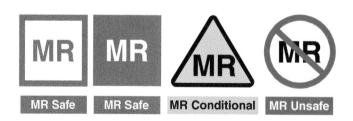

Figure 1.29   MR device labeling according to ASTM-F2503 (IEC-62570) [6]. The two MR Safe symbols are equivalent; either may be used.

CONCLUSIONS

MRI incidents can lead to injury or death. The most frequent incidents are thermal, followed by mechanical, projectile, and hearing loss. We have considered the basic elements of MRI acquisitions, the components of the scanner and the magnetic fields encountered. There is a symmetry about the magnitude and time-variance of the fields: B_0 is of the order of tesla; the imaging gradient fields a thousand times lower, typically milli-tesla; B_1 is typically one thousand times less again, in micro-tesla. At the same time the temporal variations range from zero to one hertz for movement in the static field, to kHz for the gradients, and MHz for B_1.

In the next chapter we consider the physical interactions of these fields with non-biological matter. For those wishing to become MR Safety Experts, Chapter 2 should be read in conjunction with Appendix I supplemented by reading further reading of standard electromagnetism texts.

Revision Questions

1. The Larmor frequency of a 1.5 T MRI scanner is approximately:
   A. 10 MHz
   B. 42.58 MHz
   C. 64 MHz
   D. 85 MHz
   E. 128 MHz

2. In a 1.5 T MRI scanner, if the B_{1+} amplitude required to produce a 90° flip angle is 10 μT, what B_{1+} amplitude is required in a 3T scanner if the pulse shape is unchanged?
   A. 5 μT
   B. 10 μT
   C. 20 μT
   D. 40 μT
   E. 0.01 mT

3. Which of the following is true for B_1?
   A. It is applied along the z-direction along the magnet bore
   B. It is a single sinusoid
   C. It is a radio wave
   D. It is generated by the x and y gradient coils
   E. It rotates with the magnetization precession.

4. Which of the following is untrue for the static field spatial gradient in a superconducting MRI system?
   A. It is measured in tesla per meter
   B. It is required for image acquisition
   C. It is always present
   D. It is responsible for the translational magnetic force
   E. It is reduced in extent in a self-shielded magnet.

5. If an imaging gradient system has a peak amplitude of 50 mT m^{-1} and a slew rate of 200 T m^{-1} s^{-1} what is the minimum achievable rise time for a full amplitude pulse?
   A. 10 μs
   B. 0.1 ms
   C. 0.2 ms
   D. 0.25 ms
   E. 0.4 ms

6. Which of the following is not acceptable terminology for MR safety according to ASTM-F2503?
   A. MR safe
   B. MR unsafe
   C. MR compatible
   D. MR conditional
   E. MR acceptable.

References

1. Organisation for Economic Co-operation and Development (2017). *Health care resources: medical technology*. https://stats.oecd.org/ (accessed 12 January 2019).
2. Kanal, E., Borgstede, J.P., Barkovich, A.J. et al. (2002). American College of Radiology white paper on MR safety. *American Journal of Roentenology* 178:1335–1347.
3. Delfino, J.G., Krainak D.M., Flesher S.A. et al. (2019). MRI-related FDA adverse event reports: a 10-year review. *Medical Physics* doi: 10.1002/mp. 13768.
4. International Electrotechnical Commission (2015). *Medical Electrical Equipment – Part 2-33: Particular Requirements for the Safety of Magnetic Resonance Equipment for Medical Diagnosis. IEC 60601-2-33 3.3 edn*. Geneva: IEC.
5. Lui, Y., Shen, J., Kainz, W. et al. (2013). Numerical investigations of MRI RF field induced heating for external fixation devices. *BioMedical Engineering OnLine* 12:12 doi.org/10.1186/1475-925X-12-12.
6. ASTM F2503-13 (2015). *Standard Practice for Marking Medical Devices and Other Items for Safety in the Magnetic Resonance Environment*. West Conshohocken, PA: ASTM International.

Further reading and resources

McRobbie, D.W., Moore, E.A., Graves, M.J., et al. (2017). *MRI from Picture to Proton* 3rd edn. Chapters 3, 4, 8, 9, and 10. Cambridge, UK: Cambridge University Press.

2

Let's get physical: fields and forces

BASIC LAWS OF MAGNETISM

The fundamental laws of magnetism were summarized by Scottish physicist James Clerk Maxwell in four equations. These equations are not for the faint-hearted nor for the mathematically challenged, but if you aspire to be an expert in MRI safety, then you should have a good understanding of their consequences. By comparison, if you did not understand Newton's laws of gravitation or Einstein's theory of relativity you would not become a rocket scientist. Maxwell's equations underpin *everything* in electromagnetism: the biological effects of EM fields, interactions with implants, electromagnetic modeling of field exposures and specific absorption rate (SAR), projectiles and magnet safety, magnetic shielding, fringe field gradients, and acoustic noise. A full understanding requires some knowledge of vector calculus and differential equations (see Appendix 2) but for now we will not need this. Those aspiring to be MR Safety Experts should read this chapter in conjunction with Appendix 1.

Understanding Maxwell's Equations

Maxwell's equations are given in Appendix 1. Here we describe their main consequences for MRI safety.

Electrical charge and electric fields

Gauss's Law (Maxwell's first equation) describes how electrical charges produce static electric fields E. Electric fields start at a positive charge and are directed towards their conclusion at negative charges (Figure 2.1). We are not going to use Gauss's Law much, although it has relevance in minimizing unwanted electric fields in coil design, and at some tissue boundaries where charge may accumulate.

Magnetic fields

Maxwell's second equation states that the "divergence of B is zero." This means that there is no magnetic equivalent of electrical charge – no "magnetic monopoles". Magnetic sources are not

Essentials of MRI Safety, First Edition. Donald W. McRobbie.

(a)   (b)   (c)

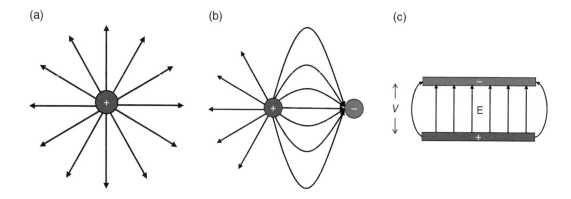

Figure 2.1 Electric field lines begin at a source of positive charge and terminate at a negative charge: (a) single point positive charge; (b) positive and negative point charges; (c) capacitor with a potential difference *V* between the plates.

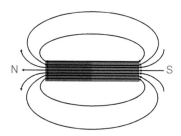

Figure 2.2 Magnetic field lines from a permanent bar magnet.

like electrostatic ones, but exist as dipoles with a north and south pole (just like the Earth). Magnetic field lines have no beginning or end, but form complete loops from north pole to south (Figures 2.2, 1.23). The nature of the B_0 fringe field depends upon this.

Electromagnetic induction

Maxwell's third equation is also known as Faraday's Law of Induction. We have met dB/dt already in Chapter 1, so clearly this equation is going to have significant implications for us. It states that a time-varying magnetic field induces an electric field; also, that the electric field lines form complete loops unlike static electric fields (Figure 2.3). The induced electric field is sometimes called "conservative" as it involves no external static charges. Faraday's Law is also responsible for the detection of the MR signal in an RF receive coil – so it's important!

Electromagnetic waves

Maxwell's fourth equation, or Ampere's Law, tells us that magnetic fields can be generated both by electric currents and by time-varying electric fields, allowing for the existence of electro-magnetic waves – everything in the electromagnetic spectrum: gamma rays, X-rays, ultraviolet, visible light, infrared, microwaves, and radiowaves (Figure 2.4). It has consequences for the more "wave-like" behavior of the B_1 excitation field at higher frequencies. It also results in field exposures from the gradients being higher than intuitively anticipated.

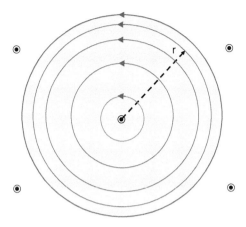

Figure 2.3   Electric fields induced by a time-varying magnetic field form complete loops (unless there are static electrical charges present); dB/dt is into the page.

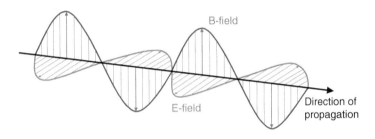

Figure 2.4   Electromagnetic wave: the magnetic and electric fields are orthogonal to each other and to the direction of propagation.

Generating magnetic fields

Maxwell's equations teach us that a magnetic field (we shall drop the proper term "flux density") is generated by an electrical current. In this section we consider the generation of magnetic fields from conductors and coils in various simple configurations. Further detail is given in Appendix 1.

B field from a long straight conductor

If we have a straight wire and pass a current I along it, then the magnetic field generated will have circular field lines (Figure 2.5). The direction of the field lines can be determined by the "right hand rule", namely that if your right hand's thumb represents the direction of current flow, then your cupped fingers will indicate the circular B field direction, denoted B_θ. The magnitude of the field at a radial distance r from the wire is proportional to $1/r$. The subscript θ (from polar coordinates- see Appendix 2) indicates that the field lines form circular paths around the wire.

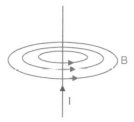

Figure 2.5 Magnetic field lines from a long straight conductor carrying current I. The direction of the lines follows the right-hand rule.

B field from loop conductors

The field on the z-axis from a circular loop of radius a is directed along the z-direction and is proportional to the current I. At the center of the loop B is proportional to $1/a$, so the field generated depends upon the radius of the coil. At long distances from the loop, it acts like a magnetic *dipole*. On-axis the field only has a B_z component with a $1/z^3$ dependence. This is often cited to represent the dropping off of the B_0 fringe field, but modern shielded MRI magnets do not exactly follow this behavior; they are not simple dipoles. Nevertheless, the $1/z^3$ dependence serves as a useful approximation of the nature of the fringe field. The spatial gradient from a dipole varies with $1/z^4$ along the z-axis. This is a very rapid decrease with distance from the iso-center and is intensely significant for projectile safety. The magnitude of B_z for a long straight wire, a loop and a dipole are plotted in Figure 2.6.

B field from a solenoidal coil

The field generated at the center of a solenoid of length d with windings of density N turns per meter - this now looks more like a MR superconducting magnet- is

$$B_z = \mu_0 NI\sin\theta \tag{2.1}$$

θ is the angle measured from the vertical at iso-center to the end of the solenoid (Figure 2.7). For very long solenoids θ tends to 90° ($\pi/2$) and the field is

$$B_z = \mu_0 NI \tag{2.2}$$

This is where the definition of magnetic field strength or intensity H in A m^{-1} (from Chapter 1) comes in, as

$$H_z = NI \tag{2.3}$$

B field from a shielded MRI magnet

The design of a MR magnet (at least for MR safety purposes) can be approximately simulated by two concentric solenoids: the inner one representing the main coil; the outer shield coil has current flowing in the opposite direction. This enables the fringe field to be significantly reduced in extent (Figure 2.8). It also results in a stronger spatial gradient of B_0, dB/dz, close to the bore entrance, but weaker at greater distance. This poses a significantly increased hazard, as the projectile force on a ferromagnetic

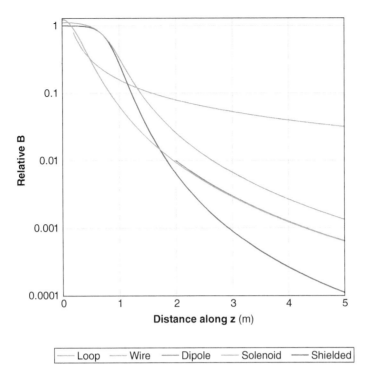

Figure 2.6 Relative magnitude of B_z along the z-axis for a long straight wire, simple loop, magnetic dipole, solenoid, and simulated self-shielded magnet with radii of 0.4 m. The iso-center is at z = 0.

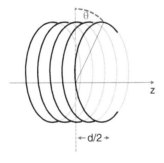

Figure 2.7 Solenoid coil showing the angle θ. For a very long solenoid θ →90°.

object may suddenly increase as you approach the bore entrance – and you only notice when it's too late. Both B and dB/dz drop off with distance more rapidly than for a dipole (Figure 2.6).

Spatial dependence of magnetic fields

Only the simplest coil geometries can be solved exactly with algebra. A generalized method of computing is given by the Biot-Savart Law (see Appendix 1). Magnet and gradient coil designers use this to numerically compute the spatial responses of B_0, $G_{x,y,z}$ and B_1 fields. It is also used in computer modeling of induced fields in tissue.

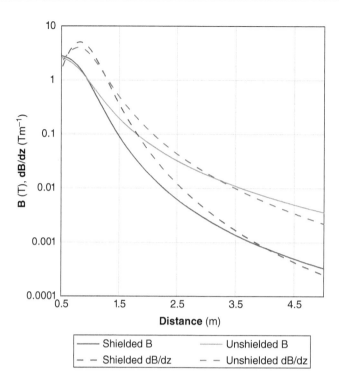

Figure 2.8   B and dB/dt along the axis of a simulated shielded and unshielded 3T MR magnet. Distances are from the iso-center, with the bore entrance at 0.8m. Simulated data for illustration only.

MAGNETIC MATERIALS

The previous section showed how a B-field can be generated in free space or air. Now we consider how materials or physical media respond to an external magnetic field. At the atomic level the electrons in their shells orbiting the nucleus have intrinsic magnetic moments. In most atoms the magnetic moments from the electrons' spin and orbital motion cancel. This is *diamagnetism*, the default "non-magnetic" state. If the cancelation is incomplete then the material is *paramagnetic*. In *ferromagnetic*[1] materials, such as iron or steel, the electron spins become aligned in large groups or *domains* and their effect is significantly greater. Figure 2.9 shows the *magnetic suscep-tibility spectrum* covering a range of materials [1]. This is an enormous range extending over ten orders of magnitude (10^{10}); each step in the chart represents a factor of ten.

When an object is placed in an external magnetic field, it becomes magnetized. Each of the types of material: dia-, para-, and ferromagnetic behave differently in the field, but because of Maxwell's equations, the underlying physics is similar. In an external field, the magnetization of the material **M** (a vector) is

$$\mathbf{M} = \chi\,\mathbf{H} \tag{2.4}$$

---

[1] Note, we do not use the term "ferrous" which means "containing iron."

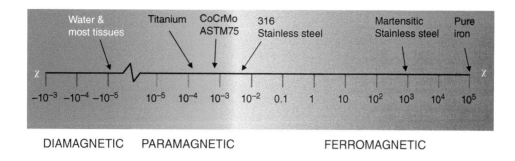

Figure 2.9 Magnetic susceptibility spectrum.

Table 2.1 Magnetic susceptibility of common materials.

Type of material	Behavior	Material	χ[1]
Diamagnetic	M opposes H and external B_0. Repulsive force.	Water and soft tissue Cortical bone De-oxygenated red blood cells Copper Superconductors	-9.05×10^{-6} -8.86×10^{-6} -6.52×10^{-6} -9.63×10^{-6} -1
Paramagnetic	M parallel to external H and B_0. Attractive force.	Air Magnesium Aluminium Titanium CoCrMo alloy	0.36×10^{-6} 11.7×10^{-6} 20.7×10^{-6} 182×10^{-6} 920×10^{-6}
Ferromagnetic	M parallel to external B_0, H anti-parallel. Strong attractive force. Can become permanently magnetized. Displays hysteresis.	Martensitic stainless steel Silicon steel Mumetal Pure iron	$\sim 10^3$ $10^3\text{--}10^4$ $10^4\text{--}10^5$ $\sim 10^5$

[1] Values from [1,2]

H is the magnetic field strength (A m^{-1}) and χ is the magnetic susceptibility which is dimensionless[2]. Table 2.1 shows some values of χ. In isotropic media χ is independent of orientation or position and is a simple scalar number. If the material is linear and isotropic we can say

$$\mathbf{B} = \mu_0\left(1+\chi\right)\mathbf{H} \tag{2.5}$$

The total field within the material is the sum of the external field plus the field resulting from the magnetization of the material.

The *relative permeability* μ_r is also used to characterize magnetic materials

$$\mu_r = 1 + \chi \tag{2.6}$$

so

$$\mathbf{B} = \mu_0\mu_r\mathbf{H} \tag{2.7}$$

for linear isotropic materials.

---

[2] Sometimes mass susceptibility is used: $\chi_\rho = \chi/\rho$ where ρ is the material's density in kg m^{-3}.

Ferromagnetism

Whilst we will consider (in Chapter 3) the possible consequences of biological effects based upon the dia- and para- magnetic properties of biological structures, ferromagnetic is the most important class of materials for safety within the MR environment due to the strong magnetic forces. Before we consider these, we need to understand more about ferromagnetism. Figure 2.10 shows how the magnetic *domains* of a ferromagnetic material may align. In the absence of a magnetic field the domains are randomly orientated with no overall magnetization. When an external B-field (or H) is applied, the domains align and the material becomes highly magnetized. Some materials will retain their magnetism once the external field is removed – these are known as *hard* ferromagnetic materials, becoming permanent magnets when magnetized. *Soft* magnetic materials do not retain their domains' alignment once the external field is removed, or do so to a minor extent which we will neglect.

The B-field in the material increases in the presence of an external field H (or B). The slope of the curve gives the magnetic permeability μ, its value depending upon the strength of H applied. For low values of external field, the magnetization is reversible. Above the *saturation point* the material becomes unable to sustain a higher magnetization no matter how large the applied field is. This material is magnetically *saturated*. For most ferromagnetic materials this occurs below 1.5 T, so it is likely that a potential projectile will be saturated when very close to the magnet bore entrance. Figure 2.11 shows the B-H curve for series 416 stainless steel, a material commonly used in domestic goods. Also shown is the dependence of its magnetic permeability μ upon the external field H.

As the applied H-field is reduced (or the material is removed from the external B_0-field of your magnet) the internal B within the material decreases. Due to *hysteresis*, it does not decrease exactly along the path of its increase (Figure 2.12). With a hard ferromagnetic material significant B remains once the external field has been reduced to zero. This is known as the *remanence*, B_{rem}. Permanent magnets have high remanence. If the H is applied in the opposite direction (i.e. is made negative) the material's B continues to fall. The intercept H_c on the -H axis is called the *coercivity*. Soft materials have low coercivity and remanence with a slim B-H (or M-H) curve. In hard ferromagnetic materials both are large and the hysteresis curve is broader. Above the *Curie temperature*, metals lose their ferromagnetic properties. Values of B_{sat}, H_c and Curie temperatures are shown in Table 2.2.

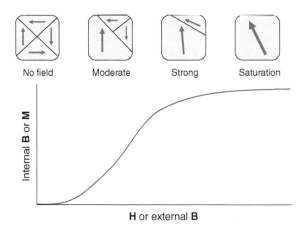

Figure 2.10   Domains in a ferromagnetic material as the external field is increased from zero to the saturation point.

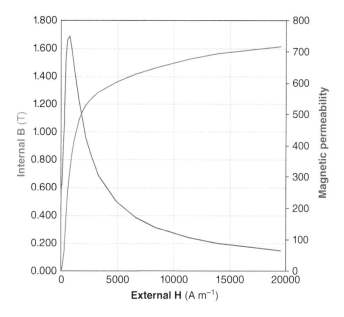

Figure 2.11   B-H curve for 416 stainless steel (blue line) and its magnetic permeability μ (red line). μ is a function of H. The metal saturates at 1.85 T. The external field $H = B_0/\mu_0$.

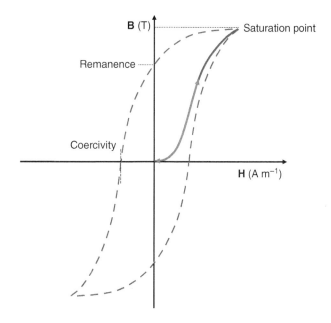

Figure 2.12   The hysteresis curve for a ferromagnetic material. The orange line represents increases in field which are reversible. Soft ferromagnetic materials have a slim curve with low remanence and coercivity. Hard ferromagnetic materials have a broader curve with higher remanence and coercivity.

Table 2.2   Properties of ferromagnetic metals.

Soft Ferromagnetic	H_c (A m^{-1})	B_{sat} (T)	Curie temperature (K)
Silicon steel	40–70	2.0	750
Mumetal (Ni-Fe alloy)	0.6–1.0	0.77	350
Iron	12–400	1.7–2.2	770
Nickel	400	0.62	358
400 series stainless steels	130–480	1.2–1.4	–
Hard Ferromagnetic			
5% Chromium steel	5×10^3	0.94	760–850
Alnico (Al-Ni-Co alloy)	50×10^3	0.56–1.35	973–1133
Supermagloy (Sm-Co alloy)	700×10^3	1.50	993–1073

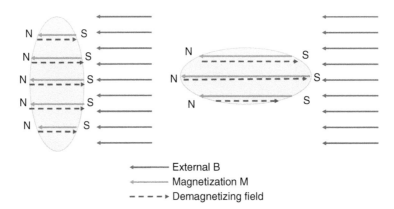

External B
Magnetization M
Demagnetizing field

Figure 2.13   Demagnetization field within objects magnetized by an external magnetic field: the flatter object (left) creates more 'virtual poles' and develops a greater degree of demagnetization.

Demagnetizing field and factors

An object's shape adds a further layer of complexity with great significance for magnetic forces and torques, and hence for MRI safety. Figure 2.13 shows how magnetization of the object in an external B_0 generates "virtual poles", resulting in a "de-magnetization field" which reduces the apparent value of susceptibility χ_{app}:

$$\chi_{app} = \frac{\chi}{1 + d_i} \tag{2.8}$$

where d_i is the *demagnetizing factor*. For simple shapes (ellipsoids of rotation, cuboids and cylinders) there are three demagnetizing factors: d_1 along the principal axis, d_2 and d_3 along the minor axes. Representative values are shown in Table A1.1 in Appendix 1. Figure 2.14 shows

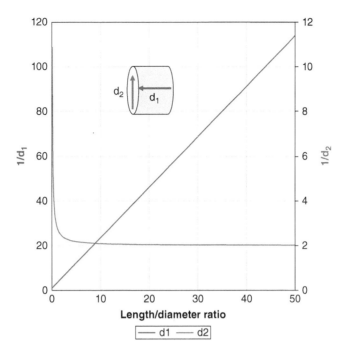

Figure 2.14 Reciprocal demagnetization factors for a cylinder: $1/d_1$ (axial, red line), $1/d_2$ (radial, blue line). For a cylinder $d_3 = d_2$.

the values of $1/d_1$ for the axial and $1/d_2$ $(=1/d_3)$ for the radial axes of cylindrical objects. It is the demagnetizing factor that determines the level of magnetization of a ferromagnetic object, rather than the value of χ. For an unsaturated sphere the internal B field is three times the external B_0. For elongated objects the internal B can be significantly greater. As a simple rule of thumb, for a cylinder whose length is aligned with B_0

$$B_{internal} = \frac{1}{d_1} B_0 \qquad\qquad (2.9a)$$

If the object is rotated 90° to B_0

$$B_{internal} = \frac{1}{d_2} B_0 \qquad\qquad (2.9b)$$

Figure 2.15 shows the theoretical internal B for ferromagnetic cylindrical objects of various length-diameter (l/d) ratios and a sphere as they approach 1.5 and 3 T shielded magnets. In each case the saturation value B_{sat} (=1.6 T) is reached at greater distances from the magnet for the more elongated objects.

Demagnetizing factors and B_{sat} are crucial for determining the force and torque on different shaped objects within the scanner's fringe field.

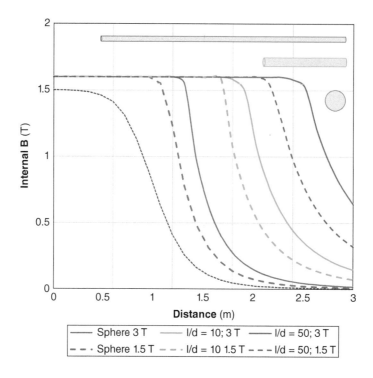

Legend:

— Sphere 3 T   — l/d = 10; 3 T   — l/d = 50; 3 T
-- · Sphere 1.5 T   -- -- l/d = 10 1.5 T   -- -- l/d = 50; 1.5 T

Figure 2.15 Predicted internal B for a ferromagnetic sphere and cylinders of differing length/diameter ratios in the approach to 1.5 and 3 T MRI magnets. The material saturates at 1.6 T. The bore entrance is at 0.8 m. The dotted gray line indicates the B_0 field strength.

MYTHBUSTER:

The internal magnetic field or degree of magnetization of a ferromagnetic object is not determined by its magnetic susceptibility but by its demagnetization factors and saturation status.

Example 2.1 Magnetization of a nickel coin

A nickel coin (length = 1 mm, diameter = 1 cm) is inadvertently brought into the MRI examination room. If the external field is 100 mT what is the field within the coin if it is: (a) lying face on to the magnet; (b) edge on to the magnet? Will the coin's metal saturate?

(a) The ratio l/d = 0.1, so from Figure 2.14 or Equation A1.31 and 2.9a

$$B_{internal} = \frac{1}{d_1} B_0 = 1.25 \times 0.1 = 0.125 \, T$$

B_{sat} for nickel is 0.62 T (Table 2.2) so, in this orientation it will be unsaturated.

(b) For the end-on orientation use d_2 and Equation 2.9b

$$B_{internal} = \frac{1}{d_2} B_0 = 9.8 \times 0.1 = 0.98 \, T$$

This exceeds B_{sat} so the internal field will saturate at 0.62 T.

Example 2.2   Iron rod in the fringe field

An iron rod of length 10 cm, diameter 2 cm is brought within the fringe field of a MR magnet with B = 100 mT. Will it be saturated if its length is aligned with the field? Iron saturates at around 2 T.
From Figure 2.14 or Equation A1.31 and 2.9a

$$B_{internal} = \frac{1}{d_1} B_0 = 12.5 \times 0.1 = 1.25\,T$$

At this point the metal will not saturate.

FORCES AND TORQUE

The forces upon ferromagnetic objects are paramount for MRI safety. "Magnet safety" should be ingrained into our behavior and consciousness. In this section we consider forces and torques on objects, conducting wires, and electrical circuits. The former is relevant for all implants, MR accessories and objects brought into the MR environment; the latter is relevant for active implants.

Translational force: non-ferromagnetic materials

For diamagnetic and paramagnetic materials where |X| is very small, we do not have to consider the demagnetizing factors. If we assume only the z-axis component, then the magnetic force on a paramagnetic object is

$$F = \frac{\chi}{\mu_0} V B_0 \frac{dB}{dz} \tag{2.10}$$

For a diamagnetic material the force will be negative, i.e. repulsive. Figure 2.16 shows plots of B, dB/dz and their product B·dB/dz along the z-axis for simulations of 1.5 and 3 T shielded magnets. Note that the locations of the maximum values of dB/dz and B·dB/dz do not necessarily coincide. For a paramagnetic or diamagnetic object the maximum force is exerted at the location of the maximum field-gradient product, near to the bore entrance. The figure shows B-field values on-axis, but in general the spatial gradient and product values are greatest around the edge of the bore circumference.

MYTHBUSTER:

The translational force within the bore is not a maximum but is close to zero.

Example 2.3   Force on a diamagnetic object

What is the force on a 1 litre bag of saline brought towards the bore of a magnet with B = 1 T and dB/dz = 5 T m⁻¹?

$$F = \frac{-0.905 \times 10^{-6}}{4\pi \times 10^{-7}} \times 0.001 \times 1 \times 5 = -0.0036\,N$$

This is a repulsive force but is 2700 times less than the force due to gravity, so is negligible.

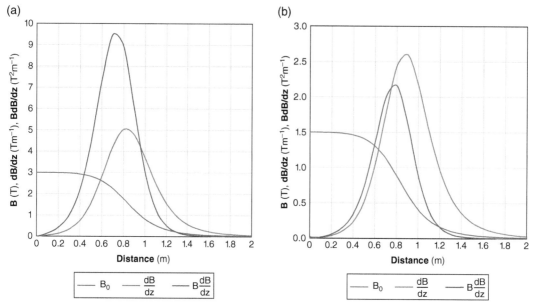

Figure 2.16   B, dB/dz and product B·dB/dz along the z-axis for: (a) a shielded 3 T magnet (b) a shielded 1.5 T magnet with bore length 1.6 m. The horizontal axis is distance from the iso-center. The bore entrance is at 0.8 m. Simulation for illustration only.

Translational force: ferromagnetic objects

The situation for a ferromagnetic object is complicated by two additional factors: *demagnetization factors* which depend strongly upon geometry, and *saturation*: the degree of magnetization sustainable by the metal. In this section we quote the final results as applied to a cylinder or ellipsoid with equal minor axes [1]. Appendix 1 provides a full derivation.

Force on a soft unsaturated ferromagnetic material

The force on an ellipsoid or cylinder aligned to B_0 (z-axis) at an angle θ, made from a soft ferromagnetic material with $\chi \gg 1$, e.g. nickel, iron, or martensitic or ferritic stainless steel, is

$$F_z = \frac{1}{\mu_0} VB_0 \left(\frac{\cos^2 \theta}{d_1} + \frac{\sin^2 \theta}{d_2} \right) \frac{dB}{dz} \tag{2.11}$$

The force is proportional to the *product* of B and dB/dz. It is striking that it does not depend upon magnetic susceptibility as long as $\chi \gg 1$, a consequence of the demagnetizing fields. As we have seen, most strongly ferromagnetic objects will saturate close to the scanner bore entrance. Figure 2.17 shows the relative forces on cylinders with length to diameter (l/d) ratios ranging from 0 (a flat disk) to 50 (like a knitting needle) and a sphere in the region where the metal is unsaturated. For a long cylinder aligned with z, the maximum force with the object aligned to B_0 is (from Equation A1.31)

$$F_z \approx \left(2.26 \frac{l}{d} + 1 \right) \frac{1}{\mu_0} VB_0 \frac{dB}{dz} \tag{2.12}$$

This formula is handy for a quick worst case estimation if you do not know the demagnetization factor or the saturation field.

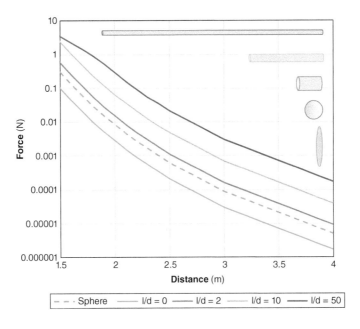

Figure 2.17 Predicted translational force (logarithmic scale) on spherical and cylindrical 0.1 kg unsaturated objects at distances remote from the iso-center along the z-axis. The bore entrance is at 0.8 m. The objects have density of 8000 kg m^{-3}, $\chi = 1000$ and $B_{sat} = 1.6$ T. The force due to gravity is approximately 1 N.

Figure 2.18 shows the effect on force of different angulations with respect to B_0. For objects with a length-diameter ratio greater than one the maximum force occurs with the greatest alignment to the field ($\theta = 0°$). For flatter objects, the greatest force occurs for an angle of 90°, that is with the planar surface perpendicular to B.

Example 2.4   Force on an unsaturated ferromagnetic object

What is the maximum force on an iron rod of length 10 cm, diameter 2 cm in the fringe field of a MRI magnet with B = 100 mT and dB/dz = 0.6 T m^{-1}? The material is unsaturated.

The material is unsaturated (see Example 2.2), so use Equation 2.12

$$F_z \approx \left(2.26 \times 5 + 1\right) \times \frac{1}{4\pi \times 10^{-7}} \times \pi \times 0.01^2 \times 0.1 \times 0.1 \times 0.6 = 18.4 \, N$$

By contrast the gravitational force is

$$F_g \approx \rho V g = 7860 \times 3.14 \times 10^{-5} = 2.4 \, N$$

The magnetic force is approximately eight times the force due to gravity at this point.

MYTHBUSTER:

For strongly ferromagnetic objects, the translational force does *not* depend upon its magnetic susceptibility, but upon its shape, the external field B_0 (or B_{sat}), and the spatial gradient dB/dz.

42

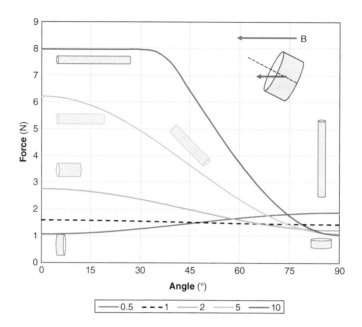

Figure 2.18 Influence of angulation of ferromagnetic objects with respect to the B_0 direction. The objects have density of 8000 kg m^{-3} weighing 0.1 kg with $\chi = 1000$ and $B_{sat} = 1.6$ T. $B = 0.1$ T and $dB/dz = 0.5$ T m^{-1}. The effect of saturation at around 30° is evident for the longest object. Simulation for illustration only.

Soft saturated ferromagnetic material

For a saturated metal the magnetization within the material is at a maximum so once saturation occurs B_0 becomes irrelevant, and the maximum force is

$$F_z \approx \frac{1}{\mu_0} V B_{sat} \frac{dB}{dz} \qquad (2.13)$$

Here, for a given object, the only variable is the gradient of the B_0 fringe field, which itself changes over distance from the magnet. The shape of the object is no longer a significant factor as it has been completely magnetized. Figure 2.19a shows the relative forces from a 1.5 and 3 T shielded magnet on 0.1 kg ferromagnetic objects which saturate at 1.6 T. State of saturation is more significant than field strength. The object's shape is a key factor. You will get closer to the magnet holding a sphere without it being wrenched from your grasp than you would with an elongated object of the same mass. Figure 2.19b, plotted on a logarithmic scale, shows the force on each object at greater distances from the iso-center, compared to the gravitational force of around 1N. A length-diameter ratio of 50 corresponds to the geometry of a Birmingham gauge 21 hypodermic needle. The force on the needle exceeds that of gravity around two meters from iso-center, half a meter further than for a spherical object of the same material and mass. Needles and scissors constitute two of the most hazardous objects around MRI scanners.

Permanent magnet

What if the object is already magnetized, i.e. is a permanent magnet? Such a situation may arise in MR if it is your institution's policy to scan patients with cochlear implants. To start, we are not

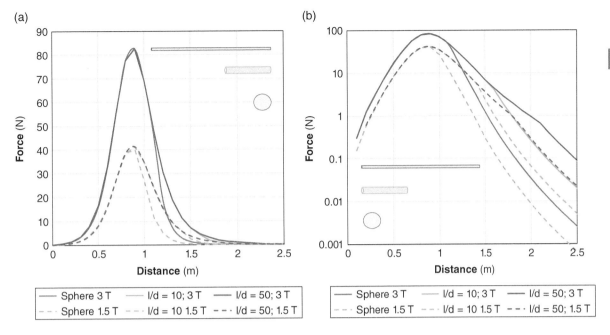

Figure 2.19 Predicted translational force on spherical and cylindrical 0.1 kg objects along the z-axis: (a) linear plot; (b) logarithmic scale. The bore entrance is at 0.8 m. The objects have density of 8000 kg m^{-3} and $\chi = 1000$ with B$_{sat}$ = 1.6 T.

Example 2.5 Force on a ferromagnetic object aligned with B$_0$

What is the maximum force on a ferromagnetic steel cylinder of length 2 cm, diameter 2 mm in the fringe field of a MRI magnet with B = 50 mT and dB/dz = 0.25 Tm^{-1}? The material saturates at 1 T.

The maximum force occurs when the object's long axis is aligned with B$_0$. Firstly determine if the object is saturated. From Figure 2.14 or Equations A1.31 and 2.9a

$$B_{internal} = \frac{1}{d_1}B_0 = 24 \times 0.05 = 1.2\,T$$

This exceeds B$_{sat}$ so use Equation 2.13

$$F_z \approx \frac{1}{\mu_0}VB_{sat}\frac{dB}{dz} = \frac{1}{4\pi \times 10^{-7}} \times \pi \times 0.001^2 \times 0.02 \times 1 \times 0.25 = 0.0125\,N$$

By contrast the gravitational force is

$$F_g \approx \rho Vg = 8000 \times 6.28 \times 10^{-8} \times 9.8 = 0.005\,N$$

The magnetic force is 2.5 times the force due to gravity at this point.

---

reliant on the external B$_0$ to magnetize the object. Whether an increase occurs close to the magnet will depend upon the hysteresis properties of the object – it may even become demagnetized- so it is virtually impossible to predict. We can say, however, that the initial translational (attractive

---

Example 2.6   Force on a ferromagnetic object side on to B₀

If the object in Example 2.5 has its long axis perpendicular to B_0. What is the attractive force on it?
  Firstly determine if the object is saturated. From Figure 2.14 or Equations A1.31 and 2.9b

$$B_{internal} = \frac{1}{d_2} B_0 = 2.09 \times 0.05 = 0.104\ T$$

In this orientation the object is not saturated so use Equation 2.11 with θ = 90°

$$F_z \approx \frac{1}{d_2}\frac{1}{\mu_0}VB_0\frac{dB}{dz} = 2.09 \times \frac{1}{4\pi \times 10^{-7}} \times 6.28 \times 10^{-8} \times 0.05 \times 0.25 = 0.0013\ N$$

(We could also have used Equation 2.13 using B = 0.1 T in place of B_{sat}).
  This is one quarter of the gravitational force. The orientation of the object matters! Twisting it towards the magnet is potentially dangerous.

---

or repulsive depending upon orientation) and twisting forces are likely to exceed those of a soft ferromagnetic object. Cochlear implants are discussed in Chapter 10.

Projectile velocity

We can estimate the velocity of ferromagnetic projectiles from the basic laws of mechanics (Figure 2.20). One non-intuitive feature of projectile velocities is that they are broadly independent of the mass of the object. For example, if the densities of two objects are equal, then the translational force will scale with the mass, but acceleration scales with its inverse. Provided

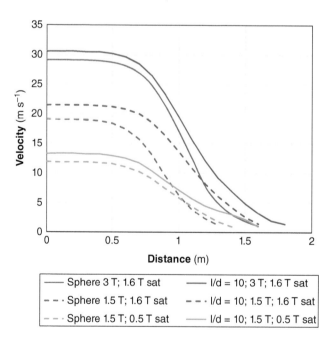

Figure 2.20   Predicted projectile velocity for the objects and magnets in Figure 2.19 saturating at 1.6 and 0.5 T.

objects are the same shape (rather than size) and made of the same material, they will fly in equally fast with velocities of tens of meters per second- in under half a second for a given magnet!

Torque

If the object is non-spherical and has an axis at an angle θ with respect to B, there will be a twisting force or torque acting to align the object with the field. Torque, **T**, is a vector (Figure 2.21) with a magnitude

$$T = mB_0 \sin\theta \tag{2.14}$$

Torque is measured in newton-meters (N m). **m** is the object's magnetic moment (= MV).

Torque on diamagnetic and paramagnetic objects

For $|\chi_m| \ll 1$ the torque is [1]:

$$T = \frac{1}{2\mu_0}\chi^2 V B_0^2 (d_2 - d_1)\sin 2\theta \tag{2.15}$$

Perhaps at odds with "common sense" is the observation that the maximum torque is exerted at 45° (Figure 2.22a), but at this angle there is the greatest product of magnetization and interaction with B. The maximum torque for a long object becomes

$$T \propto \frac{1}{4\mu_0}\chi^2 V B_0^2 \tag{2.16}$$

As $\chi \ll 1$, the torque on non-ferromagnetic objects is very small.

Torque on soft ferromagnetic objects

Of more significance is the torque on a soft ferromagnetic object. The torque on an unsaturated object is

$$T = \frac{1}{2\mu_0} V B_0^2 \frac{(d_2 - d_1)}{d_1 d_2}\sin 2\theta \tag{2.17}$$

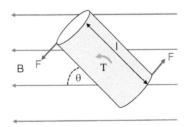

Figure 2.21 Torque T on a ferromagnetic object of length l. The force on either end is F=T/l and the total *twisting force* is double.

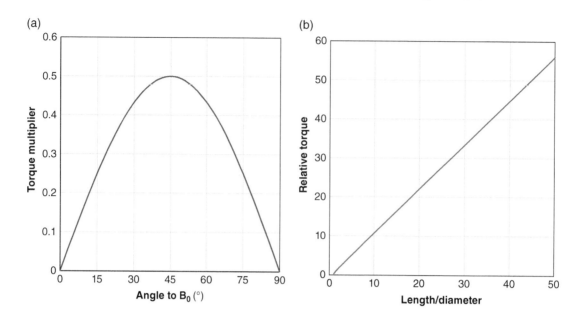

Figure 2.22 Relative torque as a function of: (a) angle; (b) ratio of length-diameter for a cylinder for unsaturated ferromagnetic objects.

Example 2.7 Torque on a weakly ferromagnetic magnetic implant

Suppose an implant of length 1 cm, diameter 0.2 cm is introduced into a 3 T scanner at 45° to the z-axis, what is the torque and twisting force if the implant has $X = 0.01$?

As X is small, treat the implant as paramagnetic. Calculate the volume and use Equation 2.15

$$V = \pi \times 0.001^2 \times 0.01 = 3.14 \times 10^{-8}\, m^{-3}$$

The torque is then

$$T = \frac{1}{4\pi \times 10^{-7}} \times 0.01^2 \times 3.14 \times 10^{-8} \times 3^2 \times (0.46 - 0.08) \times 0.5 = 4.3 \times 10^{-6}\, Nm$$

and the rotational force is

$$F = \frac{4.3 \times 10^{-6}}{0.5 \times 0.01} = 0.00086\, N.$$

This is around one third of the force due to gravity.

MYTHBUSTER:

The maximum torque does not occur when an object is at a right angle to B_0, but at 45°.

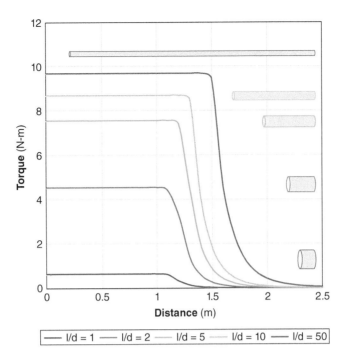

Figure 2.23 Predicted torque for ferromagnetic 0.1 kg objects of varying l/d ratios, with density 8000 kg m^{-3}, susceptibility of 1000 and B$_{sat}$ = 2 T on the axis of a 1.5 T shielded magnet. The bore entrance is at 0.8 m.

Remarkably this is also independent of susceptibility, depending upon the square of B$_0$ (so four times greater at 3 T compared with 1.5 T), with a maximum value within the magnet bore. Torque becomes larger for long needle-like objects (Figure 2.22b). For a saturated object the torque becomes proportional to B$_{sat}$^{2} and has a maximum value (Figure 2.23)

$$T_{max,sat} \approx \frac{1}{2\mu_0} V B_{sat}^2 \left(d_2 - d_1\right)$$

(2.18)

Usually an object will twist long before it reaches the bore, and hence the torque rapidly disappears, aligning the object for maximum projectile velocity. There is the possibility of serious injury if an implant is ferromagnetic.

MYTHBUSTER:

Torque on strongly ferromagnetic objects is independent of their magnetic susceptibility.

Example 2.8   Torque on a ferromagnetic cylinder

You can use Figure 2.22 and Equation 2.18 to calculate the torque on a ferromagnetic object which saturates at 1 T. Suppose a cylinder is at 30° to B_0, and is 50 cm long, 10 cm diameter.

From the figure the multiplier for the angle is 0.43 and for the l/d ratio is 5. The volume is

$$V = \pi \times 0.05^2 \times 0.5 = 0.0039 \, m^{-3}$$

The torque is then

$$T = \frac{1}{4\pi \times 10^{-7}} \times 0.0039 \times 1^2 \times (0.46 - 0.08) \times 0.43 = 514 \, Nm.$$

The force exerted on each end of the object is given by the torque divided by the length = 1028 N.

Torque v translational force

A question of some significance, especially for implants, is which is stronger, the translational or the twisting force? Figure 2.24 shows the attractive and twisting force (from the torque) for ferromagnetic objects (mass 0.1 kg, density of 8000 kg m^{-3}, $\chi = 1000$) approaching a 3 T scanner. We assume that the orientation is such to produce either the maximum torque or translation (note: that these conditions are inconsistent with each other). What is quite surprising is that, in this simulation, the force exerted from twisting is greater than that from translation at *most*

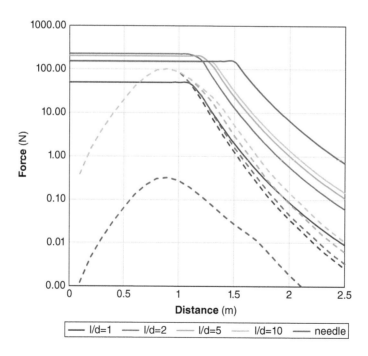

Figure 2.24   Predicted maximum twisting force (solid lines) and translational (dashed lines) from ferromagnetic 0.1 kg cylinders of varying l/d ratios and a 5 cm needle with l/d = 50, with densities 8000 kg m^{-3}, $\chi = 1000$ and $B_{sat} = 2$ T on the axis of a 1.5 T shielded magnet. The lengths of the cylinders are 11.6, 7.5, 5, and 2.5 cm.

locations. This is bad news for MR safety as the first thing to occur will be the twisting to align with the field direction which is then the optimum orientation for projectiles. Also, for ferromagnetic implants, unless they are perfectly spherical (in which case the torque will be zero) or perfectly aligned with B_0, the twisting forces will persist for the whole time spent in the bore of the magnet. In the figure the forces on a 5 cm long needle ($l/d = 50$) are shown, where the twisting can greatly exceed the projectile force. Although the attractive force on the needle appears low, remember that items tend to accelerate into the scanner with high velocities, so this situation is very dangerous.

Forces on circuits

We saw in Chapter 1 that the tesla was defined in terms of a force upon a moving charge. A moving charge is an electrical current, so it is no surprise that magnetic fields exert a force on a current-carrying conductor.

Force on a straight conductor

The force on a current-carrying conductor at an angle θ to B_0 is (Figure 2.25a):

$$F = IdB_0 \sin\theta \tag{2.19}$$

This follows Fleming's *left-hand rule*: if your forefinger points along B_0, your other fingers show the direction of current flow, then your thumb indicates the direction of the force (Figure 2.25b).

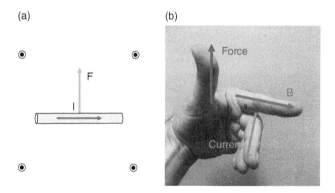

Figure 2.25   The Lorentz force on a straight conductor with (a) B into the page; (b) Fleming's left-hand rule scheme to deduce the direction of the force.

Example 2.9   Force on an electrical wire

What is the force on a 10 cm length of wire at an angle 45° to a B_0 of 1.5 T and carrying 10 A?

$$F = 10 \times 0.1 \times 1.5 \times 0.707 = 1.06 \ N$$

If the wire weighs 10 g, then this force is ten times the gravitational force on the wire.

LORENTZ AND HYDRODYNAMIC FORCES

Moving charges are subject to an additional force, the *Lorentz force*. Charge moving within an external magnetic field produces an electric field by the *hydrodynamic* or *Hall effect*.

Lorentz force

The magnitude of the Lorentz force on a charge Q possessing velocity v is given as

$$F = QvB\sin\theta \qquad (2.20)$$

The direction of the force can be determined by Fleming's left-hand rule.

Magneto-hydrodynamic effect

A similar effect is the generation of an electric field E by the flow of charge within an external magnetic field (Figure 2.26). This is analogous to the Hall effect observed in semiconductors.

$$E = vB\sin\theta \qquad (2.21)$$

In terms of induced voltage or electrical potential, *V*, where

$$V = Ed \qquad (2.22)$$

and d is the distance between charged surfaces (as in a capacitor), we have an induced voltage

$$V = dvB\sin\theta \qquad (2.23)$$

The effect is most commonly encountered in MRI as an artefact in ECG traces.

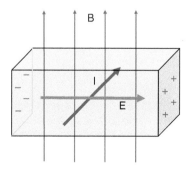

Figure 2.26   Magneto-hydrodynamic and Hall effect.

LAWS OF INDUCTION

The laws of induction follow from Maxwell's third equation or Faraday's law. If we consider a wire loop within a time-varying B-field the magnitude of the induced E-field is [3]

$$|E| = \frac{r}{2}\frac{dB}{dt} \qquad (2.24)$$

This applies for both the electric field induced by the imaging gradients responsible for peripheral nerve stimulation (PNS), and the electric field induced by the RF B_1-field responsible for SAR and tissue (and implant) heating. The direction of E follows a left-hand rule, as any magnetic field produced by the induced current in the wire opposes the rate of change of flux that induced it.

Faraday induction from the gradients

Biological tissues conduct electricity by means of water and electrolytes. Rather than considering electrical current in tissue (as in wires), we consider the *current density* **J**, a vector (Figure 2.27)

$$\mathbf{J} = \sigma \mathbf{E} \qquad (2.25)$$

σ is the tissue conductivity in siemens per meter (S m^{-1}). Some representative values are shown in Table 2.3.

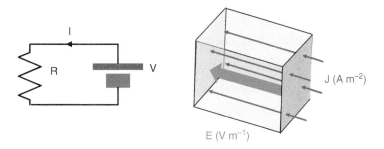

Figure 2.27   Ohm's law in a circuit and a volume conductor.

Table 2.3   Tissue conductivity at various frequencies. Electrical properties from https://itis.swiss/virtual-population/tissue-properties/database after [4].

Tissue	Conductivity (S m^{-1})		
	10 Hz	1 kHz	100 MHz
Bone (cortical)	0.02	0.02	0.064
Brain (WM)	0.028	0.063	0.32
Fat	0.038	0.042	0.068
Heart muscle	0.054	0.11	0.73
Liver	0.028	0.041	0.49
Muscle	0.20	0.32	0.71

52

In practice conductivity may be anisotropic, e.g. along a muscle fiber as opposed to across it; or, at radio frequencies, it may be *complex* with real and imaginary components. For now we shall assume the simplest situation: isotropic, non-complex but frequency dependent. Human anatomy, with irregular shapes and differing tissue conductivities, will exhibit much more complex behavior, with E-field lines and current loops being altered by tissue boundaries and electrostatic charges induced on these boundaries according to Gauss's Law.

Induced fields from movement within the static fringe field gradient

Movement through the static fringe field gradient dB/dz exposes tissue to a changing magnetic flux, and hence induces an electric field and current density. Restricting this discussion to the z-direction only

$$E = v\frac{r}{2}\frac{dB}{dz} \qquad (2.26a)$$

$$J = v\sigma\frac{r}{2}\frac{dB}{dz} \qquad (2.26b)$$

The induced E and J are greatest for the highest level of dB/dz, i.e. close the scanner bore entrance, and scale with velocity. This mechanism is thought to be the cause for some of the acute sensory effects experienced around high field magnets (see Chapter 3).

Example 2.10   Movement in the fringe field gradient

A staff member moves towards the magnet at 1 ms^{-1} in a fringe field gradient of 5 Tm^{-1}. What is the maximum induced electric field and current density around their head?
  Use Equation 2.26 with r = 0.08 m and conductivity of 0.2 Sm^{-1}

$$E = 0.5 \times 0.08 \times 1.0 \times 5.0 = 0.2\,V\,m^{-1}$$

$$J = 0.2 \times 0.2 = 0.04\,A\,m^{-2}$$

Lenz's law

The eddy currents induced by movement generate a magnetic field which opposes the change in magnetic flux. This is Lenz's law, a clarification upon Faraday's law of induction. An example of this can be observed by introducing a sheet of non-ferromagnetic metal such as aluminium or copper into the bore of the magnet. If you position the sheet vertically and transversely (normal to B_0) and then allow it to drop towards the horizontal, the flux from B_0 changes as the angle to B_0 increases and induced magnetic field will oppose B_0. The ensuing attractive force opposes the gravitational force and the sheet will tip in slow motion down towards the horizontal. Similarly, moving a non-ferromagnetic conducting object in the fringe field gradient will result in resistance to that motion. Make sure the metal you use is non-ferromagnetic.

Induction from the radiofrequency exposure

In some respects, the calculation of induced E from the RF exposure is easier than for the gradients, because to a good first approximation, we can consider B_1 as being uniform in space. The power density P_V, follows from a volumetric version of the Ohm's law relation "power equals voltage times current":

$$P_V = \mathbf{J.E} = \sigma E^2 \tag{2.27}$$

Specific absorption rate (SAR) is defined as the power deposited in tissue per unit mass given by

$$SAR = 0.5\frac{\sigma}{\rho}E^2 \tag{2.28}$$

ρ is tissue density. In the simplest case of a uniform sphere, the maximum SAR from a rectangular constant amplitude B_1 pulse repeated N times is [5]

$$SAR_{max} = 0.5\frac{\sigma\pi^2 r^2 f^2 B_1^2 D}{\rho} \tag{2.29}$$

The duty cycle D is the fraction of time for which the B_1 pulse (duration t_p) is active within the MRI sequence TR period:

$$D = \frac{t_p}{TR}N \tag{2.30}$$

The average SAR is

$$SAR_{ave} = \frac{1}{5\rho}\sigma\pi^2 f^2 B_1^2 r^2 D \tag{2.31}$$

For a sphere, the average SAR is 0.4 of the peak SAR. In terms of flip angle α, for a rectangular B_1 pulse

$$SAR_{ave} = \frac{1}{5\rho\gamma^2}\sigma\pi^2 f^2 \alpha^2 r^2 \left(\frac{N}{t_p TR}\right) \tag{2.32}$$

This illustrates the well-known result that SAR is proportional to the square of the flip angle (for a given pulse shape), increases linearly with the number of RF pulses and is inversely proportional to the pulse duration and sequence repetition time TR.

In general, calculating SAR for arbitrary geometries requires the use of numerical methods [6]. An additional issue arises as a consequence of Ampere's law (Maxwell's fourth equation) for frequencies above 10 MHz, in that the induced E, itself, induces an RF magnetic field opposed to B_1 resulting in an overestimation of SAR. Additionally, differing tissue properties, anatomical geometry, and the presence of metallic implants will alter the RF deposition pattern, often resulting in SAR hotspots. The relationship between SAR and heating is non-linear and heterogeneous and is heavily influenced by the thermal properties of tissue and cooling from perfusion and conduction. These will be considered in Chapter 5.

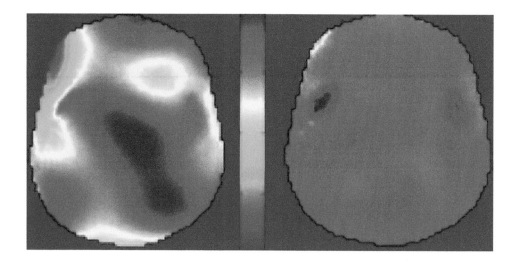

Figure 2.28 B_1 uniformity map for a head phantom at 7T showing the effect of (left) non-optimized and (right) optimized parallel transmission. Figure courtesy of Kawin Setsompop, Massachusetts General Hospital, A.A. Martinos Center for Biomedical Imaging.

Wave-like behavior of B_1

Figure 1.26 showed the uniformity of the B_1-field in air produced by a typical birdcage transmit coil. However, the presence of the patient's tissues affects the nature and amplitude of the field (Figure 2.28). In a dielectric medium the EM wavelength λ has a different value than in air or vacuum and the familiar equation for wavelength ($\lambda = c/f$) becomes

$$\lambda = \frac{c}{f\sqrt{\varepsilon_r}} \tag{2.33}$$

where c is the speed of light (3×10^8 ms^{-1}).

The "wavelength" in air is around 4.7 m at 64 MHz (1.5 T) and 2.3 m at 128 MHz (3 T) and B_1 in air is a magnetic field in the *near field* region with minimal E-field components, except close to the coil windings and tuning capacitors. However, the dielectric constant, ε_r of tissues changes the wavelength *within* the patient. Often the relative permittivity ε_r of water, with a value stated to be around 80, is used to estimate wavelength in tissue. This reduces the wavelength at 64 and 128 MHz to 0.51 m and 0.26 m. These dimensions are comparable to the patient's dimensions and also to the body transmit coil dimensions.

Near and far field

In order to better understand the RF interactions, we can consider radio antenna theory. In radio transmission for broadcasting and telecommunications, the RF field is commonly divided into different regions illustrated in Figure 2.29. Closest to the transmitter is the reactive or *inductive near field*. This is the mode of operation of the MR transmit coil, producing primarily a magnetic B_1-field. This region is said to extend to $\lambda/2\pi$ or $0.159\times\lambda$. In a 1.5 T scanner this would extend in air to 0.75 m from the iso-center and half that distance for a 3 T scanner, encompassing the entire coil volume.

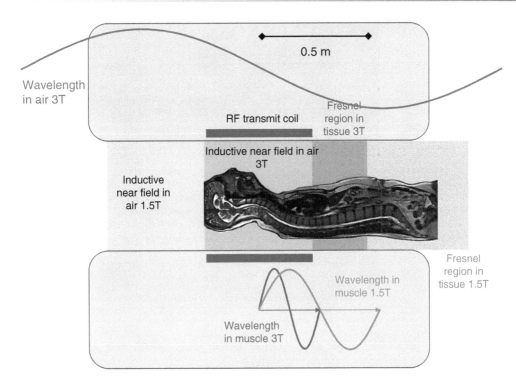

Figure 2.29   Field regions in air and within the patient's tissues. In the inductive near field zone the B$_1$ magnetic field dominates. In the radiative near field B$_1$ and E$_1$ are highly non-uniform. For comparison the wavelengths in air and muscle are shown. Top view of the scanner bore.

The *radiative near field* or Fresnel region extends between one and two wavelengths. At 3 T with a patient *in situ*, this region will extend from 0.25 to 0.5 m and double those distances in a 1.5 T scanner. In the Fresnel zone the field behavior can become very complex with local maxima and minima. This results in the B and E fields extending well beyond the end of the coil within tissue. Figure 2.23 shows measurements of B and E in a phantom where significant amounts of both fields exist up to *60 cm beyond the end of a head only transmit coil*, i.e. well beyond where we might otherwise consider the RF field to end [7]. This behavior has implications for patients with implants.

MYTHBUSTER:

With a patient lying in the bore, the RF field extends significantly beyond the confines of the transmit coil. This is a consequence of Maxwell's Equations.

λ/2 resonant length

A better-known effect of the wavelength change in tissue is the creation of standing waves or resonances when a conductor length is close to one half wavelength $\lambda/2$. This has particular importance for the avoidance of heating in active implants with lead lengths equal to or close to $\lambda/2$. Often the resonant lengths 13 cm and 26 cm are cited, but different tissues have a range of values:

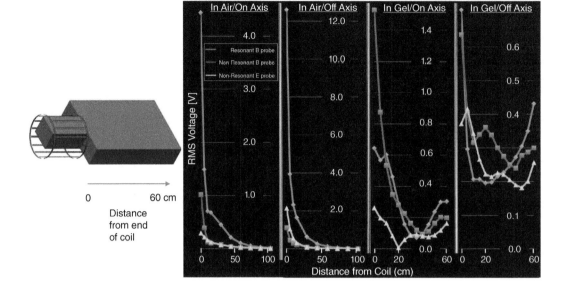

Figure 2.30 Measurements of B_1 and E_1 in a gel phantom on axis and off-axis up to 60 cm from the end of a transmit head coil in tissue equivalent material. Source [8]. Licenced under CC BY 4.0. Licensee Frontiers.

- muscle $\lambda/2 = 14.7$ cm at 128 MHz
- fat $\lambda/2 = 33.3$ cm at 128 MHz
- cancellous bone $\lambda/2 = 22.9$ cm at 128 MHz
- cortical bone $\lambda/2 = 30.6$ cm at 128 MHz.

MYTHBUSTER:

The resonant length differs from 13 or 26 cm for most tissues at 1.5 and 3 T, and much broader resonant behavior is likely.

The final zone, is the *far field* or Fraunhofer region which occurs at distances much greater than a wavelength. In this region, we have fully formed electromagnetic plane waves whose intensity decreases with the inverse square law. Their intensity is measured as power density (in W m^{-2}), but in MRI is very low – only relevant in terms of EM interference on other equipment.

Example 2.11 RF wavelength at 1.5 T

What is the RF wavelength in bone, muscle and fat at 64 MHz?

From Equation 2.33, $\lambda_{tissue} = \dfrac{\lambda_{air}}{\sqrt{\varepsilon_r}}$

ε_r *values are 16.7, 72.2 and 13.6 – so the wavelenths are 1.15 m for bone, 55 cm for muscle and 1.84 m for fat.*

CONCLUSIONS

The fields and forces associated with MRI and MRI equipment are not simple. They are all consequences of Maxwell's equations. Forces on objects may be:

- purely magnetic, relating to the shape and ferromagnetism of the material
- related to electrical current flowing in the object
- related to induction
- or movement within a field gradient.

For ferromagnetic objects the attractive or projectile magnetic force is proportional to the spatial gradient of the B_0 fringe field. The torque on an unsaturated object is proportional to the square of B_0. Most ferromagnetic objects will be saturated close to the scanner in which case the attractive force is related to $B_{sat} \cdot dB/dz$ and the torque to B_{sat}^2.

Time-varying magnetic fields from the gradients, RF, or movement within the static fringe field gradient will induce electric fields in tissue. These can lead to the stimulation of excitable tissues or to tissue heating. The RF field can exhibit unpredictable wave-like behavior. The next three chapters will look at the biological effects of the static field, gradient fields, and RF field.

Revision Questions

1. If the magnetic susceptibility χ of a diamagnetic tissue is -10^{-3} the magnetic flux density within that tissue in a 1.5 T scanner will be:
   A. 1.485 T
   B. 1.5 T
   C. 1.501 T
   D. 1.51 T
   E. 15 mT
2. The magnetic field strength H at the center of a long solenoid of length 150 cm, with 1800 turns carrying 1000 A is
   A. 1000 A m^{-1}
   B. 200 000 A m^{-1}
   C. 400 000 A m^{-1}
   D. 600 000 A m^{-1}
   E. 1 200 000 A m^{-1}
3. The magnetic flux density produced in question 2 is
   A. 500 G
   B. 0.5 T
   C. 1.0 T
   D. 1.5 T
   E. 5000 G
4. Which of the following does not affect the magnetic force on a soft ferromagnetic material with a high magnetic susceptibility?
   A. The distance to the bore opening
   B. The fringe field spatial gradient dB/dz
   C. The exact value of susceptibility χ
   D. The size of the object
   E. Its electrical conductivity.

5. A metal object saturates magnetically at 1 T. The maximum force as it approaches a 3T scanner with a spatial gradient of 5 T m^{-1} is proportional to
   A. 1 T^2 m^{-1}
   B. 3 T^2 m^{-1}
   C. 5 T^2 m^{-1}
   D. 9 T^2 m^{-1}
   E. 15 T^2 m^{-1}

6. When a previously un-magnetized ferromagnetic object is introduced into an external B field, the maximum torque occurs when the angle between the long axis of the object and the field lines is:
   A. 0°
   B. 30°
   C. 45°
   D. 60°
   E. 90°

7. The induced electric field in a circular cross section of tissue from the z-gradient is proportional to:
   A. The tissue conductivity
   B. The area of the cross section
   C. The rate of change of magnetic field
   D. The radius of the cross section
   E. Tissue density.

8. If the diameter of the heart is 8 cm, what current density would a uniform dB/dt of 100 T s^{-1} induce in it, assuming tissue conductivity of 0.2 Sm^{-1}?
   A. 1.6 mA m^{-2}
   B. 400 mA
   C. 0.8 A m^{-2}
   D. 0.4 A m^{-2}
   E. 4.0 A m^{-2}

9. If we change field strengths from 1.5T to 3T then (keeping our sequence the same)
   A. SAR will stay the same but B$_1$ will halve
   B. SAR and B$_1$ will both double
   C. SAR will double while B$_1$ remains the same
   D. Both SAR and B$_1$ will increase by four times
   E. SAR will increase by a factor of 4 while B$_1$ remains the same.

10. In a pulse sequence, if we halve the duration of the RF pulse whilst keeping the flip angle and TR the same
   A. SAR will increase
   B. SAR will not change
   C. SAR will decrease
   D. The duty cycle is doubled
   E. We cannot predict what will happen.

References

1. Schenck, J.F. (2000). Safety of strong static magnetic fields. *Journal of Magnetic Resonance Imaging* 12:2–19.
2. Kaye, G.W.C. and Laby T. H. (1995). *Tables of Physical and Chemical Constants and Some Mathematical Functions 16th edn*. Harlow, UK: Longman.
3. Budinger, T.F. (1979). Thresholds for physiological effects due to RF and magnetic fields used in NMR imaging. *IEEE Transactions on Nuclear Science* NS-26:2821–2825.

4. Payne, D., Klingenböck, A., and Kuster, N. (2018). IT'IS Database for thermal and electromagnetic parameters of biological tissues, Version 4.0, May 15, 2018. DOI: 10.13099/VIP21000-04-0.

5. Schaefer, D.J. (2014). Bioeffects of radiofrequency power deposition. In: *MRI bioeffects, safety, and patient management* (Ed. F.D. Shellock and J.V. Crues III) pp. 131–154. Los Angeles, C: Biomedical Research Publishing Group.

6. Hand, J.W. (2008). Modeling the interaction of electromagnetic fields (10 MHz–10 GHz) with the human body: methods and applications. *Physics in Medicine and Biology* 53:R 243–286.

7. Nagy, Z., Oliver-Taylor A., Kuehne A., et al. (2017). Tx/Rx head coil induces less RF transmit-related heating than body coil in conductive metallic objects outside the active area of the head coil. *Frontiers in Neuroscience* 26 January 2017. https://www.frontiersin.org/articles/10.3389/fnins.2017.00015/full

Further reading and resources

Kangarlu, A. and Schenck, J.F. (2014). Bioeffects of static magnetic fields. In: *MRI bioeffects, safety, and patient management* (Ed. F.D. Shellock and J.V. Crues III) pp. 29–63. Los Angeles, CA: Biomedical Research Publishing Group.

Panych, L.P. and Madore, B. (2018). The physics of MRI safety. *Journal of Magnetic Resonance Imaging* 47:28–43.

https://itis.swiss/virtual-population/tissue-properties/database (Accessed 9 July 2019) *Database of tissue properties.*

3

Bio-effects 1: static field

INTRODUCTION

Magnetism has been known since ancient times. As early as 1300 BCE Chinese travellers used compasses for navigation, and around 800 BCE the Greeks observed that magnetite (Fe_3O_4), a naturally occurring mineral, could attract iron. The demonstration of magnetic field lines using a compass was first made by de Maricourt in France in 1269 CE. In eighteenth century Paris the controversial physician Anton Mesmer promoted his "animal magnetism." Magnetism has long attracted pseudoscience and charlatanry. Today the "magneto-therapy" market, offering cures for all manner of aches and pains, including smoking cessation and the relief of menopausal symptoms, is worth one billion dollars globally. A feature of pseudoscience is the lack of properly designed and controlled, objective clinical trials. Hilariously, in one study which did attempt "double blinding", the supposedly unaware participants could tell that they were wearing the real magnet (rather than a sham) because their keys would stick to it in their pockets! A meta-analysis of 29 published trials concluded that there was no evidence of therapeutic benefit [1]. The National Center for Complimentary and Integrative Health (NCCIH) in the USA stated [2] *"The scientific evidence does not support the use of magnets for pain relief."* An editorial in the British Medical Journal in 2006 concluded [3]:

> Patients should be advised that magnetic therapy has no proved benefits. If they insist on using a magnetic device they could be advised to buy the cheapest- this at least will alleviate the pain in their wallet.

With more than 400 million scans performed to date, a significant proportion of the human race has undergone static magnetic field (SMF) exposures up to 60 000 times the earth's geomagnetic field of 25–65 µT. Considering that life has evolved over millions of years within the earth's field and that birds use magnetism during migration, is it inconceivable that magnets may affect life in other ways? The question is of considerable societal significance. In this chapter we review the evidence for biological effects of the static magnetic field and provide guidance on managing the acute sensory effects sometimes experienced with high field MRI.

PHYSICAL MECHANISMS

Those readers who waded through Chapter 2 will already be aware of the range and nature of magnetically induced forces on objects. Here, we will apply these results to biological structures and components. Table 3.1 summarizes the physical interactions, hypothesizes their possible

Table 3.1 Physical interactions and possible bio-effects of biological material with static magnetic fields. The magnitude of interaction is estimated for B = 3T; dB/dz =10 T m^{-1}.

Physical interaction / possible bio-effects	Dependence	Estimated maximum effect (B=3T, dB/dz =10 Tm^{-1})	
Magneto-hydrodynamic • Induced field in flowing charge (blood)	$E_i = vB\sin\theta$	3 V m^{-1}	(3.1a)
	$V = E\,d$	0.1 V	(3.1b)
Lorentz force • Movement of electrolytes • Nerve conduction velocities • Vestibular stimulation	$F = vQB\sin\theta$	$\approx 10^{-16}$ N (Na$^+$, K$^+$, Cl$^-$, Ca^{++})	(3.2)
Magneto-mechanical • Translation & orientation of molecules?	$F = \dfrac{\Delta\chi}{\mu_0}VB_0\dfrac{dB}{dz}$	$\approx 10^{-26}$N nm^{-3}	(3.3)
	$T = \dfrac{\chi^2}{\mu_0}VB^2\,\Delta d\,\sin\theta\cos\theta$	$F \approx 10^{-19}$ N nm^{-2}	(3.4)
Anisotropic susceptibility • Orientation of anisotropic paramagnetic molecules? membrane ion channels?	$T \propto \dfrac{1}{\mu_0}B^2V\,\Delta\chi\,\sin\theta\cos\theta$	$\approx 10^{-16}$ N nm^{-2} $F \approx 2\times 10^{-16}$ N for a cylindrical molecule radius 1 nm length 8 nm	(3.5)
Induced electric fields from motion in a static field spatial gradient • Sensory effects?	$E = \dfrac{r}{2}v\dfrac{dB}{dz}$	1.5 Vm^{-1} for velocity = 1 ms^{-1}	(3.6)

biological effect, and gives an indication of the strength of the interaction in a 3 T magnetic field with a 10 T m^{-1} spatial gradient. For comparison the naturally occurring electrical force on an ion crossing a nerve cell membrane is also shown. These are illustrated in Figures 3.1 and 3.2.

Magneto-hydrodynamic (Hall) effect

The magneto-hydrodynamic or Hall effect (Chapter 2) is most commonly observed as an artefact on electrocardiogram (ECG) traces (Figure 3.3a). Its origin is illustrated in Figure 3.3b where an electric field E and voltage V is induced across a vessel with conductive flowing material, such as blood, at an angle θ to the magnetic field B$_z$ (Equation 3.1).

The likely magnitude of this induced voltage was one of the earliest safety considerations in MRI. For example, if the maximum blood velocity is 0.64 m s^{-1}, then a B of 2.5 T optimally oriented across the vessel at 90° will induce an electric field of 1.6 V m^{-1} and the ensuing voltage across a 2.5 cm diameter vessel will be 40 mV. This is equal to the depolarization threshold of cardiac muscle and, for this reason, an early field limit was set at 2.5 T [4]. Of course, as we shall see, cardiac depolarization does not occur in fields up to at least 9.4 T, and this is reflected in the International Electrotechnical Commission's MRI level I exposure limit of 8 T [5]. In human anatomy, most of the major vessels: ascending and descending aorta, iliac and carotid arteries, vena cava, etc. predominantly lie closely parallel to the head-foot direction of B, so this effect is often very minor.

Lorentz force

The Lorentz force acts on electrical charges moving in a magnetic field (Figure 3.1b). The force is equal to the product of the electric field and the charge (Equation 3.2). There is the

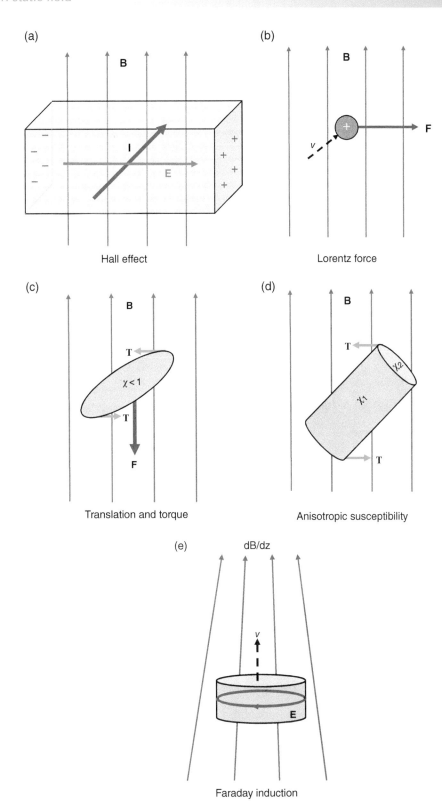

Figure 3.1 Magnetic forces in biology: (a) Hall effect; (b) Lorentz force; (c) translation and torque; (d) anisotropic susceptibility; (e) Faraday induction of electric field from motion through a field gradient.

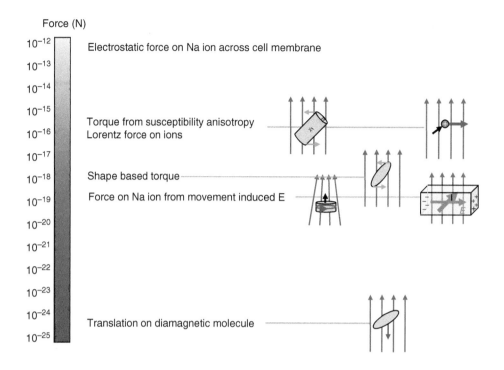

Figure 3.2 Relative strength of forces on molecules and ions.

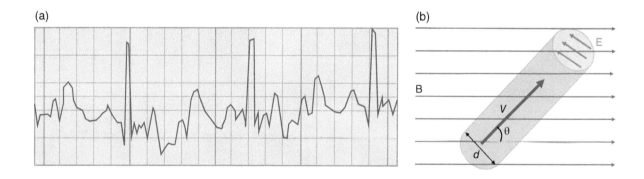

Figure 3.3 (a) Magneto-hydrodynamic (Hall effect) artefact on an MRI ECG trace; (b) the origin of the magneto-hydrodynamic effect in an artery.

possibility that this may affect ion transport across the cell membrane or affect nerve conduction velocity. However, theoretical estimation suggests that a field of 24 T would be required for a 10% change in nerve impulse conduction velocity [6]. Later in this chapter we shall see an effect of the Lorentz force on the inner ear.

Magneto-mechanical forces and torque

The attractive force and torque are key safety parameters for ferromagnetic objects and implants brought into the MR environment. However, a cursory look at Equations 3.3–3.4 shows that the

Example 3.1   Force on an electrolyte ion

What is the average force on a sodium (Na^+) ion in a 3 T field orientated perpendicular to the motion?
The thermal energy is kT (k is Boltzmann's constant, 1.38×10^{-23} J K^{-1}) and body temperature is 310 K (kelvin). The motional energy is given by

$$U = \frac{1}{2}m\bar{v}^2 = kT$$

The mass of a sodium ion is 3.8×10^{-26} kg so the average ion velocity is

$$\bar{v} = \sqrt{\frac{2kT}{m}} = \sqrt{\frac{2 \times 310 \times 1.38 \times 10^{-23}}{3.8 \times 10^{-26}}} = 475\,ms^{-1}$$

and as the electronic charge q = $1.602 \times 10^{-19}C$,

$$F_{Lorentz} = 3 \times 475 \times 1.602 \times 10^{-19} = 2.3 \times 10^{-16}\,N$$

If the membrane thickness is 8 nm (8×10^{-9}m) and there is a potential difference of 80 mV between exterior and interior, then the intrinsic force on a Na^+ ion is

$$F = \frac{V}{d}q = \frac{0.08 \times 1.602 \times 10^{-19}}{8 \times 10^{-9}} = 1.602 \times 10^{-12}\,N$$

This is 7000 times the Lorentz force on the ion.

very small diamagnetic susceptibility of biological materials (see Table 2.1) of the order of -10^{-5} renders these forces as minute and, in the context of the thermal motions and forces at work in tissues, negligible (Figure 3.1c).

For example, the magnetic force per unit mass on de-oxygenated red blood cells can be estimated from their susceptibility of -6.53×10^{-6}. For a B of 3 T and a spatial gradient of 10 T m^{-1}, this force will be 70 times less than the gravitational force (Example 3.2). The force difference between the de-oxygenated red blood cells and plasma, which tends to separate the components, will be one tenth of the separating force due to gravity alone. During MRI the field-spatial gradient product experienced is likely to be much less, and will be zero or inside the bore where the B-field spatial gradient is zero.

Example 3.2   Forces on blood cells

What is the difference in the force exerted on red blood cells (RBC) and plasma from a 3 T field with a spatial gradient of 10 T m^{-1}?
Using Equation 3.3 and remembering that density ρ equals mass m divided by volume V we can calculate the force on the red blood cells per unit mass as

$$\frac{F}{m} = \frac{\chi}{\mu_0 \rho}B_0\frac{dB}{dz} = \frac{-6.53 \times 10^{-6}}{4\pi \times 10^{-7} \times 1093} \times 30 = -0.14\,N\,kg^{-1}$$

By comparison the gravitational force on blood is around 9.8 N kg^{-1}. Similarly, the force on plasma will be -0.21 N kg^{-1} giving a difference of 0.068 N kg^{-1}.
If we have a litre of RBC and plasma with densities 1093 and 1027 kg m^{-3} respectively then the difference in gravitational force is

$$\Delta F_g = 9.8 \times (1093 - 1027) = 0.65\,N$$

Which is about ten times the force difference arising from the magnetic field.

Magnetic torque is even less significant due to its χ^2 dependence. If we consider an individual red blood cell as an 8 μm (8 × 10⁻⁶ m) diameter disk with thickness of 2 μm we can calculate the maximum force on a cell directly from Equation 3.4. For a 3 T magnet the force on a red blood cell is around one three hundredth of the gravitational force.

Example 3.3   Torque on a blood cell

What is the force due to magnetic torque on a deoxygenated red blood cell in a 3 T magnet?

We can calculate the volume of the cell by assuming it to be a cylinder of radius r = 4 μm and length l = 2 μm. As volume is equal to $\pi r^2 l$ and torque T is force times distance, we have

$$F_{rbc} = \frac{T}{r} = \frac{\left(3 \times 6.53 \times 10^{-6}\right)^2}{4\pi \times 10^{-7}} \times \frac{2 \times 10^{-6} \pi \times \left(4 \times 10^{-6}\right)^2}{4 \times 10^{-6}}$$

$$= 7.2 \times 10^{-15}\,N$$

The gravitational force is

$$F_g = 9.8 V\rho = 9.8 \times 2 \times 10^{-6} \pi \times \left(4 \times 10^{-6}\right)^2 \times 1093$$

$$= 1.08 \times 10^{-12} N$$

which is 150 times the force due to magnetic torque on the cell.

Another situation is where there is magnetic anisotropy for larger aggregations of molecules [7]. In this case the maximum torque is related to the susceptibility difference $\Delta\chi$ rather than χ^2. Using a maximum value of $\Delta\chi$ of 10⁻⁶ in a 3 T field gives a maximum torque of 3.5×10^{-6} for an object weighing 1g. The shape will be an influencing factor on the force exerted but, by contrast, the force due to gravity is 0.01 N. This anisotropy effect is seen at 0.5 T in-vitro for the red blood cells in sickle cell anaemia which aggregate together forming larger objects that twist in the field. It does not occur for healthy red blood cells, or in-vivo where other competing forces are greater.

The alignment of water molecules is often claimed to be the reason for the alleged effectiveness of magnetotherapy. However, the average dipole moment per molecule is 2×10^{-28} J I⁻¹. At 20 million times less than the molecular thermal energy at body temperature, it is hard to view this as a credible cause for any bio-effect.

A stronger force may occur where the anisotropy originates from a paramagnetic ion attached to the end of a molecule, such as those in the ion channels in the axon membrane (Figure 3.1d). The interaction is summarized by Equation 3.5, resulting in forces up to two orders of magnitude greater than those induced from shape-dependent susceptibility effects. It has been postulated that these can alter the function of sodium, potassium, and calcium ion channels over time periods of minutes in-vivo at fields as low as 100 mT [8].

Induced electric fields

The induced electric fields are not dependent upon the magnetic properties of tissue. They arise from motion within the static field spatial gradient dB/dz (Equation 3.6). It is quite easy to calculate their magnitude for an idealized model such as a sphere. Induced electric fields from motion are implicated in some of the acute sensory effects considered later in this chapter.

Example 3.4   Faraday induction from motion

What electric field is induced around a person's head if they are moving with a velocity of 1 ms⁻¹ towards the bore in a spatial gradient of 5 Tm⁻¹?

If we assume the head to be a sphere of radius 8 cm, then, from Equation 3.6, the maximum induced electric field is

$$E = 0.5 \times 0.08 \times 1 \times 5$$

$$= 0.2 \ Vm^{-1}$$

If the tissue conductivity is 0.2 Sm⁻¹, then the induced current density is 40 mA m⁻².

CELLULAR EFFECTS

Despite the very small magnetic interactions of the previous sections, the literature reports a large number of in-vitro cellular effects of SMF, and a few in animal models (Figure 3.4). These have been conducted over a vast range of fields categorized as weak (<1 mT), moderate (1 mT–1 T), strong (1-5 T), or ultra-strong (>5 T). We have seen that, theoretically, at MRI field strengths, the physical interactions between the field and biological components are weak or even negligible compared with natural thermal forces. So, how can some of the claimed effects of weak or moderate exposures occur as a direct result of the magnetic field, particularly those from exposures less than the geomagnetic field?

Whilst the analysis of the previous section on macroscopic interactions is valid, we know that alternating magnetic fields of the order of micro-tesla can have an effect on nuclear spin, although this has no effect on the chemistry (and biochemistry) at atomic and molecular levels. However, the gyromagnetic ratio of the electron is –27 204 MHz T⁻¹, over six hundred times stronger than for the proton, implying that even very small fluctuations in the magnetic field may have the ability to alter its spin state. The new scientific field of "quantum biology" attests that radical pair (RP) reactions, mediated by quantum-entangled spins, can increase the activity, concentration, and lifetime of paramagnetic free radicals, particularly oxygen and hydroxyl radicals. These reactive oxygen species (ROS) are known to cause oxidative stress, gene mutation, and apoptosis (cell death).

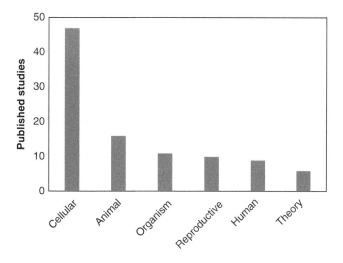

Figure 3.4   Number of published studies of bio-effects of static magnetic fields over 30 years to 2018.

Does this actually happen? This is a difficult question to answer. Figure 3.5, derived from a comprehensive review [9], indicates in-vitro studies which showed increased, decreased, or no change in the levels of ROS plotted against field strength. How do we interpret this data? The nature of the effects and the field exposure conditions that give rise to them remain controversial and the implications for MRI exposures are unclear, whether as health detriment or benefit. The International Commission on Non-Ionizing Radiation Protection (ICNIRP) noted the inconsistency of results and concluded [10]:

> Overall there is little convincing evidence from cellular and cell-free models of biologically harmful effects of exposure to magnetic fields with flux densities up to several teslas.

More significantly controlled experiments covering the magnetic field range usually implicated for the radical pair mechanism concluded that those mechanisms are unlikely (Figure 3.6) [11]. However, the European Union's Scientific Committee on Emerging and Newly Identified Health Risks (SCENIHR) reported [12]:

> In the majority of available in vitro studies, SMF above 30 mT induced effects in cellular endpoints investigated, although effects were transient in some cases. Gene expression was affected in all studies, with predominantly up-regulated outcomes. Findings from these new studies are consistent with previous results.

Whilst there may be an underlying biological process which is affected, either aided or hindered, by the presence of SMFs, these effects have only been observed for in-vitro cell studies rather than in animal models. They are also usually accompanied by a chronic or repeated exposure to the magnetic field over a time period comparable with the duration of cell cycle or several cycles. In a more MRI relevant situation exposure to 7 T alone and 7 T plus MRI gradients and RF showed no DNA damage or cell proliferation on isolated human mononuclear blood cells [13].

Another class of experiments showed subtle changes in electrophysiological properties of nerve cells as low as 10 mT, and a small reduction in sodium channel current amplitude at 125 mT [14]. Whilst by no means proven, magnetic torque on diamagnetic molecules that terminate with

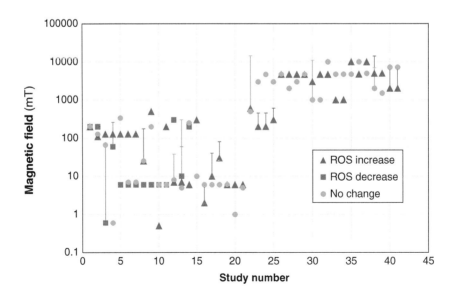

Figure 3.5   Reactive oxygen species (ROS) results from in-vitro studies. Derived from [9].

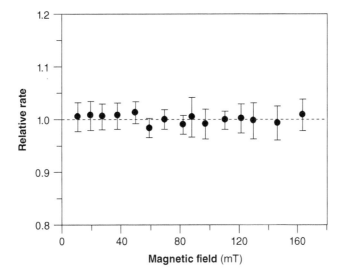

Figure 3.6   Magnetic field dependence of the kinetics of flavin oxidation in P2O from *Trametes multicolour* showing that radical pair mechanisms are unlikely in redox enzymes. Source [11]. Licensee: the Royal Society Society under CC BY 4.0.

a paramagnetic ion as discussed earlier in the chapter appears to offer the most plausible explanation.

However, in MRI we are looking at *acute*, *short-term* exposures where any of these claimed effects, for good or ill, will not have time to manifest. Additionally, all the reported effects, whether affecting ion transport or oxidization, were noted as reversible when the field was removed. They are unlikely to constitute a hazard in MRI.

ANIMAL EFFECTS

Various animal experiments have demonstrated biological effects from static magnetic fields. The mere phenomenon of avian navigation during migration indicates that a specific bio-effect from the earth's field exists, and it has been hypothesized that the RP mechanism may be implicated in this [16]. Other reported effects include bone damage and vitamin A depletion from movement by rodents in a static field gradient, changes to nerve firing parameters in various models, behavioral changes, developmental abnormalities, and skin blood flow changes, again principally in rodents. Mice bred for 28 days in static fields up to 12 T showed no effect on weight, blood indicators, or organ morphology [17]. A review of mouse model studies concluded that both acute and chronic moderate exposure levels have no substantial effect on cardiovascular dynamics, hematological indices, skeletal health, nerve activity, cognitive function, behavioral activity, and immune response [18]. For stronger fields (>1 T) ion transport and gene expression may be affected, but only transiently and are reversible when the field is removed. A human MR exposure of short duration is therefore highly unlikely to result in any deleterious health outcome.

The published evidence and claims of each study need to be examined closely. ICNIRP noted that many studies suffer from poor dosimetry and design, and many results are contradictory lacking replication. SCENIHR concluded [12]:

A number of studies report that effects of SMF exposures occur in animals at levels ranging from mT to T. However, since many findings are limited to single studies, they do not provide a firm foundation for risk assessment.

Reported effects on nerve electrical properties at higher fields appear consistent with human studies. Studies at 7 T have demonstrated abnormal locomotive behavior in rats, where they walk in circles in the static field gradient of an MRI magnet, but move normally in the uniform field at the iso-center [18]. This behavior disappeared following labrynthectomy [19], supporting the findings of studies on the human vestibular system.

Most importantly, no credible carcinogenic effects have been observed.

EPIDEMIOLOGY

Epidemiological studies of MRI-level exposures to SMF have not been conducted. The conclusions from ICNIRP [10] are:

Overall, the few available epidemiological studies have methodological limitations and leave a number of issues unresolved concerning the possibility of risk of cancer or other outcomes from long-term exposure to static magnetic fields. These studies do not indicate strong effects of static magnetic field exposure of the level of tens of mT on the various health outcomes studied, but they would not be able to detect small to moderate effects. Other occupations with a potential for higher magnetic field exposures have not been adequately evaluated, e.g. MRI operators.

MRI has been available as a clinical tool since the 1990s with more than 400 million examinations. It would appear highly improbable that any carcinogenic effect has remained undetected so far, although studies to confirm this do not exist. Studies relating to effects on the fetus will be considered in Chapter 7.

HUMAN PHYSIOLOGICAL EFFECTS

Human physiological effects of high field exposures have been studied as a necessary step in the evaluation of high field MRI as a potential clinical modality. No change in temperature, respiratory rate, pulse rate, blood pressure, finger oxygenation, or any blood flow reduction were observed in a 9.4 T magnet [20]. A study of 538 workers in an MRI manufacturing facility reported a cautious possible link of prolonged cumulative exposure to static magnetic fields with hypertension [21]. Specific dosimetry data was unavailable and the conclusions are tentative, but warrant further investigation.

ACUTE SENSORY EFFECTS

Acute effects arising from the higher SMF exposures afforded by modern MR systems include vertigo, nausea, nystagmus, and metallic taste.

Metallic taste

Human experiments with an unshielded 7 T magnet found that approximately 50% of subjects experienced "metallic taste" when shaking their heads left-right vigorously at the bore entrance with a periodicity of 1.5 s. The mean dB/dt was $2.3\pm 0.3\ T\ s^{-1}$ with a minimum threshold of $1.3\ T\ s^{-1}$ [22].

The effect was unrelated to the presence or absence of dental fillings and it was hypothesized that it arose from either direct stimulation of taste buds or from electrolysis of saliva. Only one subject experienced the sensation from head-nodding. A study of occupational exposure involving 361 MR workers in the Netherlands [23] reported metallic taste in only 0.4% and 0.8% of participants working at 1.5 and 3 T but rising to 19.4% at 7 T (Figure 3.7). The effect disappeared quickly and there was no suggestion or evidence of a health risk. It has been described as being like "licking a battery." Metallic taste was reported in 5.5% of 3457 examinations at 7 and 9.4 T [24]. Animal studies at 14 T have also demonstrated taste disturbances [18].

Vertigo and nystagmus

Vertigo is a well-documented acute effect of exposure to strong magnetic fields. Up to 19% of more than 1400 patients questioned experienced vertigo whilst moving into a 7 or 9.4 T scanner with other effects less prevalent. Only 2% reported this whilst lying within the bore [24]. MRI-related symptoms were reported during 4% of the measured shifts from 104 MR workers in the UK. These were slight dizziness after cleaning the bore, dizzy feeling for 30s, slight or mild headache, and eye strain [25]. Another study reported vertigo at 7 T but not 1.5 T [26]. When introduced into the field of a 7 T scanner in total darkness 85% of subjects experienced an illusionary sense of horizontal rotation lasting less than one minute [27]. Significantly higher occurrences of vertigo (84%) were reported in a modern actively-shielded 7 T system in a study of 124 patients and research volunteers [28].

The effect has been linked to involuntary eye movement or nystagmus. The vestibular ocular reflex (VOR) links head rotational movement to eye viewing direction. If your head moves in one direction, then your eyes automatically move in opposition. This enables us to have a consistent

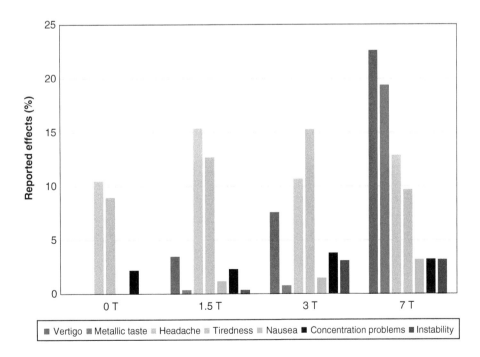

Figure 3.7   Acute sensory effects reported in the Netherlands occupational exposure study. Those showing a credible dose-response relationship include vertigo and metallic taste. Data from [23].

visual field when moving, otherwise the act of head rotation would give you a visual experience akin to changing orientation in street view mode in Google Maps. Roberts et al. [29] asserted that all subjects with an intact labyrinthine function experienced nystagmus when inside the bore of either a 3 T or 7 T scanner. The movement commenced at the start of the field exposure, persisted whilst within the magnet and ceased when the subject was removed from the field. The direction of eye movement reversed when the subjects entered the bore feet first. Moreover, there was a linear dose response relationship (Figure 3.8) with field strength. The detection of the effect required the subjects to be introduced into the scanner in total darkness which explains why this effect was undetected previously. For long exposures (of a few minutes) the effect gradually decreases with an adaptation time constant of 39.3 seconds (Figure 3.9) [30].

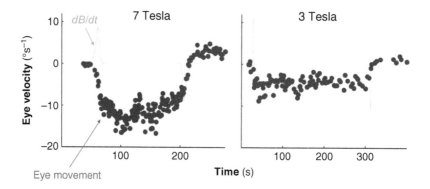

Figure 3.8 Nystagmus caused by 7 and 3 T static magnetic fields: blue dots = eye movement; green line dB/dt. Source [29]. Reproduced with permission of Elsevier.

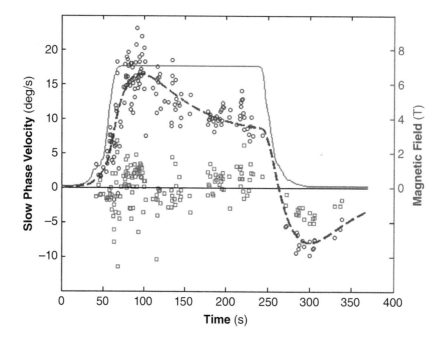

Figure 3.9 Temporal response of nystagmus at 7 T: horizontal movement (blue points); vertical movement (green points); model fit (blue line); magnetic field (red line). Source [30]. Reproduced with permission of Wiley.

The internal chambers of the labyrinth are filled with endolymph, a fluid with a high concentration of potassium (K^+) ions in contact with the hair cells that provide the vestibular sensitivity. Movement of this fluid within the SMF is subject to the Lorentz force and it is postulated that this exerts a force on the semi-circular canal cupula to induce nystagmus. The nystagmus threshold pressure is around 0.1 mPa (milli-Pascals), whereas the maximum pressure exerted by the Lorentz force at 7 T is estimated as 1.6 mPa [31]. Other potential mechanisms related to the spatial gradient field or to motion are improbable [32]. A consistent nystagmus threshold has been determined as 1.7 T ±0.6 T and for vertigo as 5.1 T ±1.1 T (Figure 3.10). To avoid vertiginous sensations patients should keep their eyes open within the bore as the involuntary eye movement can be overridden by attention to visual cues, i.e. looking at things.

MYTHBUSTER:

Magnetic vertigo is not related to motion within the B_0 spatial gradient but to B_0 directly. Patients should keep their eyes open during MRI.

Nausea

Feelings of nausea experienced in an around MR scanners can be attributed to a reaction to the vestibular disturbances. The Nottingham study reported only two nausea reactions (one subject vomited) from 164 volunteers exposed at 7 T [22]. The Netherlands study reported nausea rates

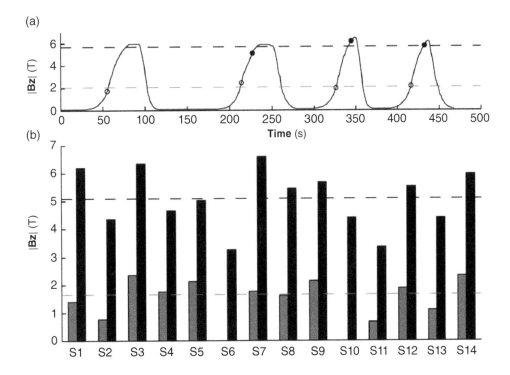

Figure 3.10   Vertigo and nystagmus: (a) B field variation with time showing onset (hollow circles) and fictitious motion perception (solid circles) for one subject; (b) thresholds for nystagmous and motion perception for 14 subjects, group means shown as lines. Source [27]. Licensee: PlosOne under CC BY 4.0.

in MR personnel as 1.2, 1.5 and 3.2% at 1.5, 3 and 7 T with no instances of vomiting [23]. Studies at 8 and 9.4 T reported nauseous sensations from 2.2% of a total of 3457 MR examinations [24]. Nausea as a consequence of MRI exposure is rare.

COGNITIVE EFFECTS

The occurrence of cognitive effects from static field exposures is perhaps more controversial with an enduring "myth" regarding "mag lag." Various experiments have been conducted in and around MR scanners to look for cognitive effects. No change in immediate and delayed working memory or processing speed was seen for healthy volunteers undergoing 9.4 T sodium MRI [20], whilst none were detected in a study of MR factory workers [25]. A more comprehensive battery of tests and improvements in experimental design allowed the detection of small field dependent changes from 0.5 and 1 T exposures relating to attention and concentration in 5 out of 33 psychometric parameters investigated [33]. Whatever the underlying mechanism we can conclude that, in MRI, these effects are extremely subtle, transient, and not harmful. After all, if you conducted intensive psychometric testing on this author before and after morning coffee, you would detect a significant change in mental performance.

STATIC FIELD EXPOSURE LIMITS

Various national and international safety organizations have published SMF exposure limit guidelines. These do not apply to patients. Patient exposures are covered by the International Electrotechnical Commission (IEC) standard *Medical Electrical Equipment – Part 2–33: Particular Requirements for the Safety of Magnetic Resonance Equipment for Medical Diagnosis*, usually abbreviated to "IEC 60601-2-33". Under this standard's three tiers of exposure levels, patients can be routinely scanned in the "Normal Mode" at field strengths of up to and including 3 T. The "First Level Controlled Mode" requires that there be medical supervision for exposures above 3 T but less than 8 T. This covers the current range of commercial clinical MR systems. A Second Level Controlled Mode allows for research scanning at fields greater than 8 T but requires institutional research board (IRB) or medical ethics committee (MEC) approval. The adoption of the IEC limits has harmonized exposure limits internationally as all major jurisdictions have adopted them including the FDA in the US, member nations of the European Union, Australasia, Japan, South Korea, etc. National and international standards and guidance are considered in Chapter 14.

ICNIRP offers guideline limits for MRI of 4 T for the normal mode, 8 T for the first level, and above 8 T as the second level, again with research approval restrictions [34]. For non-MR exposures ICNIRP has suggested a 2 T occupational exposure limit for head and trunk exposures, but allowing up to 8 T for "controlled situations" such as for MR workers. A general public limit of 400 mT is prescribed [10]. Static field exposure limit values are given in Table 3.2.

ICNIRP has also defined limits for movement within the static field for the avoidance of acute sensory effects [35]. For movement lasting one second or more the *basic restriction* is a peak B of 2 T or a field change ΔB of 2 T. Alternatively an induced electric field limit is 1.1 V m^{-1}. A *reference level* in terms of dB/dt is 2.7 T s^{-1}. Reference levels are used in various guideline limits to demonstrate compliance with a basic restriction. This is discussed further in Chapter 13.

CONCLUSIONS

Despite a large scientific literature purporting biological effects from static magnetic field exposures, there remain few that have been observed in human experiments. It is highly unlikely that MRI exposures can instigate carcinogenic processes. At higher fields, an awareness of acute

Table 3.2 Limits for static magnetic field exposures.

Standard	Patients			Staff		Public
	Normal mode	Level 1 controlled mode	Level 2 controlled mode	Head & trunk	Limbs	Any
IEC [5] (MRI exposures)	3 T	8 T	>8 T	8 T	8 T	
ICNIRP [10,34]	4 T	8 T	>8 T	2 T (8 T controlled)	8 T	0.4 T
ICNIRP [35]				2 T or 2.7 T s^{-1}		

sensory effects may help to improve patient comfort, cooperation, and tolerance of the procedure. Rapid head movements close to the scanner bore should be avoided, and patients should keep their eyes open in the scanner. Research is ongoing into possible cognitive effects but these are extremely subtle and reversible.

Revision questions

1. The magneto-hydrodynamic effect only induces an electric field across blood vessels
   A. parallel to the direction of the magnetic field
   B. perpendicular to the direction of the magnetic field
   C. at an angle to the direction of the magnetic field
   D. which are arteries
   E. only when they are moving with respect to the static field spatial gradient.
2. Alignment of biological molecules with the static magnetic field due to the molecules' diamagnetic magnetic susceptibility is
   A. responsible for acute sensory effects
   B. insignificant compared with thermal motions in tissue
   C. likely to cause blood pressure changes
   D. very small because of the small, positive susceptibility
   E. of concern because of the large, negative susceptibility.
3. Which of the following physical interactions is least likely to lead to biological effects from exposure to static magnetic fields?
   A. Magneto-hydrodynamic (Hall) effect
   B. Lorentz force on moving electrical charges
   C. Peripheral nerve stimulation
   D. Induced electric field from movement within the static field spatial gradient
   E. Magnetic translational forces on diamagnetic molecules.
4. Which of the following is most likely to be experienced in a high field MRI scanner?
   A. Magneto-phosphenes
   B. Nystagmus
   C. Raised temperature
   D. Vertigo
   E. Blurred vision.
5. Which of the following is/are true? MRI induced vertigo is
   A. carcinogenic
   B. caused by motion within the fringe field spatial gradient
   C. caused by electrolysis
   D. related to nystagmus
   E. more likely if patient close their eyes.

6. The static magnetic field limits contained in the IEC 60601-2-33 standard 3rd edition are:
   A. Normal mode 1.5 T; first level controlled mode 3 T
   B. Normal mode 2 T; first level controlled mode 3 T
   C. Normal mode 2 T; first level controlled mode 4 T
   D. Normal mode 3 T; first level controlled mode 8 T
   E. Normal mode 4 T; first level controlled mode 4 T.

References

1. Pittler, M.H., Brown, E.M., and Ernst, E. (2007). Static magnets for reducing pain: systematic review and meta-analysis of randomized trials. *Canadian Medical Association Journal* 177:38–742.
2. National Center for Complimentary and Integrative Health (2017). *Magnets for Pain* https://nccih.nih.gov/Health/magnets-for-pain. (accessed 27 December 2018).
3. Finegold, L. and Flamm, B.L. (2006). Magnet therapy: extraordinary claims, but no benefits. *British Medical Journal* 332:4.
4. National Radiological Protection Board (1983). Revised guidance on acceptable limits of exposure during nuclear magnetic resonance clinical imaging. *British Journal of Radiology* 56:974–977.
5. International Electrotechnical Commission (2015). *Medical Electrical Equipment – Part 2–33: Particular Requirements for the Safety of Magnetic Resonance Equipment for Medical Diagnosis*. IEC 60601-2-33 3.3 edn. Geneva: IEC.
6. Wikswo, J.P. and Barach, J.P. (1980). An estimate of the steady magnetic field strength required to influence nerve conduction. *IEEE Transactions on Biomedical Engineering* BME-27:722–723.
7. Schenck, J.F. (2000). Safety of strong static magnetic fields. *Journal of Magnetic Resonance Imaging* 12:2–19.
8. Hashemi, S. and Abdolali, A. (2017).Three-dimensional analysis, modeling, and simulation of the effect of static magnetic fields on neurons. *Bioelectromagnetics* 38:128–136.
9. Okano, H. (2008). Effects of static magnetic fields in biology: role of free radicals. *Frontiers in Bioscience* 13:6106–6125.
10. International Commission on Non-Ionizing Radiation Protection (2009). Guidelines on limits of exposure to static magnetic fields. *Health Physics* 96:504–514.
11. Messiha, H.L., Wongnate T., Chaiyen P. et al. (2015). Magnetic field effects as a result of the radical pair mechanism are unlikely in redox enzymes. *Journal of the Royal Society.* Interface 12: 20141155. http://dx.doi.org/10.1098/rsif.2014.1155
12. Scientific Committee on Emerging Newly Identified Health Risks (2015). SCENIHR opinion on potential health effects of exposure to electromagnetic fields. *Bioelectromagnetics* 36:480–484.
13. Reddig, A., Fatahi, M., Friebe, B., et al. (2015). Analysis of DNA double-strand breaks and cytotoxicity after 7 tesla magnetic resonance imaging of isolated human lymphocytes. *PLoS One.* 10(7):e0132702. doi: 10.1371/journal.pone.0132702.
14. Rosen, A.D. (2003). Effect of a 125 mT static magnetic field on the kinetics of voltage activated Na+ channels in GH3 cells. *Bioelectromagnetics* 24:517–523.
15. Ritz, T., Adem, A. and Schulten, K. (2000). A model for photoreceptor-based magnetoreception in birds. *Biophysical Journal Volume* 78:707–718.
16. Wang, S., Luo J., Lv, H., et al. (2019). Effects of whole-body exposure to high static magnetic fields (2 T–12 T) on mice for 28 days. *Magnetic Resonance in Medicine.*
17. Yu, S. and Shang, P. (2014). A review of bioeffects of static magnetic field on rodent models. *Progress in Biophysics and Molecular Biology* 114:14–24.
18. Houpt, T.A., Carella, L., Gonzalez, D. et al. (2011). Behavioral effects on rats of motion within a high static magnetic field. *Physiology & Behavior* 102:338–346.
19. Cason, A.M., Kwon, B., Smith, J.C. et al. (2009). Labyrinthectomy abolishes the behavioral and neural response of rats to a high-strength static magnetic field. *Physiology & Behavior* 97: 36–43.
20. Atkinson, I.C., Renteria, L., Burd H. et al. (2007). Safety of human MRI at static fields above the FDA 8 T guideline: sodium imaging at 9.4 T does not affect vital signs or cognitive ability. *Journal of Magnetic Resonance Imaging* 26:122–1227.

21. Bongers, S., Slottje, P., and Kromhout, H. (2018). Development of hypertension after long-term expo-sure to static magnetic fields among workers from a magnetic resonance imaging device manufacturing facility. *Environmental Research* 164:565–573.

22. Cavin, I., Glover, P.M., Bowtell, R. et al. (2007). Thresholds for perceiving a metallic taste at large magnetic field. *Journal of Magnetic Resonance Imaging* 26:1357–1361.

23. Schaap, K., Christopher-DeVries, Y., Mason, C.K., et al. (2014). Occupational exposure of healthcare and research staff to static magnetic stray fields from 1.5-7 tesla MRI scanners is associated with reporting of transient symptoms. *Occupational & Environmental Medicine* 71:423–439.

24. Rauschenberg, J., Nagel, A.M., Ladd, S.C., et al. (2014). Multicenter study of subjective acceptance during magnetic resonance imaging at 7 and 9.4 T. *Investigative Radiology* 49:249–259.

25. De Vocht, F., Batistatou, E., Mölter, A., et al. (2015). Transient health symptoms of MRI staff working with 1.5 and 3.0 Tesla scanners in the UK. *European Radiology* 25:2718–2726.

26. Theyson, J.M., Kraff, O., Eilers, K., et al. (2014). Vestibular effects of a 7 tesla MRI examination compared to 1.5 T and 0 T in healthy volunteers. *PLoS ONE* 9(3): e92104. doi:10.1371/journal.pone.0092104

27. Mian, O., Li, Y., Antunes, A., et al. (2013). On the vertigo due to static magnetic fields. *PLoS ONE* 8(10): e78748. doi:10.1371/ journal.pone.0078748

28. Hansson, B., Höglund, P., Markenroth, B.K., et al. (2019). Short-term effects experienced during examinations in an actively shielded 7 T MR. *Bioelectromagnetics* 40:234–249.

29. Roberts, D.C., Marcelli, V., Gillen, J.S., et al. (2011). MRI magnetic field stimulates rotational sensors of the brain. *Current Biology* 21: 1635–1640.

30. Glover, P.M., Li, Y., Antunes, A. et al. (2014). A dynamic model of the eye nystagmus response to high magnetic fields. *Physics in Medicine and Biology* 59:631–645.

31. Antunes, A., Glover, P.M., Li Y. et al. (2012). Magnetic field effects on the vestibular system: calcula-tion of the pressure on the cupula due to ionic current-induced Lorentz force. *Physics in Medicine and Biology* 57:4477–4487.

32. Glover, P.M., Cavin, I., Qian, W. et al. (2007). Magnetic-field-induced vertigo: a theoretical and experi-mental investigation. *Bioelectromagnetics* 28:349–361.

33. Van Nierop, L.E., Slottje, P., van Zandvoort, M.J. et al. (2015). Simultaneous exposure to MRI-related static and low-frequency movement-induced time-varying magnetic fields affects neurocognitive per-formance: A double-blind randomized crossover study. *Magnetic Resonance in Medicine* 74:840–849.

34. International Commission on Non-Ionizing Radiation Protection (2009). Amendment to ICNIRP statement on medical magnetic resonance procedures: protection of patients. *Health Physics* 97:259–261.

35. International Commission on Non-Ionizing Radiation Protection (2014) ICNIRP guidelines for limiting exposure to electric fields induced by movement of the human body in a static magnetic field and by time-varying magnetic fields below 1 Hz. *Health Physics* 106:418–425.

Further reading and resources

International Commission on Non-Ionizing Radiation Protection (2004). ICNIRP statement on medical magnetic resonance (MR) procedures: protection of patient. *Health Physics* 87:197–216.

Kangarlu, A. and Robitaille, P-M. L. (2000). Biological effects and health implications in magnetic reso-nance imaging. *Concepts in Magnetic Resonance* 12:321–359.

Kangarlu, A. and Schenck, J.F. (2014). Bioeffects of static magnetic fields. In: *MRI bioeffects, safety, and patient management* (Ed. F.D. Shellock FD and J.V. Crues JV III) pp. 29–63. Los Angeles, CA: Biomedical Research Publishing Group.

World Health Organization (2006). *Environmental Health Criteria 232: Static Fields*. Geneva: WHO.

4

Bio-effects 2: time-varying gradient fields

INTRODUCTION

In 1775 Charles Le Roy attempted a cure of blindness using electric pulses passed through a wire round the patient's head (Figure 4.1a) [1]. The patient was not cured, but experienced flashes of light (in addition to severe burns). At the end of the nineteenth century D'Arsonval [2] used a sinusoidally-varying magnetic field applied to the head (Figure 4.1b) to induce artificial visual sensations, magneto-phosphenes (MP). Since then bio-effects of time-varying magnetic fields (TVMF) have been used in bone-healing and depression therapies, and neuro-stimulation. Conversely, there has been concern about the negative health effects of chronic exposure to electric and magnetic fields from high voltage AC power transmission cables. This chapter provides a detailed review of the effects most pertinent to MRI, namely respiratory, cardiac, and peripheral nerve stimulation. We will briefly review the evidence for other bio-effects.

PHYSICAL INTERACTION

The physical interaction between a time-varying magnetic field and tissue is the induction (Faraday's law) of an electric field E and accompanying current density J in tissue. In a uniform medium [3]

$$E = \frac{r}{2}\frac{dB}{dt} \qquad (4.1)$$

where r is the radius of a circular loop and dB/dt is the rate of change of magnetic field (T s^{-1}). If σ is the tissue's electrical conductivity (S m^{-1}), the current density (A m^{-2}) is

$$J = \sigma\frac{r}{2}\frac{dB}{dt} \qquad (4.2)$$

Example 4.1   Electric field induced from a gradient pulse

What electric field will be induced around a head of radius 8 cm in a uniform time-varying magnetic field of 50 T s⁻¹?
From Equation 4.1

$$E = 0.5 \times 0.08 \times 50 = 2\ V\ m^{-1}$$

If the conductivity of tissue is 0.2 S m⁻¹, the maximum current density (Equation 4.2) is

$$J = 0.2 \times 2 = 0.4\ A\ m^{-2}.$$

(a)   (b)

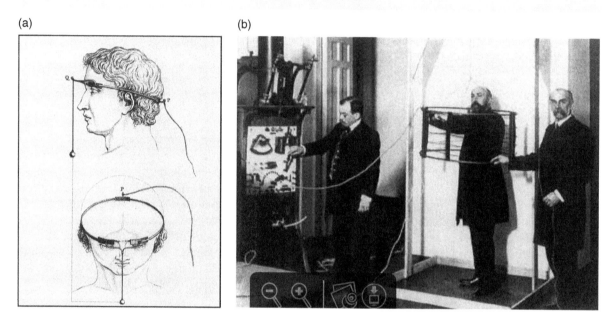

Figure 4.1   Early phosphene research: (a) Charles Le Roy's "cure for blindness", 1775; (b) Arsene D'Arsonval's magnetophosphene experiments, 1896. Source [1]. Reproduced with permission of Wolters Kluwer Heath, Inc.

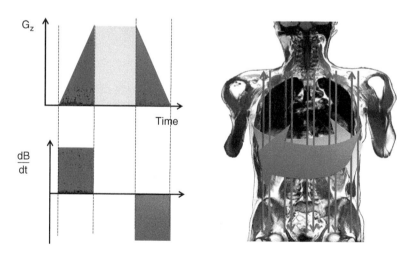

Figure 4.2   Induced E-field and current density J from a uniform time-varying magnetic field dB/dt.

MRI gradient waveforms usually have a trapezoidal shape. The rising (or falling) slope is a changing magnetic field, effectively a rectangular dB/dt pulse, which induces an electric field and current density within the patient. The falling (or rising) slope produces a dB/dt pulse of the opposite polarity, inducing E and J in the opposite direction (Figure 4.2).

A more realistic model for the body is an elliptic cylinder. The maximum current density around an elliptical cross section is [4,5]

$$J_{max} = \frac{a^2 b}{a^2 + b^2} \sigma \frac{dB}{dt} \qquad (4.3)$$

where a and b are semi major and semi minor axes of an elliptical cross section (Figure 4.3). In a supine body the maximum will be on their front or back.

Example 4.2   Induction in an ellipse

Calculate the maximum induced current density in an elliptical cross section with semi-major axes 0.2 and 0.1 and conductivity 0.2 Sm^{-1} in a time varying field of 100 T s^{-1}.
From Equation 4.4

$$J_{max} = \frac{0.2^2 \times 0.1}{0.05} 0.2 \times 100 = 1.6 \; A \; m^{-2}.$$

The geometric factor 0.08 can be used for a standard sized adult, positioned supine within the bore of an MRI magnet.

The basic equations can be understood looking at Figure 4.4 which shows the amplitude of G_z relative to a patient position. E and J will be induced in axial planes and their strengths depend upon:

- Gradient strength and slew rate
- The position along the gradient axis
- The size of "induction loop" available.

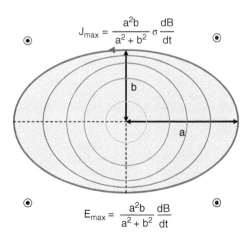

Figure 4.3   Induced E-field and current density J in an elliptical cross section with uniform dB/dt into the plane of the page.

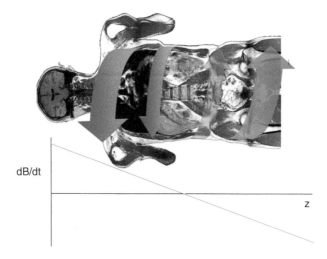

Figure 4.4   B and dB/dt magnitude for G_z relative to a supine patient. dB/dt is primarily along the z-axis.

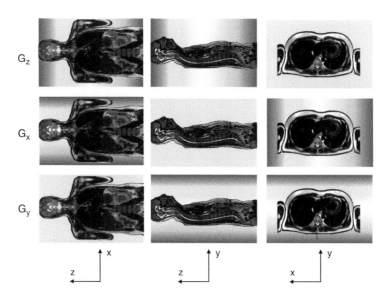

Figure 4.5   Variation of B and dB/dt from gradients G_x, G_y, and G_z. Field magnitude is represented by the shading.

   The current density also depends upon the conductivity of tissue.
   These equations are adequate for a uniform dB/dt applied in the z-axis, but do not describe the E-field and current density distributions arising from G_x and G_y whose amplitudes vary within the patient cross-section (Figure 4.5). They do not even fully apply to the z-gradient. Figure 4.6 illustrates why. In order to generate a linear field gradient of B_z, it is necessary for the lines of force relating to the field produced by the gradient to converge. In other words, G_z cannot exist in isolation and there must be additional, or *concomitant*, field components in x and y, a consequence of Maxwell's equations. This is not especially important for image formation as only the z-component is effective. However, it matters for MR safety as the actual field experienced by a

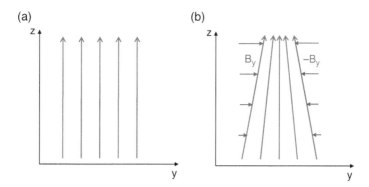

(a)

(b)

Figure 4.6   (a) A uniform magnetic flux density B_z; the strength of the field is represented by the spacing of lines. (b) From Maxwell's equations generating a z-gradient must involve other directions, in this example B_y components (in red).

patient from the gradients will vary in both direction and magnitude from the simple model. For more detailed and anatomical maps, it is necessary to employ numerical, computer simulations [6,7] (Figure 4.7).

ELF TIME-VARYING MAGNETIC FIELD EFFECTS

The most robust and consistent biological effects from TVMF are those which relate to excitable tissues, particularly those causing acute sensory and muscular activities. There is also much research into the effects of chronic exposure to time-varying electromagnetic fields arising from power frequency (50–60 Hz) transmission and distribution in the domestic setting. These frequencies lie in the Extremely Low Frequency (ELF) range defined as 0–3000 Hz.

Cellular effects

In vitro studies report changes in the outward flux of calcium (Ca^{++}) ions across the cell membrane, attributed to time varying electromagnetic field exposures in the extremely low frequency range, typically 60 Hz or less. There are claims of malignant cell growth inhibition with very low amplitude TVMF– of the order of micro- or even nano-tesla. On the other hand, exposures at 1.5 T show the opposite effect. Attempts to isolate and demonstrate the mechanism for low frequency, low field effects have proved elusive. More relevant to MRI, exposure of human peripheral blood monocytes cells to both the static field and static field plus gradients and RF in a 7 T MRI scanner showed no DNA damage or cell proliferation [8].

Do electromagnetic fields in the frequency range 50–60 Hz cause cancer?

Since the 1980s there has been concern about the incidence of childhood leukaemia in children living in the proximity of power lines. A World Health Organization report [9] recognized a weak correlation for magnetic field exposures above 0.4 μT at power transmission frequencies with leukaemia incidence. This does not necessarily mean that magnetic fields are the cause.

(a)

84

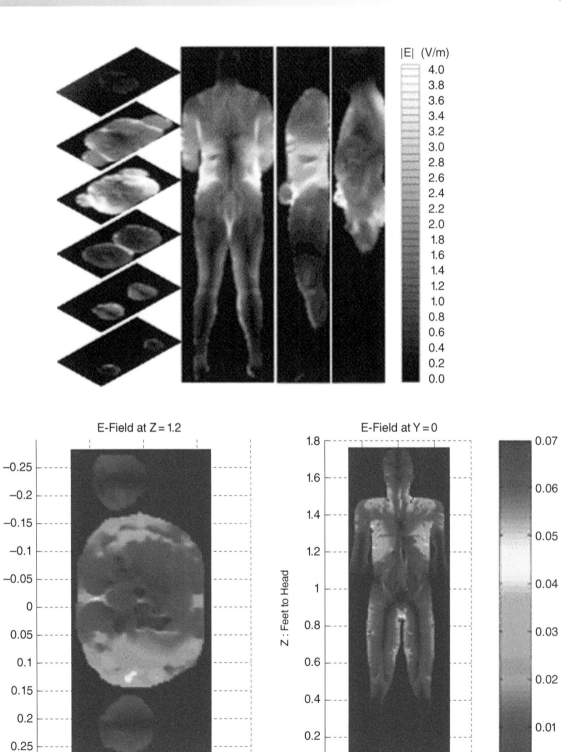

Figure 4.7 Modeling of induced electric fields: (a) from the y-coil for dB/dt=100 T s⁻¹. Source [6]. Reproduced with permission of Elsevier; (b) from z-gradient coil [7]. Used with permission of IEEE.

Table 4.1   Typical electric and magnetic field exposure from electrical wiring and appliances. Induced electric fields in the brain calculated using 2.2 mV m⁻¹ per kV m⁻¹[11].

Source	External E $(V\,m^{-1})$	Induced E in the brain $(mV\,m^{-1})$	B (μT)
Overhead HV power line	3000	6.6	5
TV monitor	1500	3.3	1
Laptop computer	1500	3.3	0.08
Refrigerator	1000	2.2	0.4
Hairdryer	40	2.0	70
Electrical appliances 1 m distant	80–300	0.18–0.66	<0.1
Domestic wiring	3–30	0.007–0.07	0.05–0.15
MRI gradients		0–1000	0–5000

For example, you could correlate ice cream consumption with weight gain, but that does not mean that hot sunny weather makes you fat. Most importantly, in-vitro cell experiments and animal study results do not show any carcinogenic effect. In human studies, no other cancer is implicated from EMF exposures. Nevertheless, the International Agency for Research into Cancer (IARC) has declared electromagnetic fields (ELF) as a "possible carcinogen" [10].

The short-term acute TVMF exposures in MRI are very dissimilar to chronic, prolonged, i.e. potentially life-long, exposures to electric and magnetic fields from power transmission lines. Table 4.1 shows the range of exposures from various sources of electric and magnetic fields. The induced E-field is several orders of magnitude smaller than the external electric field [11]. Also shown for comparison are the field exposures from MRI gradients.

Therapeutic magnetic stimulation

Bone healing

Electrical stimulation to promote bone growth and healing has been practised since the 1980s. The stimulation is achieved either by direct electric currents, capacitive coupling, or by induced electric fields from TVMF. B values are 0.01–1 mT, with frequencies of 20–200 kHz, inducing electric fields of 1–100 mV cm⁻¹. The efficacy of this treatment is still uncertain. A review of 105 clinical studies [12] noted "promise" in the technique but also poor study design. Mixed results have been achieved for slow-healing fractures, the principal clinical application. It is arguable that the extended immobilization of the limb required during the treatment or associated tissue heating may contribute to any therapeutic benefit.

Transcranial Magnetic Stimulation

Transcranial magnetic stimulation (TMS) arose from MRI-directed research into the biological effects of TVMF [13]. Since then TMS has developed into a key tool for neuroscience research with a vast and varied literature covering aspects of neurological function, stimulation mechanism, and therapeutic applications [14]. In a TMS machine large electrical current pulses are discharged into a small coil, often in a figure-of-eight or "butterfly" configuration to generate dB/dt pulses of the order of thousands of T s⁻¹ to stimulate the cerebral cortex. Repetitive TMS (rTMS) has been used to treat psychiatric conditions with varying degrees of success [15], but it appears established in the treatment of depression [16].

MAGNETIC STIMULATION

Magneto-phosphenes

The word "phosphene" derives from the Greek for light "phos" and "phainein", meaning "to show". Phosphenes are perceived by the subject as faint flashes of light, thought to originate from direct stimulation of retinal receptors or of the optic nerve, rather than from an actual optical source. Much of the published literature in the early twentieth century lacks sufficient technical details, making the dosimetry difficult to assess. Figure 4.8 shows the composite results from a number of studies [17]. The onset of phosphenes has a minimum value of around 12 mT RMS (root mean square) corresponding to a peak-to-peak stimulus of around 34 mT in the frequency range 15–45 Hz, depending upon the ambient light conditions and dark-adaption of the subjects [18]. For pulsed fields the threshold dB/dt is around 2 T s^{-1} [19].

The MP-sensitive frequency range is not usually present in MR exposures, hence reports of phosphenes in MRI are rare, arising occasionally from movement close to high field systems rather than as a consequence of the imaging gradients. An incidence of 0.8, 1.5, and 0.0% occurred in a survey of 361 MR staff working with 1.5, 3 T, and 7 T scanners [20]. A multicentre study at 7 T and 9.4 T reported an incidence of 1.6% from 1400 scanned subjects [21]. In each case, movement with respect to the static field spatial gradient appears to be the physical cause.

The importance of magneto-phosphenes is neither their occurrence nor their (minimal) health consequence, but their use in the determination of occupational exposure limits. Phosphenes are considered by various organizations, including the International Commission on Non-Ionizing

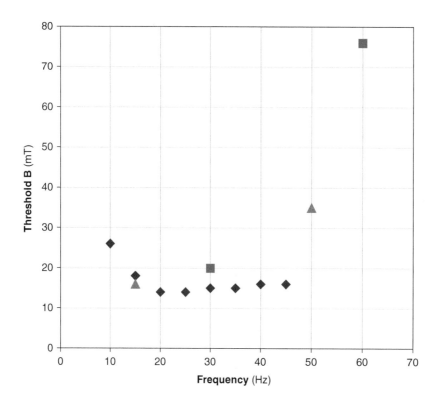

Figure 4.8 Magneto-phosphene threshold v frequency; data from various sources [17,18]. The threshold is given as RMS value of a sinusoidal stimulus.

Radiation Protection (ICNIRP) as being the most sensitive acute sensory effect from TVMF, and their onset serves as a precautionary level for the avoidance of any other stimulation effects [11].

MYTHBUSTER:

In terms of B-field exposures peripheral nerve stimulation, not magneto-phosphenes, is the most sensitive bio-effect of TVMF.

Example 4.3   Magneto-phosphene threshold

What is the maximum magnitude of dB/dt for the minimum MP threshold of 12 mT RMS at 30 Hz?
The field waveform is

$$B(t) = \sqrt{2}B_{RMS}\sin \omega t$$

The magnitude of the rate of change is

$$\left|\frac{dB}{dt}\right| = 2\pi f B = \sqrt{2} \times 2 \times \pi \times 30 \times 12 \times 10^{-3} = 3.2 \ T \ s^{-1}$$

Using Equation 4.1, a dB/dt exposure of 3.2 T s⁻¹ to the head will induce a maximum electric field and current density of

$$E = \frac{0.08}{2} \times 3.2 = 0.128 \ Vm^{-1}$$

If tissue conductivity is 0.2 Sm⁻¹, then the maximum induced current density is

$$J = 0.2 \times 0.128 = 0.026 \ A \ m^{-2} \ or \ 26 \ mA \ m^{-2}.$$

Nerve and muscular stimulation

Magnetic nerve stimulation was initially demonstrated on an excized frog muscle [22]. The first in-vivo stimulation in humans was achieved via capacitor discharge into a small topical coil [23]. The technique would be finessed further for use in TMS. The basic magneto-physiological relationship is the strength duration (SD) curve (Figure 4.9) [24]. This shows that the minimum threshold, known as the *rheobase (Rh)*, occurs for long stimulus durations. As the stimulus duration becomes shorter, the threshold rises. The *chronaxie (Ch)* is the stimulus duration for which the threshold is double the intensity of the rheobase. These early investigations utilized small solenoidal coils placed on or close to the limbs of the subjects. Stimulation of peripheral nerves by MRI equipment was subsequently reported [25,26].

Basic electrophysiology of nerves

Magnetic nerve stimulation is often considered to be analogous to electrical stimulation, so a good place to start is with the electrophysiology of nerves. We are particularly interested in the larger peripheral myelinated nerves that are distal to the root and plexus. These consist of bundles of fibers conveying motor, touch, and proprioceptive impulses. Figure 4.10a shows a schematic of the axon of a nerve cell or neuron. The myelin sheath acts as insulation with gaps called *nodes of Ranvier* where the excitation occurs. This structure enables the nerve impulse or action

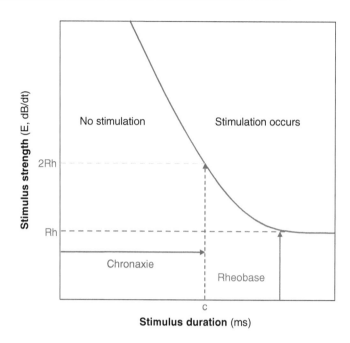

Figure 4.9 Strength duration curve showing the rheobase (the minimum threshold for long stimuli) and the chronaxie (the stimulus duration for a threshold double the rheobase). The stimulus can be given as dB/dt, induced E field or current density, J.

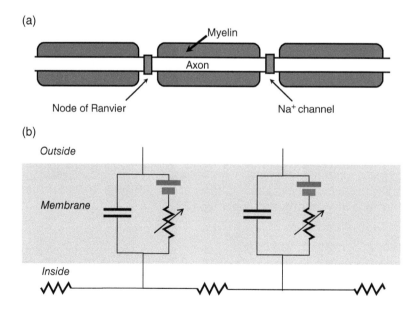

Figure 4.10 (a) Structure of a myelinated nerve axon; (b) electrical, transmission cable model of an A-fiber.

potential to propagate rapidly along the fiber. The underlying bio-physical mechanism is complex, sufficiently so to justify the awarding of the 1963 Nobel Prize for Physiology and Medicine to Huxley and Hodgkin. For our purposes, a simpler understanding will suffice.

The basis of the action potential is shown in Figure 4.11. At rest, the interior of the axon has a negative potential compared to the exterior. This resting potential is maintained by a balance of electrical and osmotic forces upon electrolytes, particularly sodium (Na$^+$), potassium (K$^+$), chloride (Cl$^-$) ions and negatively charged molecules (A$^-$). The resting potential is typically −70 mV, but if it can be raised locally by around 15 mV (to −55 mV), then sodium channels in the cell membrane open, allowing Na$^+$ ions to flow in, raising the interior potential. At some point above 0 V, potassium channels open, allowing the egress of K$^+$ ions, reducing the internal potential. After a refractory period, the resting potential (and distribution of ions) is restored. Once triggered, the action potential propagates the full length of the axon. Non-myelinated, or C-fiber, nerves convey autonomic and chronic pain impulses. They have a slower conduction velocity than myelinated fibers.

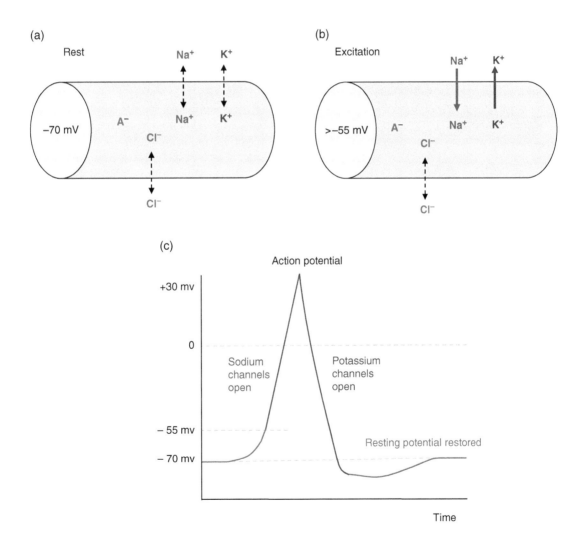

Figure 4.11   Nerve ion dynamics (a) at rest; (b) during excitation; (c) and the action potential.

Forms of the strength-duration curve

Two basic forms of SD curve for electrical stimulation are used. The *hyperbolic* form is [27]:

$$I_{thresh}(t) = I_{Rh}\left[1 + \frac{Ch}{t}\right]$$

(4.4)

where I_{thresh} is the generator current (applied via electrodes) for threshold stimulation, t is the stimulus duration for a rectangular pulse and Ch is the chronaxie. The other form of the SD curve is exponential [28]:

$$I_{thresh}(t) = I_{Rh} / \left(1 - e^{-t/\tau}\right)$$

(4.5)

where τ is the tissue or membrane time constant.

One theoretical advantage of the exponential form is that it produces the predicted response of a simple equivalent circuit of the nerve under the action of a rectangular current stimulus. Moreover, the tissue time constants can be theoretically derived from the fiber diameters. Table 4.2 shows the electrical properties of various excitable tissues.

The function of nerves has been described using the analogy of electrical circuit components. In the spatially extended non-linear node (SENN) model [29], the cell membrane is considered as a resistor and a voltage source in parallel with a capacitor at each node, whilst the nodes are connected internally by a series of resistors (Figure 4.10b). This model has been used to predict many of the features of electrical stimulation, such as the rheobase, the tissue time constant and waveform dependence. It has been used to estimate the threshold for cardiac stimulation by time-varying magnetic fields [30]. However, whilst it is a useful starting point, it has some inadequacies in describing magnetic stimulation phenomena, including the predicted time constants and waveform dependence [24,31,32].

Properties of magnetic stimulation

Unlike electrical stimulation which involves a chemical reaction between the electrodes and the skin, magnetic stimulation makes use of the endogenous ions in tissue. The mechanism is usually attributed to a change in the induced electric field along the axon, i.e. from an electric field gradient, or a change in the direction of the axon in a constant electric field. Such a model has

Table 4.2 Electrical properties of excitable tissue.

	Fiber type	Diameter (μm)	Conduction speed (m s⁻¹)	Time constant τ (ms)
Motor nerve	A	12–20	15–120	0.12
Pain & temperature (nociceptors)	A δ	2–5	12–30	0.25
Pain & temperature	C	1	0.5–2	1
Skeletal muscle		10–100	1–5	0.5
Cardiac muscle		10–100	0.5–4	2.9

worked well for electrical stimulation, but there is controversy around this as the sole mechanism for magnetic stimulation.

B-field change step size

It is common to consider stimulation in terms of either the external field – dB/dt, or the internal induced electric field, E. One can consider a *stimulus rheobase* in T s^{-1} or a *physiological rheobase* in V m^{-1}. In the hyperbolic form the SD curve is

$$\left(\frac{dB}{dt}\right)_{thresh}(t) = \left(\frac{dB}{dt}\right)_{Rh}\left[1+\frac{Ch}{t}\right] \tag{4.6}$$

By considering the step change in B, or ΔB, the SD curve can be made linear [33]:

$$\Delta B_{thresh} = \Delta B_{min}\left[1+\frac{\Delta t}{Ch}\right] \tag{4.7}$$

From this an estimated theoretical minimum ΔB for PNS is 12.5 mT (Figure 4.12) and 480 mT for cardiac stimulation.

On a practical level, this provides a simple means of determining whether the stimulation threshold is likely to be exceeded, and this model is often used in the scanner's stimulation monitor. On a more philosophical level, it shifts the perceived cause of stimulus from dB/dt to just the *change* in B. Is this physically meaningful? By comparison with electrical stimulation, the analogue of ΔB is a change in electric charge, which is the underlying agent of the action potential. In other words, move a sufficient amount of charge within a timescale determined by

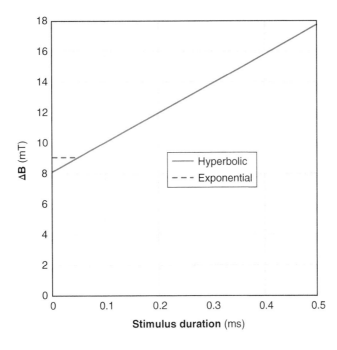

Figure 4.12   Linearizing of the SD curve in terms of ΔB. The exponential form of the SD curve (red line) flattens out for very short stimulus duration.

the tissue time constant, and stimulation will occur. If the B-field change is less than ΔB_{min}, nothing happens. This also implies that a bi-phasic change in B or the peak-to-peak value of a constantly changing B is more relevant than the amplitude or RMS value.

Applying a similar analysis to the exponential SD curve results in a larger minimum B (Figure 4.12). For t << τ

$$\Delta B_{thresh} \approx \tau \left(\frac{dB}{dt} \right)_{Rh} \tag{4.8}$$

Which shape of SD curve is the correct one? Electrophysiologists have been arguing over this since the 1900s, so it is perhaps optimistic to think that MR safety will provide the answer. Figure 4.13 shows a curve fit to extensive data from topical magnetic nerve stimulation [24]. The hyperbolic fit results in a lower rheobase. Various other studies have not definitively distinguished between the two. The IEC standard 60601-2-33 "hedges its bets", using the hyperbolic model for peripheral nerve stimulation prediction, and the exponential model for cardiac stimulation [34].

MYTHBUSTER:

It is the change in B rather than dB/dt that is most fundamentally responsible for PNS.

Strong stimuli

For stimuli with amplitudes above the threshold, the response increases as more and more fibers are recruited, until they are all firing, and the response is supra-maximal (Figure 4.14). Perception will occur first, followed by muscular twitching. It is harder to stimulate the Aδ and C fibers that convey pain as they are smaller.

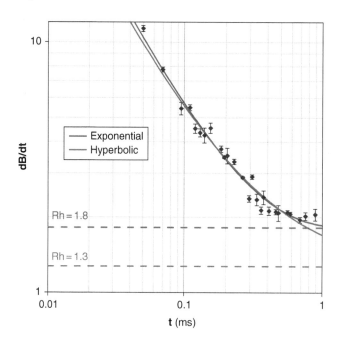

Figure 4.13   Fitted exponential and hyperbolic SD curves to real data from topic stimulation of the human ulnar nerve. Redrawn from [24]. The exponential fit predicts a higher rheobase.

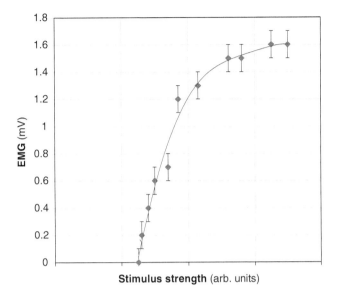

Figure 4.14   Increasing the stimulus strength above the threshold to a supramaximal response. Strength of response was measured using electromyography (EMG). Redrawn from [24].

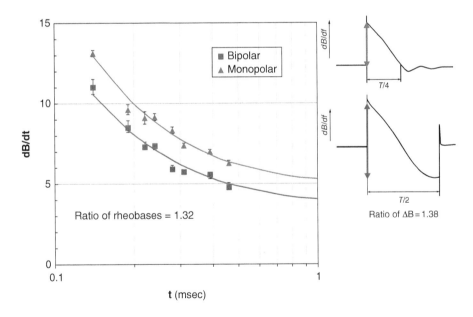

Figure 4.15   Waveform dependence: bi-phasic or bipolar stimuli display lower thresholds than monopolar. The dB/dt waveforms are shown on the right. The ratio of rheobases is similar to the ratio of ΔB values. Redrawn from [24].

Waveform dependence

The other important property of magnetic stimulation is the waveform dependence. The prediction of the SENN model is that unipolar stimuli should have lower thresholds than bipolar stimuli. This is not the case in magnetic stimulation (Figure 4.15) [24]. This result is confirmed by numerous transcranial magnetic stimulation studies [1].

Very short stimuli

As the stimulus duration decreases or the frequency increases, the PNS threshold increases. It has been estimated that nerve stimulation is possible up to 100 kHz [35]. At frequencies above 25 kHz the SD curve departs from the usual hyperbolic or exponential form, with elevated thresholds (Figure 4.16) [36]. Figure 4.17 shows the extension of the IEC PNS curve for stimulus durations of less than 20 µs using exposure data from magnetic particle imaging experiments [37] and MRI [38]. The increase in threshold may be attributed to leakage currents across the cell membrane.

Respiratory and cardiac stimulation

Magnetic stimulation affecting respiration or the cardiac cycle is not possible with MRI scanner gradients for four reasons:

1. The available conduction loop around the heart is significantly smaller than around the trunk, and so PNS will always occur first. The absence of PNS ensures that cardiac stimulation cannot happen.

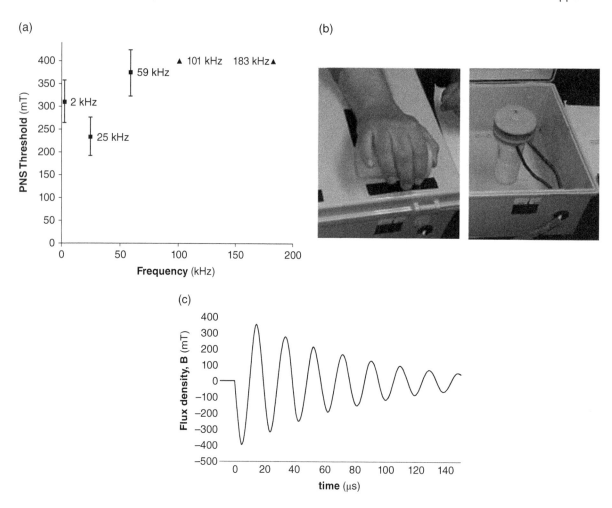

Figure 4.16 Stimulation at very high frequencies (very short period stimuli): (a) Strength-duration curve showing a departure from the usual forms at high frequencies; (b) the stimulus apparatus; (c) stimulus used. Source [36]. Reproduced with permission of Wiley.

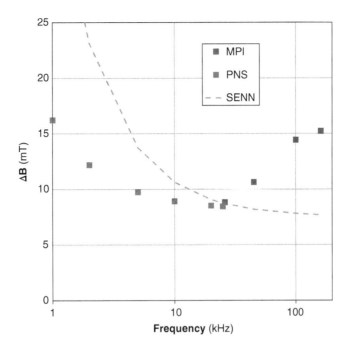

Figure 4.17   A combined SD curve for ΔB using published PNS data for MRI (Table 4.4) and PNS data from magnetic particle imaging [37] and MRI [38]. Rather than limiting at ΔB$_{min}$, the threshold increases for very high frequencies (short stimulus durations). The dotted grey line shows the SENN prediction [29].

2. The time constant of heart muscle (3 ms) is significantly longer than that of peripheral nerves (0.5 ms) making the generation of a suitable stimulating pulse harder.
3. The gradients cannot generate sufficient ΔB. The theoretical field required is more than an order of magnitude greater than the maximum gradient output.
4. The scanner's stimulation control software will prevent this.

Respiratory stimulation has been demonstrated in dogs using a capacitor discharge system via a topical coil [39]. The estimated B was 2.2 T with a 1.17 ms pulse duration and dB/dt of 11 000 T s^{-1}. Two further canine studies have demonstrated cardiac stimulation with ΔB =1.43 T, or dB/dt = 2700 T s^{-1} and estimations of the induced electric field in the range 50–340 V m^{-1} [40,41]. These exposures are orders of magnitude beyond the capabilities of MR gradient systems.

Example 4.4   Induction in the heart

Using a simple model for a 20 T s^{-1} dB/dt exposure from trapezoidal z-gradient pulse with a ramp duration of 1 ms, what electric field is induced around the trunk periphery and the heart?
Use Equation 4.4 for the body cross section with a = 0.2 and b = 0.1 m.

$$E_{max} = \frac{0.2^2 \times 0.1}{0.05} \times 20 = 1.6\,Vm^{-1}$$

Assume a spherical heart of radius 4 cm, then

$$E_{max} = \frac{0.04}{2} \times 20 = 0.4\,Vm^{-1}$$

PERIPHERAL NERVE STIMULATION IN MRI

Table 4.3 shows the results of a range of human PNS threshold experiments conducted using MRI gradient systems [26,33,42–44]. These were carried out using physically different gradient coil designs, pulse waveforms and numbers of subjects (N). The weighted mean from these studies for the dB/dt rheobase is 19.4 T s^{-1} with a chronaxie of 0.42 ms. The mean ΔB_{min} is 8.1 mT. The chronaxie differs significantly from the value expected from electrical stimulation of around 100 µs [29,30].

It has been shown that the y-gradient has the lowest thresholds. Looking at Figure 4.5 you can see that G_y produces a strong field the entire H-F length of the patient, maximizing the likelihood of stimulation. By contrast, the z-gradient has maximal values only towards the ends of the scanner bore and is the least likely to stimulate. A stimulus at 150% of the threshold is "uncomfortable", whilst at 200% the response becomes "intolerable" [26]. Figure 4.18 shows subjects' reporting of three levels of stimulation (threshold, uncomfortable, and intolerable) fitted to the hyperbolic form.

In Table 4.3 the parameters are given in terms of ΔB and dB/dt. These are not immediately relatable to the MR scanner gradient specifications of amplitude $G_{x,y,x}$ and slew rate. The law of stimulation in terms of the imaging gradient parameters can be expressed as [45]:

$$\Delta G(t) = SR_{min}Ch + \Delta G_{min}. \tag{4.9}$$

where SR_{min} is the smallest stimulating slew rate for infinitely long pulse durations, ΔG_{min} is the smallest stimulating gradient excursion for infinitely short pulse durations, and Ch is the chronaxie. This is represented in Figure 4.19 where the gradient coil technical performance is shown in terms of its slew rate limitation and its amplitude limitation. The PNS threshold has a linear form and can easily be used to predict the PNS-limited region of the gradient's operation. Table 4.4 collates stimulation results using this approach [43,45–49]. The weighted mean minimum slew rate is 59.3 Tm^{-1}s^{-1}, and the minimum stimulating gradient amplitude is 35.4 mT m^{-1}. The chronaxies are slightly longer than in the previous table, although they may be skewed by a few long values.

The results from Tables 4.3 and 4.4 were obtained by exceeding the usual PNS limits encountered in clinical MR systems. One study examined the occurrence of PNS in patients when operating the scanner in the Level II mode at 120% of the median perception threshold. From 210 patients, only 16.7% experienced stimulation and only 2.9% rated the experience as very uncomfortable [50].

Table 4.3 PNS from MRI gradient coils.

Waveform	N	Axis	Rheobase dB/dt (T s^{-1})	ΔB_{min} (mT)	Chronaxie (ms)	Reference
Sinusoid	1	Z	18.0	9.9	0.55	[33]
Trapezoid, 128 lobes	84	Y	14.9	5.4	0.37	[26]
	84	Z	26.2	9.9	0.38	
Trapezoid	153	Y	18.8	6.8	0.36	[42]
Trapezoid 64, lobes	20	XY	24.7	11.1	0.53	[43]
Trapezoid, 128 lobes	65	Y	16.3	8.6	0.52	[44]
	65	XY	18.6	8.7	0.47	
	65	XYZ	20.1	10.2	0.51	
MEAN			**19.4 ± 3.9**	**8.1 ± 1.9**	**0.42 ± 0.14**	

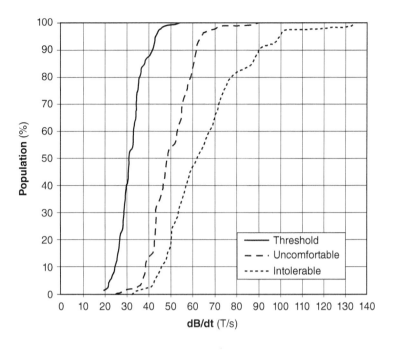

Figure 4.18   Population response for PNS from MRI gradients for three levels of stimulation: threshold, uncomfortable, and intolerable. Source [26]. Used with permission of Wiley.

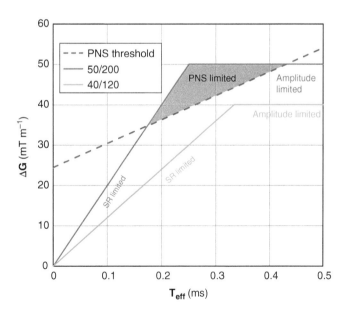

Figure 4.19   Gradient specification formulation of the SD curve showing areas that are slew rate-limited or amplitude-limited for two systems: 40/120 (amplitude/slew rate) and 50/200. The shaded area is likely to be limited by PNS. The 40/120 system is unlikely to cause PNS.

Table 4.4   PNS in terms of MRI gradient coil parameters.

Waveform	N	Axis	SR_{min} (T m^{-1} s^{-1})	G_{min} (mT m^{-1})	Chronaxie (ms)	Reference
Sinusoid	4	Z	41.5	34	0.81	[46]
Trapezoid 64 lobes	20	XY	66.8	24.7	0.37	[43]
	20	XY	75.4	34.0	0.45	
	20	XY	77.0	40.5	0.53	
Trapezoid	14	Y	26.0	20.8	1.03	[47]
Trapezoid	20	XY	62.2	44.4	0.77	[45]
Trapezoid	18	XY	50.1	48.5	1.054	[48]
Trapezoid	14	X	252	218	0.87	[49]
	14	Y	222	147	0.66	
	14	Z	210	133	0.63	
MEAN			**59.3 ± 14**	**35.4 ± 8.6**	**0.69 ± 26**	

Predicting and avoiding PNS

Peripheral nerve stimulation in MRI is not harmful, and rarely intolerable. Nevertheless, its avoidance is clearly desirable for maximum patient cooperation and comfort. The strength duration behavior in MR systems is well categorized and hence the scanner's software is able to predict the likely onset of stimulation.

The likelihood of PNS occurrence is related to the type of pulse sequence. Figure 4.20 shows the relative magnitude of dB/dt from various sequences. Sequences with high dB/dt include echo planar imaging (EPI) and balanced steady state free precession (SSFP) gradient echo (e.g. TruFISP, b-FFE, FIESTA). Echo planar imaging has the additional feature of the rapid train of opposed polarity readout lobes, resulting in a longer stimulus duration which is more likely to cause PNS.

Example 4.5   PNS predicition

Use the linear SD plot (Figure 4.12) to predict whether stimulation will occur in the following cases:

Case 1: A single y-gradient lobe, with a maximum amplitude of 5 mT, rise time 0.1 ms.
Case 2: A single y-gradient lobe, with a maximum amplitude of 10 mT, rise time 0.2 ms.
Case 3: Two opposing y-gradient lobes, with a maximum amplitude of −10 mT and +10 mT, rise time 0.4 ms.

In each case dB/dt = 50 T s^{-1}. Case 1 amplitude is below ΔB_{min} and therefore cannot stimulate irrespective of rise time and slew rate. Case 2 is above ΔB_{min} but falls below the line of stimulation on account of its duration. Case three has a t_{eff} of 0.4 ms and lies above the line of stimulation. PNS is possible.

PNS is more likely to occur for:

• rapid sequences, such as EPI (echo planar imaging)
• when the y-gradient has the greatest gradient activity: e.g. if used for frequency-encoding in EPI
• diffusion imaging, where stronger gradient amplitudes are used
• high resolution images, which require higher gradient amplitudes
• oblique slices.

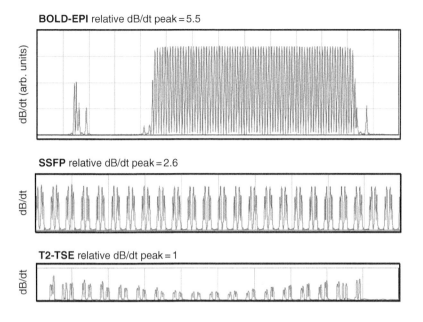

Figure 4.20 Combined for all gradients dB/dt from different sequences: BOLD EPI, Steady State Free Precession (SSFP) GRE, and T_2-weighted TSE. Although the dB/dt units are arbitrary, all the waveforms are at the same scale.

EXPOSURE LIMITS

In order to comply with IEC 60601-2-33 requirements [34], each manufacturer may calibrate their PNS monitor either from the results of actual volunteer exposures on the system, or by using predefined default SD curves. The IEC default SD curve is characterized by the parameters given in Table 4.5 and follows the hyperbolic form.

Gradient weighting-factors are applied to the scanner's stimulation predictions to account for the different sensitivities of each axis:

- W_{AP} = 1.0, patient anterior–posterior, i.e. for the y-gradient
- W_{LR} = 0.8, for patient left–right, i.e. for the x-gradient
- W_{HF} = 0.7, for patient head–feet, i.e. for the z-axis.

This results in a modified SD curve, where the gradients are summed:

$$\sqrt{\sum \left(W_i \left(\frac{dB}{dt} \right)_i \right)^2} < 20 \left(1 + \frac{0.36}{t_{eff}} \right).$$

(4.10)

Table 4.5 Default IEC rheobase and chronaxie values [34].

Type of gradient system	Chronaxie (ms)	Rh expressed as dB/dt (T s^{-1})	Rh expressed as E (V m^{-1})
Whole-body gradient system (cylindrical magnet)	0.36	20	2.2
Special purpose gradient system	0.36	(not applicable)	2.2

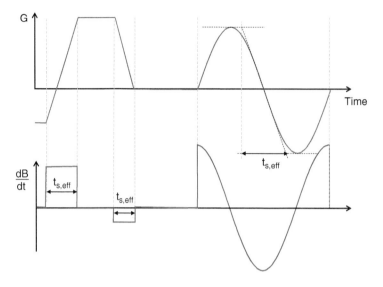

Figure 4.21　Effective stimulus durations ($t_{s,eff}$) defined in IEC-60601-2-33 [34].

The vector sum of the weighted dB/dt from each axis must be less than the PNS threshold. The effective stimulus duration t_{eff} is defined according to Figure 4.21.

The IEC PNS limits apply to both patients and MRI staff and are:

- **Normal mode**: 80% of the median perception threshold of the population (either from direct measurement[1] or from the parameters in Table 4.5):

$$L_{01} = 0.8\,Rh\left(1 + \frac{0.36}{t_{eff}}\right)$$
(4.11a)

- **First level controlled mode (L1)**: 100% of the median perception threshold or

$$L_{12} = 1.0\,Rh\left(1 + \frac{0.36}{t_{eff}}\right)$$
(4.11b)

- **Second level controlled mode (L2)**: up to 120% of the median perception threshold or

$$L_2 = 1.2\,Rh\left(1 + \frac{0.36}{t_{eff}}\right)$$
(4.11c)

The second level is only accessible as a research mode, subject to IRB or ethics committee approval. ICNIRP defines the modes in a similar manner with identical limits [51]. Using the median value from a population entails that stimulation is not inevitable if a limit is exceeded. This is borne out by the relative infrequency of PNS in clinical practice.

The IEC cardiac limit uses the exponential version of the SD curve:

$$\frac{dB}{dt} < 20 / \left(1 - e^{-\frac{t_{eff}}{3}}\right)$$
(4.12a)

---

[1] From the mean PNS threshold from at least 11 healthy adult volunteers of both sexes.

or in terms of induced electric field

$$E < 2 / \left(1 - e^{-\frac{t_{eff}}{3}} \right)$$ (4.12b)

These limits are shown in Figure 4.22.

Example 4.6   Cardiac stimulation

Calculate the dB/dt required for cardiac stimulation for a trapezoidal gradient pulse with a rise time of 0.5 ms and the amplitude of B required:

$$\frac{dB}{dt} > 20 / \left(1 - e^{-\frac{0.5}{3}} \right) = 130\, T\, s^{-1}$$

and the ΔB amplitude will be

$$\Delta B = t_{eff} \times \frac{dB}{dt} = 0.5 \times 130 = 65\ mT.$$

Assuming a 50 cm FOV (±0.25 m), this would indicate a gradient specification of 260 mT m⁻¹ and a slew rate of 520 T m⁻¹s⁻¹ – well beyond the capabilities of MR gradient systems.

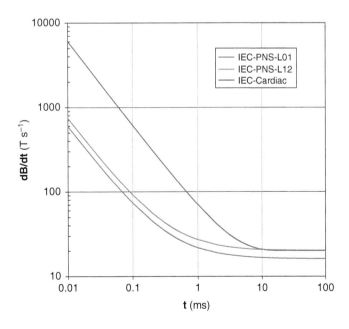

Figure 4.22   IEC limits for peripheral nerve and cardiac stimulation [34].

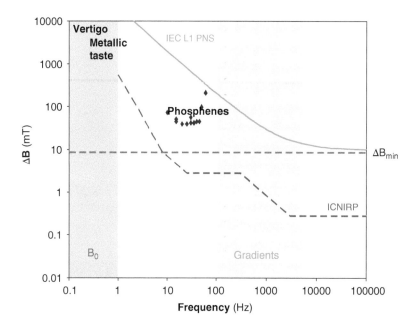

Figure 4.23 Bio-effects spectrum showing the principal sensory effects and frequency ranges relevant to MRI. The ICNIRP occupational limit (dashed red line) is shown as a peak value.

CONCLUSIONS

The only substantiated effects of time-varying magnetic fields in the ELF region are related to the stimulation of excitable tissues. Figure 4.23 shows the "bio-effects spectrum" from 0–100 kHz along with the IEC PNS threshold (1st Level) and the current ICNIRP occupational exposure reference level [11]. Magneto-phosphenes rarely occur in MRI and direct respiratory or cardiac stimulation are impossible with today's and future envisaged MRI systems. Peripheral nerve stimulation occurs for the lowest B-field stimuli but is harmless and well controlled by the scanner. Through the IEC operating modes, the MRI operator is alerted to the possibility of inducing PNS in the patient. PNS is most likely to occur for rapid sequences, diffusion, or for high resolution imaging, particularly with oblique slices.

Revision questions

1. Which bio-effect of time-varying magnetic fields has the lowest threshold in terms of the peak-to-peak change in B?
   A. Magneto-phosphenes
   B. Cardiac stimulation
   C. Respiratory stimulation
   D. Peripheral nerve stimulation
   E. Vertigo.
2. The limit of the Normal Operating Mode for the time-varying gradient magnetic fields is defined as ____ of the median perception threshold for peripheral nerve stimulation
   A. 50%
   B. 80%

C. 100%
D. 120%
E. 200%
3. In the strength duration curve for PNS:

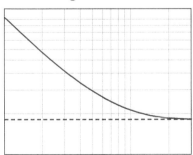

   A. Vertical axis is dB/dt, horizontal is stimulus duration, and the dotted line is the rheobase
   B. Vertical axis is B, horizontal is stimulus duration, and the dotted line is the chronaxie
   C. Vertical axis is B, horizontal is stimulus duration, and the dotted line is the rheobase
   D. Vertical axis is dB/dt, horizontal is stimulus duration, and the dotted line is the chronaxie
   E. Vertical axis is B, horizontal is chronaxie, and the dotted line is the rheobase.
4. The likelihood of inducing PNS from the MRI gradients depends upon which of the following?
   A. Larmor frequency
   B. Gradient lobe length
   C. Gradient pulse rise time
   D. Gradient amplitude
   E. The current Mode of operation.
5. Which of the following gradient exposures is most likely to induce PNS?
   A. 6 mT, 0.1 ms rise time
   B. 12 mT, 0.2 ms rise time
   C. 12 mT, 0.2 ms rise time, bipolar pulses
   D. All of the above
   E. None of the above.
6. What is the maximum current density induced in the brain from a dB/dt of 100 T s^{-1} if the brain is considered to be a sphere of diameter 15 cm with conductivity 0.2 S m^{-1}?
   A. 0.75 A m^{-2}
   B. 1.5 A m^{-2}
   C. 3 A m^{-2}
   D. 3.75 A m^{-2}
   E. 7.5 A m^{-2}

References

1. Marg, E. (1991). Magnetostimulation of vision: direct and non-invasive stimulation of the retina and the visual brain. *Optometry and Vision Science* 68:427–440.
2. D'Arsonval, A. (1896). Dispositifs pour la mesure des courants alternatifs de toutes frequences. *Comptes Rendus Hebdomadaires des Seances et Memoires de la Societe de Biologie* 3:450–451.
3. Budinger, T.F. (1979). Thresholds for physiological effects due to RF and magnetic fields used in NMR imaging. *IEEE Transactions in Nuclear Science* NS-26:2821–2825.
4. McRobbie, D. and Foster, M.A. (1985). Pulsed magnetic field exposure during pregnancy and implications for NMR foetal imaging: a study with mice. *Magnetic Resonance Imaging* 3:231–234.

5. McRobbie, D.W. (1987). Relationship between changing B and induced electric and physiological effects. In *Safety Assessment of NMR Imaging* (ed. K. Schmidt), Georg Thieme Verlag: Stuttgart, pp 64–70.

6. So, P.P., Stuchly, M.A., and Nyenhuis, J.A. (2004). Peripheral nerve stimulation by gradient switching fields in magnetic resonance imaging. *IEEE Transactions in Biomedical Engineering* 51:1907–1914.

7. Liu, F. and Crozier, S. (2004). A distributed equivalent magnetic current based FDTD method for the calculation of E-fields induced by gradient coils. *Journal of Magnetic Resonance* 169:323–327.

8. Reddig, A., Fatahi, M., Friebe, B., et al. (2015). Analysis of DNA double-strand breaks and cytotoxicity after 7 tesla magnetic resonance imaging of isolated human lymphocytes. *PLoS One* 10(7):e0132702. doi: 10.1371/journal.pone.0132702.

9. World Health Organization (2007). *Environmental Health Criteria 238: Extremely Low Frequency (ELF) Fields*. Geneva: WHO.

10. International Agency for Research into Cancer (2011). *Press release no. 201*. Geneva: World Health Organization. https://www.iarc.fr/wp-content/uploads/2018/07/pr208_E.pdf (accessed 11 July 2019).

11. International Commission on Non-Ionizing Radiation Protection (2010). ICNIRP statement on the "Guidelines for limiting exposure to time-varying electric, magnetic, and electromagnetic fields (up to 300 GHz)". *Health Physics* 93:257–258.

12. Griffin, M. and Bayat, A. (2011). Electrical stimulation in bone healing: critical analysis by evaluating levels of evidence. *Journal of Plastic Surgery* 11:303–353.

13. Barker, A.T., Freeston, I.L., Jalinous, R. et al. (1987). Magnetic stimulation of human brain and peripheral nervous system: an introduction and the results of an initial clinical evaluation. *Neurosurgery* 20:100–109.

14. Klomjai, W., Katz, R., and Lackmy-Vallee, A. (2015). Basic principles of transcranial magnetic stimulation (TMS) and repetitive TMS (rTMS). *Annals of Physical and Rehabilitation Medicine* 58:208–213.

15. Basil, B., Mahmud, J., Mathews, M. et al. (2005). Is there evidence for effectiveness of transcranial magnetic stimulation in the treatment of psychiatric disorders? *Psychiatry* 2:64–69.

16. Conolly, K.R., Helmer, A., Cristancho, M.A., et al. (2012). Effectiveness of transcranial magnetic stimulation in clinical practice post-FDA approval in the United States: results observed with the first 100 cases of depression at an academic clinical center. *Journal of Clinical Phsychiatry* 73:e567–e573.

17. Kavet, R., Hailey, W.H., Bracken, T.D. et al. (2008). Recent advances in research relevant to electric and magnetic field exposure guidelines. *Bioelectromagnetics* 29:499–525.

18. Lovsund, P., Oberg, P.A., and Nilsson, S.E.G. (1980). Magnetophosphenes: a quantitative analysis of thresholds. *Medical and Biological Engineering and Computing* 18:326–334.

19. Glover, P.M., Cavin, I., Qian, W. et al. (2007). Magnetic-field-induced vertigo: a theoretical and experimental investigation. *Bioelectromagnetics* 28:349–361.

20. Schaap, K., Christopher-DeVries, Y., Mason, C.K. et al. (2014). Occupational exposure of healthcare and research staff to static magnetic stray fields from 1.5–7 tesla MRI scanners is associated with reporting of transient symptoms. *Occupational & Environmental Medicine* 71:423–439.

21. Rauschenberg, J., Nagel, A.M., Ladd, S.C. et al. (2014). Multicenter study of subjective acceptance during magnetic resonance imaging at 7 and 9.4 T. *Investigative Radiology* 49:249–259.

22. Oberg, P.A. (1973). Magnetic stimulation of nerve tissue. *Medical and Biological Engineering and Computing* 11:55–64.

23. Polson, M.J.R., Barker, A.T., and Freeston, I.L. (1982). Stimulation of nerve trunks with time-varying magnetic fields. *Medical and Biological Engineering and Computing* 20:243–244.

24. McRobbie, D. and Foster, M.A. (1984) Thresholds for biological effects of magnetic fields. *Clinical Physics and Physiological Measurement* 5:67–78.

25. Budinger, T.F., Fischer, H., Hentschel, D. et al. (1991). Physiologic effects of fast oscillating magnetic field gradients. *Journal of Computer Assisted Tomography* 15:609–614.

26. Bourland, J.D., Nyenhuis, J.A. and Schaefer, D. (1999). Physiologic effects of intense MR imaging gradient fields. *Neuroimaging Clinics of North America* 9:363–377.

27. Weiss, G. (1901). Sur la possibility de rendre comparables entre eux les appareils servant a l'excitation electrique. *Archives of Italian Biology* 35:413–446.

28. Lapicque, L. (1907). Recherches quantitatifs sur l'excitation electrique des nerfs traites comme un polarisation. *Journal of Physiology– Paris* 9:622–35.

29. Reilly, J.P. and Diamant, A.M. (2011). Electrostimulation: Theory, Applications, and Computational Mode. Norwood, MA: Artech House.

30. Reilly, J.P. (1993). Safety considerations concerning the minimum threshold for magnetic excitation of the heart. *Medical and Biological Engineering and Computing* 31:651–654.
31. Recoskie, B.J., Scholl, T.J., and Chronik, B.A. (2009). The discrepancy between human peripheral nerve chronaxie times as measured using magnetic and electric field stimuli: The relevance to MRI gradient coil safety. *Physics in Medicine and Biology* 54:5965–5979.
32. Recoskie, B.J., Scholl, T.J., Zinke-Allmang, M. et al. (2010). Sensory and motor stimulation thresholds of the ulnar nerve from electrical and magnetic field stimuli: implications to gradient coil operation. *Magnetic Resonance in Medicine* 64:1567–7159.
33. Irnich, W. and Schmitt, F. (1995) Magnetostimulation in MRI. *Magnetic Resonance in Medicine* 33:619–23.
34. International Electrotechnical Commission (2015). Medical Electrical Equipment – Part 2–33: Particular Requirements for the Safety of Magnetic Resonance Equipment for Medical Diagnosis. IEC 60601-2-33 3.3 edn. Geneva: IEC.
35. Bohnert, J. and Dössel, O. (2010). Effects of time varying currents and magnetic fields in the frequency range of 1 kHz to 1 MHz to the human body - a simulation study. *Conference Proceedings of the IEEE Engineering in Medicine and Biology Society* 2010:6805–6808.
36. Weinberg, I.N., Stepanov, P.Y., Fricke, S. et al. (2012). Increasing the oscillation frequency of strong magnetic fields above 101 kHz significantly raises peripheral nerve excitation thresholds. *Medical Physics* 39:2578–2583.
37. Schmale, I., Gleich, B., Rahmer, J. et al. (2014). Patient safety in future magnetic particle Imaging: First experimental study of PNS thresholds. Safety in MRI: Guidelines, Rationale & Challenges, Washington DC, 5–7 September 2014. Berkeley: International Society for Magnetic Resonance in Medicine.
38. McRobbie, D.W. (2016). Does trans-membrane stimulation occur in peripheral nerve stimulation: why the SENN does not fit the data? Proceedings of 24th Annual Scientific Meeting of the International Society for Magnetic Resonance in Medicine. Berkeley, CA:ISMRM, p24.
39. Mouchawar, G,. Bourland, J.D., Voorhees, W.D., et al. (1990) Stimulation of inspiratory motor nerves with a pulsed magnetic field. *Medical and Biological Engineering and Computing* 28:613.
40. Bourland, J.D., Mouchawar, G, Geddes L.A. et al. (1990). Trans chest magnetic (eddy current) stimulation of the dog heart. *Medical and Biological Engineering and Computing* 28:196–198.
41. Yamaguchi, M., Andoh, T., Goto, T. et al. (1994). Effects of strong pulsed magnetic field on the cardiac activity of an open chest dog. *IEEE Transactions in Biomedical Engineering* 41:1188–1191.
42. Den Boer, J.A., Bourland, J.D., Nyenhuis, J.A. et al. (2002). Comparison of the threshold for peripheral nerve stimulation during gradient switching in whole body MR systems. *Journal of Magnetic Resonance Imaging* 15:520–525.
43. Zhang, B., Yen, Y.F., Chronik, B.A. et al. (2003). Peripheral nerve stimulation properties of head and body gradient coils of various sizes. *Magnetic Resonance in Medicine* 50:50–58.
44. Hebrank, F.X. and Gebhardt, M. (2007). SAFE-Model – a new method for predicting peripheral nerve stimulation in MRI. In: Proceedings of the Joint Annual Meeting of the International Society for Magnetic Resonance in Medicine and the European Society for Magnetic Resonance in Medicine and Biology, 19–25 May 2007, Berlin. Berkeley CA: ISMRM.
45. Chronik, B.A. and Rutt, B.K. (2001). Simple linear formulation for magnetostimulation specific to MRI gradient coils. *Magnetic Resonance in Medicine* 45:916–919.
46. Ham, C.L., Engels, J.M., van de Wiel, G.T. et al. (1997). Peripheral nerve stimulation during MRI: effects of high gradient amplitudes and switching rates. *Journal of Magnetic Resonance Imaging* 7:933–937.
47. Hoffman, A., Faber, S.C., Werhahn, K. et al. (2000). Electromyography in MRI: first recordings of peripheral nerve stimulation caused by fast magnetic field gradients. *Magnetic Resonance in Medicine* 43:543–539.
48. Chronik, B.A. and Ramachandran, M.J. (2003). Simple anatomical measurements do not correlate significantly to individual peripheral nerve stimulation thresholds as measured in MRI gradient coils. *Magnetic Resonance Imaging* 17:716–721.
49. Feldman, R.E., Hardy, C.J., Aksel, B., et al. (2009). Experimental determination of human peripheral nerve stimulation thresholds in a 3-axis planar gradient system. *Magnetic Resonance in Medicine* 62:763–770.

50. Vogt, F.M., Ladd, M.E., Hunold, P. et al. (2004). Increased time rate of change of gradient fields: effect on peripheral nerve stimulation at clinical MR imaging. *Radiology* 233:548–554.
51. ICNIRP (International Commission on Non-ionizing Radiation Protection). (2004). Medical magnetic resonance (MR) procedures: protection of patients. *Health Physics* 87:197–216.

Further reading and resources

Glover, P.M. (2009). Interaction of MRI field gradients with the human body. *Physics in Medicine and Biology* 54:R99–R115.

McRobbie, D.W. (2014). Bioeffects of gradient magnetic fields. In: *MRI bioeffects, safety, and patient management* (Ed. F.D. Shellock and J.V. Crues III) pp. 64–87. Los Angeles, CA: Biomedical Research Publishing Group.

Panych, L.P. and Madore, B. (2018). The physics of MRI safety, *Journal of Magnetic Resonance Imaging* 47:28–43.

Schaefer, D.J., Bourland, J.D., and Nyenhuis, J. A. (2000). Review of patient safety in time-varying gradient fields. *Journal of Magnetic Resonance Imaging* 12:20–29.

5

Bio-effects 3: radio-frequency fields

INTRODUCTION

The radio-frequency (RF) region of the electromagnetic (EM) spectrum covers the range 3 kHz to 300 GHz. Most MRI falls within the Very High Frequency (VHF) range, 30–300 MHz. In addition to MRI, the RF region hosts radio and television transmission, Wi-Fi, mobile telephony, therapeutic diathermy, and microwave heating. The RF region occupies the lowest frequencies, and hence energies, of the EM spectrum (see Figure 1.1). With low photon energy and long wavelength, it lacks the potential for ionization, unlike X- and gamma rays. Figure 5.1 shows the relative energy of an X-ray and a 128 MHz RF photon compared with molecular thermal energy in living tissue and the energy of a hydrogen bond. A RF photon in MRI is 11 orders of magnitude (100 billion times) less energetic than a diagnostic X-ray photon, possessing a million times less energy than that required to break the hydrogen bonds in proteins. The existence of direct causative bio-effects other than those that are heating-related is highly improbable. So-called "non-thermal" effects are not considered in this chapter.

PHYSICAL INTERACTION

We considered the physical interaction of the RF with tissues in Chapter 2. The main interaction is Faraday induction of an electric field E by the time-varying B_1 RF magnetic field, leading to tissue heating.

Radiofrequency in MRI

It is a misnomer to refer to the RF pulses in MRI as "radio waves," as EM waves possess orthogonal electric and magnetic fields and propagate with an inverse square law. Rather, the B_1 pulse is a magnetic field, orientated at right angles to the B_0 z-direction. It is usually generated by a birdcage coil driven in *quadrature* mode to produce a *circularly polarized* B_1 field that rotates at the precession frequency along with the patient's magnetization. Older MRI systems utilized linear RF transmit coils which produced a stationary B_1 field in one direction at a time, but their use meant that half the RF power was wasted, deposited in tissue, but ineffectual for manipulating the magnetization.

Essentials of MRI Safety, First Edition. Donald W. McRobbie.
© 2020 John Wiley & Sons Ltd. Published 2020 by John Wiley & Sons Ltd.

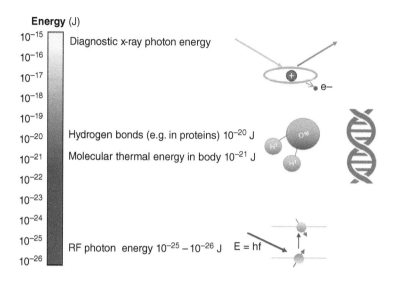

Figure 5.1 Relative energies: 128 MHz RF photon 8.48×10^{-26}J; 100 kV$_p$ diagnostic X-ray 5×10^{-15}J.

Table 5.1 Attributes of RF pulses.

Parameter / attribute	Symbol	Value	Units	Key relationship	Comments
Frequency	f	10–300	MHz	$f_o = \gamma B_o$	f_o is the "carrier" frequency
Bandwidth	Δf	0–100	kHz	$\Delta f = sw\,\gamma G_{ss}$	Δf depends upon slice width sw
Envelope / pulse shape	$B_1(t)$	Sinc (sinθ)/θ, Gaussian, rectangular, other	µT	$B_1(t) = B_1 e^{-i(\omega t + \phi)}$ Or for linear transmit $B_1(t) = B_1 \cos(\omega t + \phi)$	Amplitude and phase modulated; frequency modulated for adiabatic pulses.
Peak amplitude	B_{1+pk}	0–50	µT	Flip angle $\alpha = \gamma \int B_{1+}dt$	$\alpha = \gamma B_{1+}t_p$ for a rectangular pulse.
Root mean square value	B_{1+RMS}	0–10	µT	$B_{1+RMS} = \sqrt{\dfrac{\int_0^t (B_1(t))^2 dt}{t}}$	The "average" B_{1+} over a 10s duration.

Some important pulse metrics are:

- The peak B_1 amplitude in µT – denoted B_{1+pk} to indicate its rotation
- The duty cycle (D) – the fraction of time for which B_1 is transmitted
- B_{1+}RMS – the root mean square of B_{1+}, a type of average
- B_{1-}, a counter-rotating RF field which exists for *linear* transmit coils and does not interact with the magnetization
- The shape of the pulse: rectangular, Gaussian, sinc, etc.

Table 5.1 shows the principal properties of B_1 pulses.

Specific Absorption Rate

The RF energy deposition in tissue is given by the *Specific Absorption Rate* (SAR) defined as the power absorbed per unit mass measured in watts per kilogram (W kg^{-1}). SAR depends upon (Equation 2.28):

- The electric field E (squared) induced in tissue
- The tissue's electrical conductivity σ
- The tissue density ρ.

The maximum and average SAR for a uniform sphere were calculated in Equations 2.29– 2.31 showing that SAR:

- is not uniform throughout the patient.
- is a maximum towards the periphery of the patient.
- is strongly related to patient size.
- increases with the square of frequency, and hence with B_0^2.
- increases with the square of B_1: i.e. for a constant pulse shape, with the square of the flip angle.
- depends upon the number of RF pulses per second.

SAR is also related to the tissue properties of conductivity and density (Table 5.2 and Figure 5.2). Tissues with higher conductivity or lower density will experience higher SAR. Conductivity increases with frequency, contributing to higher SAR for 3T scanners, in addition to the B_0^2 dependence.

Example 5.1   SAR from linear and quadrature transmission

Calculate the maximum SAR from a linear body transmit coil with B_{1+} orientated in the y-direction on a patient of elliptical shape and uniform conductivity. How does this differ if B_{1+} is orientated along x?
From Equations A1.71, 2.28 and because a linear field of twice B_{1+} is required

$$E_{max} = 2\frac{a^2 b}{a^2 + b^2}\frac{dB_1}{dt}$$

$$SAR_{max} = 2\frac{a^4 b^2}{\left(a^2 + b^2\right)^2}\frac{\sigma\omega^2 B_1^2 D}{\rho}$$

Suppose a=0.3 m and b=0.2 m for a coronal body section corresponding to B_{1y} along the y-axis, then the geometric term is 0.019. If B_{1x} is directed along x, then consider a sagittal section for the induced E field with a=0.3 and b=0.1 in which case the geometric factor is 0.0081. The maximum SAR from B_{1y} is 2.4 times that from B_{1x}. For a circularly polarized B_1 this difference will be smeared out, resulting in a more uniform SAR distribution.

SAR hotspots

As the physical properties of tissue differ, SAR is not uniform throughout the body even if B_1 is perfectly uniform (which it is not). Differences in conductivity and permittivity (Table 5.2) between tissues and the presence of metal can result in SAR hotspots. A simple analytical solution [2] considers two situations: an organ surrounded by fat, or a fatty infiltration in an

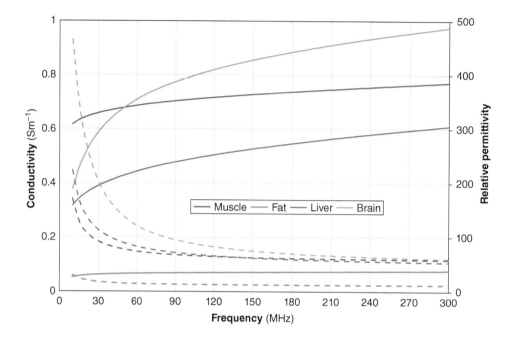

Figure 5.2 Tissue conductivity (solid lines) and relative permittivity (dashed lines). Data from [1].

Table 5.2 Physical properties of human tissues. Electrical properties from https://it is.swiss/virtual–population/tissue–properties/database [1].

Tissue /substance	Density ρ (kg m^{-3})	Conductivity σ (S m^{-1})		Relative Permittivity ε_r	
		64 MHz	128 MHz	64 MHz	128 MHz
Air	1 ± 0	0	0	1	1
Saline/water	1000 ± 0	1.55	1.55	84.6	84.6
Blood	1050 ± 17	1.21	1.25	86.4	73.2
Bone (cancellous)	1178 ± 149	0.161	0.180	30.9	26.3
Bone (cortical)	1908 ± 133	0.060	0.067	16.7	14.7
Brain (WM)	1041 ± 6	0.292	0.342	67.8	52.5
Eye (lens)	1076 ± 21	0.286	0.313	50.3	42.8
Fat	911 ± 53	0.066	0.070	13.6	12.4
Heart muscle	1081 ± 36	0.678	0.766	107	84.3
Kidney	1066 ± 56	0.714	0.852	119	89.6
Liver	1079 ± 53	0.448	0.511	80.6	64.3
Muscle	1090 ± 52	0.688	0.719	72.2	63.5
Skin (dry)	1109 ± 14	0.463	0.523	92.2	65.4
Testes	1082 ± 54	0.885	0.926	84.5	72.1
Uterus	1105 ± 74	0.911	0.961	92.1	75.4

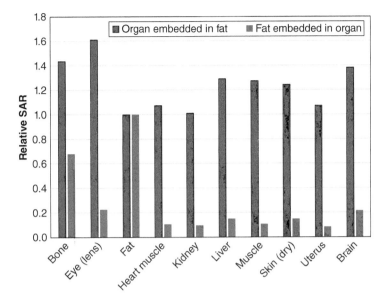

Figure 5.3   SAR hotspot formation due to electrical properties for idealized geometries: a sphere of tissue within fat, or a sphere of fat within tissue.

organ – albeit with unrealistic spherical geometries. The first situation results in an increase in SAR, whilst a blob of fat inside an organ will result in a lower SAR (Figure 5.3).

Additionally, the interdependence of electric and magnetic field components from Maxwell's fourth equation can result in very uneven SAR arising from "wave-like" properties considered below. Solving the SAR distribution for real anatomies requires sophisticated EMF modeling and anatomically realistic models [3].

On the scanner SAR monitoring is usually of the average head SAR or whole-body SAR. These quantities do not take account of SAR hotspots, or even the maximum SAR in peripheral tissues, so it is common in electromagnetic modeling to use a local SAR calculated for every 10 g of tissue. Figure 5.4 shows some results of such modeling [4].

B_1 non-uniformity

The B_1 field in air produced by a typical birdcage transmit coil is highly uniform (see Figure 1.26). However the presence of the patient's tissues distorts the RF field (e.g. as in Figure 2.28). The "wavelength" in air is around 4.7 m at 64 MHz (1.5 T) and 2.3 m at 128 MHz (3 T). However, the dielectric constant, ε_r of tissues changes the wavelength *within* the patient. From the data in Table 5.2 we can calculate values for different tissues using Equation 2.33 (See Table 9.4).

An effect of the wavelength change in tissue is the creation of standing waves or resonances when either the patient dimension or a conductor length is close to one half wavelength $\lambda/2$. This has particular importance for the avoidance of heating in active implants with lead lengths equal to or close to $\lambda/2$. Another consequence of the wave-like behavior of the RF in tissue is the propagation of the B_1 field beyond the limit of the transmit coil [5] (Figures 2.29, 2.30).

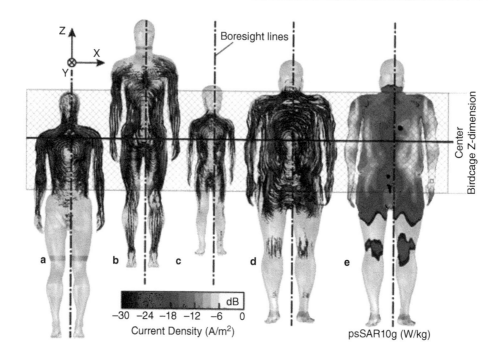

Figure 5.4 Human body models in a 1.5 T whole-body RF coil (shaded region): (a-d) induced current density streamlines from $B_1 = 1\ \mu T$; 0 dB corresponds to 100 A m^{-2}; (e) peak spatial SAR averaged over any 10 g of tissue from 4 W kg^{-1} whole-body SAR; 0 dB corresponds to 80 W kg^{-1}. Source [4]. Used with permission of Wiley.

MYTHBUSTER:

Half wavelength values in tissue are not 13 cm or 26 cm at 1.5 and 3 T as commonly supposed, but vary substantially according to tissue type.

TISSUE HEATING

SAR is the rate of energy deposition in tissue. However, what we really want to know is the absolute *temperature* of tissue as this is the cause of thermal injury and other adverse biological effects. This is not straight forward, but we can establish some simple principles to describe heating in a qualitative manner.

SAR and temperature rise without cooling

The basic heat equation gives the amount of energy U in joules (J) required to raise the temperature of a material by ΔT:

$$U = Cm\Delta T \qquad (5.1)$$

where C is the specific heat capacity of the material (J kg^{-1} °C^{-1}) and m is the mass (kg).

Table 5.3 Tissue properties and heating in the absence of thermal conduction. Electrical properties from https://it is.swiss/virtual–population/tissue–properties/database after [1].

Tissue /substance	Specific heat capacity C (J kg^{-1} °C^{-1})	Blood flow (perfusion) rate F_b (ml min^{-1} kg^{-1})	Thermal conductivity K (W m^{-1} °C^{-1})	Relative local SAR $\frac{1000\sigma_t}{0.54\rho_t}$	Temperature rise ΔT_r for average whole-body SAR=4 W kg^{-1} No conduction (°C)
Air	1004 ± 3	0	0.026	0	0
Saline (0.9% NaCl)	4178	0	0.6 ± 0.01	2.87	0.089/min
ASTM phantom	4140	0	0.0538		
Blood	3617 ±301	10000	0.52 ± 0.03	2.2	0.01
Bone (cancellous)	2274 ±234	30 ± 20	0.31 ± 0.03	0.28	0.60
Bone (cortical)	1313 ±295	10	0.32 ± 0.03	0.07	0.41
Brain (WM)	3583 ±78	212 ±24	0.48 ± 0.03	0.61	0.18
Eye (lens)	3133 ±297	0	0.43 ± 0.06	0.54	0.032/min
Fat	2348 ±372	33± 13	0.21 ± 0.02	0.14	0.27
Heart muscle	3686 ±62	1026 ±307	0.56 ± 0.04	1.31	0.08
Kidney	3763 ±120	3795 ±544	0.53 ± 0.02	1.48	0.02
Liver	3540 ±119	860 ±170	0.52 ± 0.03	0.88	0.06
Muscle	3421 ±460	37 ±13	0.49 ± 0.04	1.22	2.09
Skin (dry)	3391 ±233	106 ±37	0.37 ± 0.06	0.87	0.52
Testes	3778	200 ±24	0.52	1.58	1.19
Uterus	3676	458 ±408	0.53 ± 0.02	1.61	1.11

In terms of SAR,

$$\Delta T = \frac{SAR\, t}{C} \tag{5.2}$$

The material will keep on heating up unless there is a cooling mechanism to bring it into thermal equilibrium. Values of tissue specific heat capacities are shown in Table 5.3.

Example 5.2   Heating of the lens

How much energy is required to heat the lens of the eye by 2 °C assuming a mass of 250 mg and no cooling mechanism? If a MR acquisition runs for 100 s, what local SAR is required?
  The lens' specific heat capacity is 3133 J kg^{-1} °C^{-1}. From Equation 5.1:

$$U = 3133 \times 250 \times 10^{-6} \times 2 = 1.57\,J$$

Power = Joules per second = 0.0157 W
  The SAR is 0.0157/250 × 10^{-6} = *62.7 W kg^{-1}.*

Temperature rise with perfusion cooling

In tissue there are various cooling and thermal regulation mechanisms. Perfusion of tissues by blood is the most important. The temperature rise ΔT in the presence of perfusion is [6]

$$\Delta T = \Delta T_f \left(1 - e^{-t/\tau}\right) \tag{5.3}$$

ΔT_f is the final or steady state temperature increase (Figure 5.5) given by

$$\Delta T_f = 15.8 \times \frac{SAR}{F_b} \tag{5.4}$$

where F_b is the blood flow (ml min⁻¹ kg⁻¹). Some values of F_b are shown in Table 5.3. The tissue undergoes a rapid initial temperature rise, plateauing as thermal equilibrium is achieved with the cooling effect of perfusion (and conduction). Tissues with lower perfusion (fat, bone, muscle) will achieve the highest temperatures.

The time constant τ is:

$$\tau = 15.8 \times \frac{C_t}{F_b} \tag{5.5}$$

Not all tissues will heat up at the same rate. Those with lower specific heat capacity C_t and greater perfusion will equilibrate more quickly. Fortunately, the tissues that display the highest

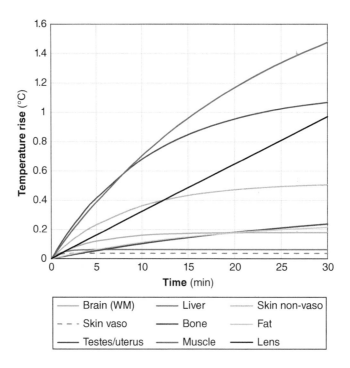

Figure 5.5 Temperature increase versus time for various tissues exposed to a whole-body SAR of 4 W kg⁻¹ with cooling by perfusion only. Derived from [6].

temperature rise have longer time constants and the restriction of heating can be achieved by avoiding long scan times. For example, the temperature rise in cortical bone can be kept to 1 °C if the scan does not exceed 15 minutes.

This model was developed for head only exposures and assumed a constant blood temperature of 37 °C. In a whole-body exposure with the body-transmit coil, a significant fraction of the blood may experience a temperature rise too. Consequently Equations 5.3–5.5 and Figure 5.5 should be considered as illustrative only.

Other cooling mechanisms

Other cooling mechanisms are thermal conduction, convection, evaporative, and radiative heat loss.

Thermal conduction

For a small spherical region or radius r (it's always a sphere!) with poor perfusion the only way to lose heat is by thermal conduction. In this case the equilibrium temperature rise is [6]

$$\Delta T = \frac{\rho r^2}{6K} \, SAR \qquad (5.6)$$

Values of thermal conductivity K (W m^{-1} °C^{-1}) are given in Table 5.3. Most tissues have K in the region of 0.5 W m^{-1} °C^{-1}. However, fat and bone will reduce any hotspot less rapidly than other tissues.

Radiative cooling

Radiative cooling depends upon the difference between surface temperature T_s and the ambient temperature T_a to the 4th power and also upon the surface area. The Stefan–Boltzmann Law gives the power of the heat loss:

$$P = s\,e\,A \left(T_s^4 - T_a^4 \right) \qquad (5.7)$$

where s is the Stefan–Boltzmann constant = 5.67 × 10^{-8} W m^{-2} K^{-4} and the emissivity of skin e = 0.98. The skin surface area A can be calculated from the height d (m) and mass m (kg) [7].

$$A = \sqrt{dm} / 6 \qquad (5.8)$$

This formula has been shown to work for all ages down to neonates [8].

A small child will radiate less heat than an adult, but will experience a lower SAR on account of their smaller volume, but also will have a greater fraction of their body within the RF transmit field. Figure 5.6 shows some theoretical values of absorbed power (W) from SAR compared with radiative heat loss assuming a difference between skin temperature and ambient temperature of 10 °C based upon an adult SAR of 2 W kg^{-1} and neglecting the insulating effect of clothing. Whilst it appears that a baby is less likely to be affected by RF heating, the baby is likely to be more heavily clothed or swaddled in blankets and hence the radiative heat loss will be significantly less effective than shown in the figure. Ambient temperature also plays and important role. Figure 5.7 shows the relative loss in radiative cooling over the temperature range 20–30 °C.

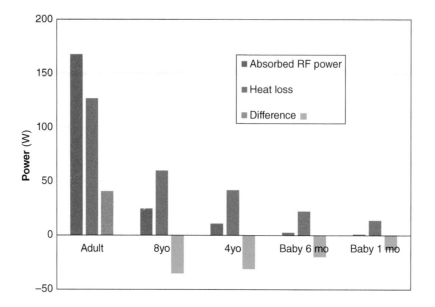

Figure 5.6 Nett power absorption differences with age: the red bars indicate the absorbed power from a whole-body SAR of 2 W kg⁻¹: the blue bars indicate radiative cooling from the skin surface area.

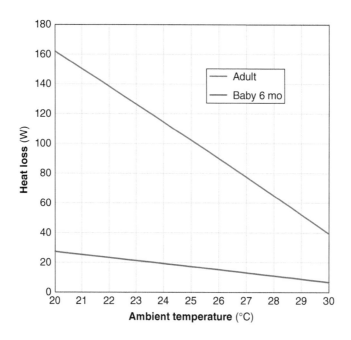

Figure 5.7 Effect of ambient temperature on radiative cooling rates.

Other cooling mechanisms

Other cooling mechanisms include evaporative losses from respiration and perspiration, contact conduction, and convection.

> ### Example 5.3   Radiative cooling
>
> Calculate the radiative cooling from a 1.8 m tall, 80 kg adult in an ambient temperature of 22 °C using the Stefan–Boltmann Law.
>   *Body surface area A, can be calculated from $A = \sqrt{dm}\,/\,6 = 2m^2$.*
>   *Expressing temperature in Kelvin, skin temperature = 273 + 33 K, ambient temperature = 273 + 22 K, the heat loss is therefore*
>
> $$P = 5.67 \times 10^8 \times 0.98 \times 2 \times \left(306^4 - 295^4\right) = 133\,W$$
>
> *If the SAR is 2 W kg⁻¹, the additional heat power is 2 × 80 = 160 W and radiative losses alone are insufficient to maintain a constant temperature.*

Thermal regulation

Humans are endotherms or "warm-blooded" generating and maintaining their core body temperature at 37 °C, with fluctuations of about ± 0.5 °C. Skin temperature is typically 33 °C but may fluctuate over a range of 15 °C depending upon the environment. The core temperature is maintained by metabolic activity, with the basal metabolic rate being around 1.4 W kg⁻¹. Vigorous exercise can result in 3 W kg⁻¹ whilst elite athletes can produce several times that.

Physiological mechanisms for heat removal are increased blood flow and peripheral vessel dilation. A model for thermoregulation [9] is illustrated in Figure 5.8. Vasomotor adjustment occurs within the "thermal neutral zone" (TNZ). Below an ambient temperature less than the

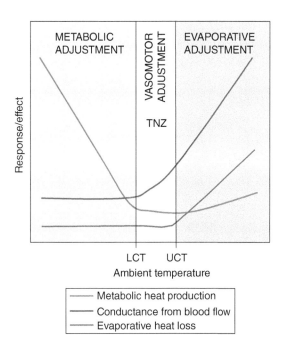

Figure 5.8   Temperature regulation. TNZ is temperature neutral zone. Below LCT (lower critical temperature) more heat must be generated by metabolism. Above UCT (upper critical temperature) evaporative cooling is required. Redrawn from [9].

lower critical temperature, thermoregulation is maintained primarily by metabolic activity. For ambience above the upper critical temperature, full vasodilation has already occurred and evaporative cooling from sweating and respiration come into play. Heating from RF exposure will be additive to that from metabolism – requiring some thermo-regulatory response to maintain thermal balance.

If the thermal load is too large, a greater demand is made on cardiac output and organ blood pressure may reduce. Both could have serious consequences for the patient. Patients requiring caution with regard to heating include those with fever, compromised thermal regulation (perhaps caused by diuretics or other drugs), the elderly, the obese, pregnant patients and fetuses, and neonates.

BIOLOGICAL EFFECTS

Temperature is known to have a significant effect upon chemical reactions, so it is not surprising that RF induced tissue heating can have biological consequences. Much of the research relates to RF and microwave exposures at broadcast and telecommunications frequencies.

Cellular studies

In-vitro studies have shown changes in cell morphology, water and electrolyte content, and cell membrane function. Of some interest is the observation that amplitude modulated (AM) VHF exposures, with modulation frequencies of 6–60 Hz, may increase Ca^{++} flow from cells. However, many results have not been replicated, so there remains significant doubt about the veracity of this effect.

The UK's National Radiological Protection Board concluded that microwaves are not mutagenic [10]. Regarding non-thermal effects, the International Commission for Non-Ionizing Radiation Protection (ICNIRP) stated [11]:

> Overall, the literature on athermal effects of AM electromagnetic fields is so complex, the validity of reported effects so poorly established, and the relevance of the effects to human health is so uncertain, that it is impossible to use this body of information as a basis for setting limits on human exposure to these fields.

Animal studies

Body temperature rises of 1–2 °C have been shown to affect neural and muscular function, increased blood–brain barrier permeability, disrupt the immune system, reduce sperm production, and increase teratogenicity [12]. Cataract formation can occur for temperatures of 41–43 °C in addition to corneal abnormalities [13]. RF hyperthermia, utilizing temperatures of 40–45 °C has been trialed extensively as a cancer therapy [14]. Protein denaturing occurs at temperatures of 45 °C. Thermal ablation therapies involve temperatures in the range 75–90 °C.

CEM43

Cumulated Equivalent Minutes at 43 °C, or CEM43, is a model for thermal damage used extensively in hyperthermia studies. A series of thermal exposures can be converted to an equivalent number of minutes of heating at 43 °C using the formula:

$$CEM43 = \sum_{i}^{n} t_i R^{(43-T_i)} \tag{5.9}$$

Table 5.4   CEM43 values for tissue damage [15].

| Tissue/organ | Cumulated equivalent minutes at 43°C (CEM43) | | Effects |
	Reversible damage	Irreversible damage	
Bone		16	
Brain	10		BBB, perfusion changes
Eye (lens)		2.4	Opacity
Fat	15		Apidocyte cell death
Muscle	41	80	Acute hemorrhage, chronic necrosis
Skin	41	288	Erythema, necrosis

where T_i is the average temperature for the ith treatment of duration t_i. R is related to the rate of cell death, equal to ¼ for T<43 °C and ½ for higher temperatures [15]. CEM43 values have been estimated for a wide range of tissues from a range of species including humans (Table 5.4). For example, blood brain barrier (BBB) changes would occur for 10 minutes at 43 °C or the CEM43 equivalent exposure. Skin erythema could occur after 41 minutes. Tissues with poor perfusion, e.g. bone and fat, are particularly sensitive to thermal injury. Figure 5.9 shows the relationship between temperature and exposure time for damage.

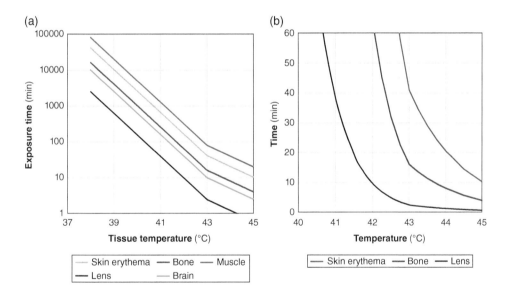

Figure 5.9   CEM43: (a) Cumulative equivalent minutes at 43 °C for damage to various tissues; (b) expanded region most relevant to MRI.

Example 5.4   CEM43 and time to cause a skin burn

How long would a MRI scan that raised skin temperature locally to 45 °C need to last to cause a burn?
   Use Figure 5.9 or Equation 5.9. Using the equation, CEM43 for skin is 41 min. The value of R for T>43 °C is ½. So, the time required is

$$t = \frac{41}{0.5^{(43-45)}} = 41 \times 0.5^2 = 10.25 \; min.$$

Carcinogenic effects

With the advent of mobile telephony, new research has been conducted into the possibility of cancer induction from exposure to phone frequencies. One major study is the National Toxicology Project (NTP): Toxicology and Carcinogenicity Studies of Cell Phone Radiofrequency Radiation [16, 17]. In this study 90 male and 90 female rats experienced nine hours RF exposure per day lifelong from conception to death. The irradiation was either 0, 1.5, 3 or 6 W kg^{-1} at 900 and 1800 MHz with two signal modulations: Code Division Multiple Access (CDMA) and Global System for Mobile Communications (GSM).

There was no difference between the four groups in littering, size, or sex distribution of the litters, or pup survival. A lower birth weight was observed for the RF exposed rats, but this returned to normal after a few weeks. The incidence of heart (malignant schwannoma) and brain tumors (malignant glioma and glial cell hyperplasia) showed a slight increase with the higher RF exposures, particularly for the males. However, on average the RF exposed animals, particularly the males, *outlived* the non-exposed rats, suggestive of both possible detrimental and beneficial effects of RF.

This type of equivocal result is fairly typical in research into the bio-effects of EMF. Of course, the exposure conditions are fairly extreme – the rodents practically living inside a super-powered phone! At these frequencies the RF penetrates much deeper into the rats' tissues than it can in humans, making extrapolation of the results to human exposures problematical.

Human studies and epidemiology

Concerns about the possible carcinogenicity of RF exposures first arose in the 1980s. A study of nearly 500 000 adult male deaths over 32 years showed increased mortality rates from leukemia and non-Hodgkins lymphomas for workers in EMF-related occupations compared with others [18]. However, this study did not include any dosimetry and the author's conclusions were tentative. Nevertheless, the International Agency for Research into Cancer (IARC) of the World Health Organization (WHO) has declared ELF electromagnetic fields as a "possible carcinogen" [19].

Do mobile phones cause cancer?

The rapid adoption of mobile telephony since the 1980s has raised concern about possible consequences of their use including the induction of malignant gliomas in the brain and non-malignancies such as meningioma and acoustic neuroma. There have been several large studies of potential cancer induction and phone usage. Most of these do not show a correlation, although many suffer from methodological difficulties such as gaining accurate dosimetry and usage data.

The INTERPHONE study [20] of 5000 users in 13 countries found no link between brain tumor risk and the frequency of calls, call time, or phone use over ten years. A small association of extreme phone usage with the incidence of gliomas, acoustic neuromas, and meningiomas was suggested, but biases and error margins precluded a causal explanation. However, a longer-term study in Denmark of 420 000 phone users detected no increased risk for any brain or salivary gland tumours, ruling out a link with heavy use [21]. The Million Women study in the UK, with 792 000 participants, also found no link with brain tumors but did indicate a possible link between high usage and acoustic neuromas [22].

In the USA the Food and Drug Administration [23] concluded:

"Based on our ongoing evaluation of this issue, the totality of the available scientific evidence continues to not support adverse health effects in humans caused by exposures at or under the current radiofrequency energy exposure limits. We believe the existing safety limits for cell phones remain acceptable for protecting the public health."

The mobile phone SAR limit in the USA, set by the Federal Communications Commission (FCC), is 1.6 W kg^{-1} in any one gram of tissue. The European Committee for Electrotechnical Standardization (CENELEC) limit is 2 W kg^{-1} in any 10 g of tissue.

Microwave hearing

An unusual effect of RF is "microwave hearing" whereby a clicking sound is heard from exposure to pulsed 2450 MHz microwaves [24]. The mechanism is attributed to thermal expansion in the auditory system stimulating the hair cells in the cochlea. The phenomenon has also been demonstrated in MRI transmit head coils operating in the range 2.4–170 MHz with pulses of duration 3 –100 µs and pulse energies of 16 mJ [25]. A peak RF transmitter power of 30 kW was proposed to avoid the noise being excessive.

RF burns in MRI

The most common detrimental bio-effect from the RF exposure in MRI is burns. In the UK, where there is mandatory reporting of injuries, Department of Health figures indicate that 95 RF burn incidents from 21 million scans occurred between 1995 and 2011 – a rate of 0.00045% of all examinations, or 1 incident per 220 000 exams. More recent is a report of 10 RF burns from 1.3 million examinations – or 0.00075% – with RF burns accounting for 1.5% of all incidents [26]. In the USA RF-related thermal injuries account for 59% of all MRI incidents reported to the FDA [27].

Figure 5.10 shows the anatomy of the skin. The pain threshold is 43 °C but a burn is caused if the basal layer of the epidermis reaches 44 °C. Above this temperature the rate of tissue damage increases logarithmically with a linear increase in temperature. An epidermal erythema,

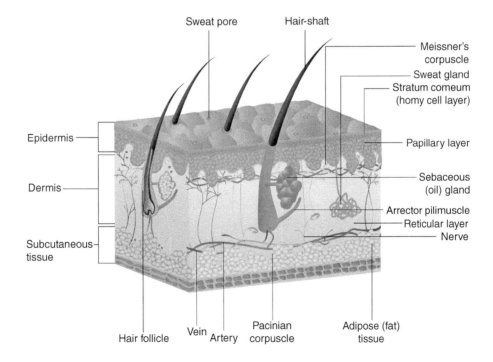

Figure 5.10   Skin anatomy. Source: stockshoppe/Shutterstock.

or first-degree burn, will resolve itself within a few days. A dermal or second-degree burn is deeper, more painful and may last for two weeks, but without permanent scarring. A third- or fourth-degree burn extends beyond the dermis resulting in extensive scarring and necrosis. Tissue damage thresholds may be lower for children [28].

Skin burns [29] can arise from:

- The use of inappropriate non-MRI physiological monitoring leads and electrodes
- Inappropriate scanning of external fixation devices
- Receive coil faults
- Contact or proximity of the patient's skin to the inner surface of the bore
- Larger conduction paths, e.g. from larger patients
- Other reasons in specific cases whose causes are hard to determine.

Leads, electrodes, and fixation

Inappropriate lead use allows the RF to induce large currents in the cables or electrodes potentially leading to a burn (Figure 5.11a). The presence of the metal can result in a magnification of the local SAR. The same is true of external fixation devices (Figure 5.11b). Some sports clothing items contain metal threads which may also heat up. Contact with an object accounts for at least 28% of MRI-thermal injuries [27].

Coil faults

In normal operation a receive only coil is insensitive to the large RF B_1 pulses. This is achieved using detuning circuitry during transmission. If this circuitry fails, then B_1 will induce large currents in the receive coil, further amplified because the coil is now tuned to the same frequency as B_1. Skin in close proximity to the coil can heat up significantly, leading to a burn.

(a)   (b)

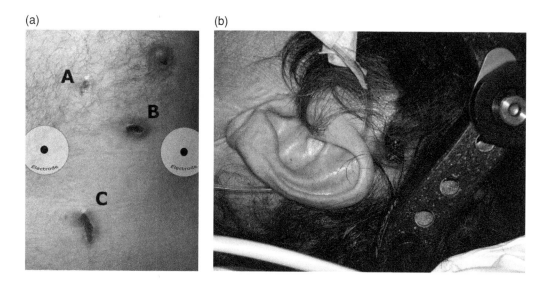

Figure 5.11   RF burns: (a) from inappropriate ECG electrodes. Source [29]. Licensee NobleResearch Publishers under CC BY 4.0; (b) from heating of cervical traction tong pins.

Contact with or proximity to the bore

Larger patients whose skin may be in contact with or very close to the inner surface of the scanner bore are more likely to experience burns for several reasons: the B_1 field may be stronger close to the coil windings, the conduction paths in tissue are greater, and the proximity to the coil windings and tuning capacitors may result in the electric field coupling directly with tissue, adding to the SAR induced by B_1. Additionally, the greater volume of fat and the reduced opportunity for cool air flow make it harder for heat to dissipate from the skin surface. Bore contact accounts for 10% of RF thermal injuries [27].

123

For no apparent reason

RF burns do rarely occur for reasons other than those listed above. It may be that the patient's geometry, particularly in the inner thigh region, results in an unexpected concentration of RF energy leading to burn. Patient sweating may be a contributing factor (or it may not!).

Avoiding RF burns

The best way to avoid the possibility of RF burns is to limit SAR. Some MR systems may default to the higher SAR First Level Controlled Mode and you should be aware when this happens. Care is required especially at 3 T or above. Patients should be asked not to clasp their hands or cross their legs at the ankle (even if this is more comfortable) as these will produce greater conduction paths leading to higher SAR (Figure 5.12). The region between the upper thighs is often a hot-spot for SAR so it is advisable to ensure there is non-conductive material between the legs. Padding between the shoulders and the bore wall is also advisable for larger patients. Ensure a good airflow through the bore and maintain verbal contact with the patients most at risk: the

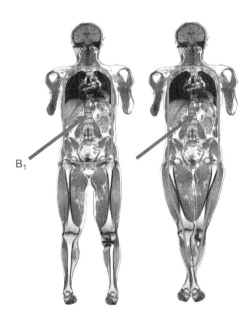

Figure 5.12 RF conduction paths. Crossing legs at ankle level increases the RF induced current path, potentially increasing SAR.

elderly, obese, pregnant, very young, those on medications that affect thermal regulation, those with fever or poor cardiac or vascular function, the sweaty, and those with metallic implants.

RF EXPOSURE LIMITS

One of the most important clinical tasks for the MR professional is to limit, control and monitor SAR. In this section we will review RF limits, the influence of pulse sequence parameters upon SAR, and how to monitor SAR.

Temperature and SAR Limits

In most jurisdictions patient RF exposure limits are set by the International Electrotechnical Commission's 60601-2-33 standard [30]. In the USA this has been recognised by the FDA since December 2017 as a voluntary standard.

Temperature limitation

With RF heating in MRI the fundamental physical insult is *temperature*, rather than temperature rise or SAR. Thermal injuries are avoided by limiting the maximum temperature in tissues. Table 5.5 shows the IEC temperature limits. In the Normal Mode, a maximum temperature of 39 °C or core temperature rise of 0.5 °C is not expected to cause any physiological stress. In the 1st Level Controlled Mode the limit is 40 °C and some physiological stress may occur. In this mode medical supervision is required and the patient should be warned of the possibility of heating. The 2nd Level is a research only mode, requiring IRB or ethical approval to unlock it and to determine levels of risk.

SAR limits

As in-vivo temperature is hard to monitor, limits are also given in terms of SAR (Table 5.6). By adhering to the SAR limits, temperature *should* be sufficiently limited to avoid tissue damage, provided significant SAR hotspots do not occur. SAR measurements are averaged over six minutes. For short durations of less than 10 seconds the SAR may be double the average limit. *Partial body* SAR is calculated according to the ratio of the mass of the exposed region to the total patient mass (Example 5.5). If the ambient temperature exceeds 25 °C, the 1st Level limit reduces by 0.25 W kg^{-1} per degree (Figure 5.13). The Normal Mode limit remains unchanged.

Table 5.5   IEC temperature limits [30]. Higher temperature values are permitted, but subject to clinical risk–benefit decisions.

Operating Mode	Maximum temperature limits (°C)		Maximum core temperature rise (°C)
	Core	Local	
Normal	39	39	0.5
1st Level Controlled	40	40	1.0
2nd Level Controlled	>40	>40	>1.0

Table 5.6   IEC SAR limits [30]. $m_{exposed}$ denotes mass of patient exposed (%), $m_{patient}$ is patient mass. SAR may exceed these limits by 100% over a 10s duration.

Operating mode	Whole-body (W kg⁻¹)	Partial body (W kg⁻¹)	Head (W kg⁻¹)	Local transmit coils		
				Head (W kg⁻¹)	Trunk (W kg⁻¹)	Extremity (W kg⁻¹)
Normal	2	$10-8\dfrac{m_{exposed}}{m_{patient}}$	3.2	10	10	20
1st Level Controlled	4	$10-6\dfrac{m_{exposed}}{m_{patient}}$	3.2	20	20	40
2nd Level Controlled	>4	$>10-6\dfrac{m_{exposed}}{m_{patient}}$	3.2	>20	>20	>40

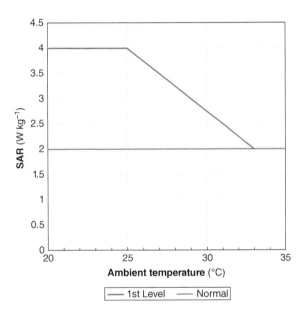

Figure 5.13   SAR derating for the First Level Controlled Mode for ambient temperature above 25 °C.

SAR limits are also specified for local transmit coils. These are defined as coils which are not volume coils. A transmit–receive knee coil would *not* count as a local transmit coil, but the appropriate partial body SAR could be used. For local transmit coils, the SAR is to be calculated over each 10 g of tissue. Local transmit coils are not commonly used in routine clinical practice. Their SAR characteristics are described by [2].

Example 5.5   Partial body SAR

What is the Normal Mode partial body SAR limit for a 70 kg adult patient whose lower limbs only are in the scanner?
The lower limbs comprise approximately 30% of body mass (trunk ≈ 50%, head and neck ≈ 10%, upper limbs ≈ 10%). So the SAR partial body limit is

$$SAR = 10-8\times\frac{0.3}{1} = 7.6 \ W \ kg^{-1}.$$

Specific Energy Dose

The Specific Energy Dose (SED) is defined as the RF energy absorbed per kilogram of patient mass. It has units of joules per kg (J kg^{-1}) and is equal to the average SAR times the scan duration. It can be summed for all the sequences in an examination, making it a convenient exposure metric for patient records:

$$SED = \sum_{all\, sequences} SAR_i t_i \qquad (5.10)$$

The total energy absorbed is equal to the SED times patient weight. The IEC-60601-2-33 [30] limit for SED is 14.4 kJ kg^{-1}, equivalent to 4 W kg^{-1} for one hour (240 W min kg^{-1}). The system will disable scanning above this value. SED can be used along with equation 5.1 to crudely estimate the thermal load or maximum core body temperature rise (assuming no cooling mechanisms).

Example 5.6   SED for an examination

What is the SED and total energy absorbed by an 80 kg patient who underwent the following examinations?

Localizer/scout:	0.1 W kg^{-1},	scan duration: 20 s;
T_1-w SE (pre-contrast):	0.9 W kg^{-1},	scan duration: 120 s;
T_2-w TSE/FSE:	1.6 W kg^{-1},	scan duration: 40 s;
Diffusion EPI:	0.3 W kg^{-1},	scan duration: 360 s;
T_1-w SE (post-contrast):	0.9 W kg^{-1},	scan duration: 120 s.

$$SED = 0.1 \times 20 + 0.9 \times 120 \times 2 + 1.6 \times 40 + 0.3 \times 360 = 390\, J\, kg^{-1}$$

And the total absorbed energy is 80 × 390 = 31.2 kJ. From Equation 5.1 using a specific heat capacity of 3500 J kg^{-1} °C^{-1}, the maximum core temperature increase is unlikely to exceed

$$\Delta T = \frac{31.2 \times 10^3}{3500 \times 80} = 0.11\ °C.$$

Other limits

The FDA "Criteria for Significant Risk Investigations of Magnetic Resonance Devices" [31] specifies a whole-body SAR as 4 W kg^{-1} averaged over 15 minutes and a head SAR exceeding 3.2 W kg^{-1} averaged over 10 minutes as requiring control and approval.

ICNIRP limits [32] are essentially similar to IEC60601-2-33 but with slightly different terminology: the modes are "Normal", "Controlled" and "Restricted". The head SAR limit is stated as 3 W kg^{-1}, and the short-term SAR over 10 seconds should not exceed *three* times the relevant limit.

In the UK the Health Protection Agency (HPA) guidance [33] uses the terminology "Routine", "Controlled" and "Experimental", with numerical limits identical to ICNIRP. Temperature limits for ICNIRP and HPA are the same as IEC-60601-2-33, with the HPA making the proviso that core temperature rise in the Experimental Mode be less than 2 °C.

CONTROLLING SAR IN PRACTICE

SAR depends strongly upon patient size, increases with the square of B_0 and B_1, increases with the number of RF pulses per unit time, is not uniform, with maximum values for peripheral tissues and those with high electrical conductivity. Now we wish to express this behavior in terms of scanning parameters.

The flip angle is

$$\alpha = \gamma A |B_1| t_p \qquad (5.11)$$

where B_1 is the pulse amplitude, A is constant which accounts for the pulse shape (and is unity for a rectangular or "hard" pulse), and t_p is the pulse duration. SAR for a given patient, assuming a constant RF pulse shape, is

$$SAR \propto B_0^2 \alpha^2 \frac{N_{echoes} N_{slices}}{t_p \, TR} \qquad (5.12)$$

We can use this to predict how SAR will change when we manipulate the scanning parameters, in particular to achieve SAR reductions– we wouldn't want to increase SAR!

Flip angle

The α^2 dependence of SAR suggests that the most effective means of reducing SAR is to reduce the flip angle. It might surprise you that this is not generally the case. Figure 5.14 shows the reduction in SAR (relative to a 180° pulse) for RF pulses with durations t_p of 1, 1.5 and 2 ms. Changing the RF pulse duration, if possible, may be a more effective means of reducing SAR.

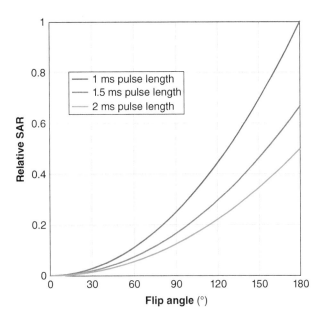

Figure 5.14   SAR reduction: flip angle and RF pulse type. Changing the RF pulse type can result in a greater reduction in SAR than reducing the flip angle.

Reducing the flip angle will also result in a loss in signal-to-noise ratio and may affect the image contrast. As a rule of thumb, each 10° of flip angle reduction (for a nominally 180° pulse) reduces SAR by 10–15%.

RF pulse type

Some scanners allow the choice of RF pulse type with options such as: fast, normal or low SAR. The selection of a low SAR pulse increases the pulse duration t_p but decreases B_1, giving a SAR reduction. Using a low SAR pulse may lengthen TE or increase inter-echo spacing, but if that is not a problem, this is one of the most efficient ways to reduce SAR. See figure 5.14.

MYTHBUSTER:

Reducing flip angle may not be the most efficient way to reduce SAR. Changing the RF pulse type may be more effective.

Example 5.7   SAR reduction strategies

What SAR reduction can be gained by (a) reducing a 180° pulse by 20° and (b) increasing the RF pulse length from 1 to 1.5 ms?

   Either from Figure 5.14 or Equation 5.12

$$(a)\ Relative\ SAR = \frac{160^2}{180^2} = 0.79$$

$$(b)\ Relative\ SAR = \frac{1}{1.5} = 0.67$$

Increasing the RF pulse length by 50% is the more effective means of SAR reduction. A flip angle of 147° would be required to gain the same reduction.

Number of echoes / number of slices

SAR varies linearly with the number of RF pulses per TR (Figure 5.15). Reducing the number of echoes in a TSE/FSE echo train is an effective way to reduce SAR without affecting contrast or SNR, but it will increase scan time. Reducing the number of slices has a similar effect but will reduce anatomical coverage.

Changing TR

Increasing TR also reduces SAR, but inversely proportional to TR (Figure 5.15). It is therefore more efficient to decrease the number of echoes or slices, or both. A 50% reduction in $N_{echo} \times N_{slices}$ will halve the SAR, whilst a 50% increase in TR will reduce SAR by only a third. In practice the number of slices is determined by the anatomical coverage required. Increasing TR is not recommended for T_1–weighted sequences as this affects the image contrast.

Hyperechoes

As an alternative to changing the RF pulse type or flip angle, *hyperechoes* (if available) are a very effective means of reducing SAR. In a TSE sequence with hyperechoes enabled, an RF pulse train with much smaller flip angles is used, but is periodically "topped up" with a full amplitude

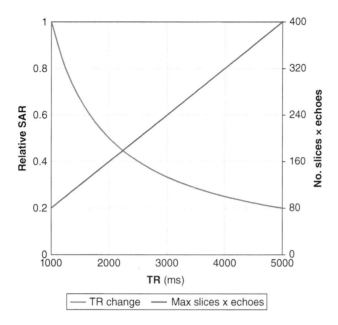

Figure 5.15   SAR reduction: the relative reduction in SAR (with respect to TR = 1000 ms, no. of echoes (TF) = 10, no. of slices = 40).

RF refocusing pulse (Figure 5.16). Hyperechoes are available on some 3 T scanners and can reduce SAR by around 50% with only a minor effect on SNR and contrast.

Preparation and restoration pulses

All RF pulses within the sequence will contribute to SAR. This includes magnetization preparation such as inversion pulses, fat saturation ("fatsat"), magnetization transfer (MT), spatial saturation ("sat bands"), and driven equilibrium (DE) or longitudinal magnetization restoration pulses.

Scan time and delay

As SAR is averaged over six minutes, what happens for a three-minute sequence? The short–term SAR limit over 10 seconds may not be exceeded. As this is twice the usual SAR limit, the scanner can operate at up to double this – but it will have to restrict further scanning with a time delay to bring the six-minute average within the limit. To avoid these delays, it is a good strategy to alternate high SAR sequences with low SAR ones in the examination.

Parameters which do not affect SAR

Because SAR is related to the RF power, i.e. the absorbed energy per unit time, a number of parameters do not directly affect SAR but may change the SED. Notably, field of view (FOV), slice width and bandwidth have no effect on SAR, unless changing them involves other parameter changes that do influence SAR. Image matrix, number of signal averages and the use of parallel imaging do not directly affect SAR, but will alter SED and the total absorbed energy.

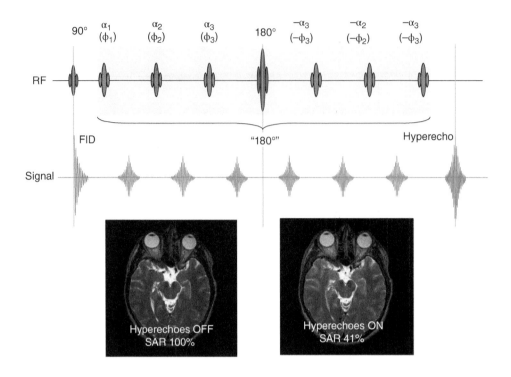

Figure 5.16   Hyperechoes use a train of small flip angle pulses with variable RF phase in place of 180° pulses in TSE sequences, resulting in significant SAR reduction.

MYTHBUSTER:

Using parallel imaging does not necessarily reduce SAR but it reduces the overall RF energy absorbed by the patient.

Getting a feel for SAR

It can be quite hard to get a feel for the impact of these changes without actually scanning. A SAR calculator is located at https://drdonaldmcrobbie.com/sar–and–b1rms–calculator/ (accessed 31 July 2019). This enables you to see the effect of parameter changes such as flip angle, TR, RF pulse type, sequence type, etc. It even allows you to change B_0, something you can't do on your scanner! It will also allow you to experiment with different patient weights and heights. Just be aware that the values are indicative only. It is not a real scanner with a real patient!

Example 5.8   SAR exercise

Use the SAR calculator (https://drdonaldmcrobbie.com/sar–and–b1rms–calculator/) starting with the default parameters but try to reduce the SAR to 1 W kg^{-1} without adversely affecting the anatomical coverage.
   Alternatively attempt the same using the maths. If you aspire to be an MRSE, then you should try the maths!

Controlling B_{1+}RMS

B_{1+}RMS was introduced in the IEC 60601–2–33 standard in 2015. It is a measure of the average B_{1+} over each 10 second period. It is a useful metric for active implant manufacturers to determine appropriate scanning conditions for MR Conditional devices, and it can be used to ensure compliance with these when scanning. How does it relate to SAR?

The formula for B_{1+}RMS was given in Table 5.1. Using the flip angle equation 5.11 we can show that for a given patient and a specific RF pulse waveform and the same B_0:

$$B_{1+RMS} \propto \sqrt{SAR} \qquad\qquad (5.13)$$

The advantage of B_{1+}RMS is that it is defined by the incident B_1 in μT and can be calculated from the transmitter voltage required for a given flip angle.

Example 5.9   SAR and B_{1+}RMS

Using the SAR calculator (https://drdonaldmcrobbie.com/sar-and-b1rms-calculator/) verify that parameter changes that affect SAR change B_{1+}RMS values in proportion to the square root of SAR. Do not change patient weight or height. What happens when you change B_0? Why?

Monitoring SAR

In some circumstances it is important to monitor the SAR.

Patient registration

The first step in scanning is always patient registration where demographic details are entered at the console or fetched from a radiology or hospital information system (RIS, HIS) or picture archiving and communications system (PACS). All scanners require you to enter a patient weight (in kg or lb). It is essential that you enter the appropriate value as this is used by the scanner to determine the safe limits of RF exposure.

Some scanners require entry of patient height as well. This is because they use a slightly more realistic (but still very approximate) body model. This can improve the estimation of the induced electric field and will change the estimated volume of tissue. The advantages are that a more accurate SAR estimation is achieved. Additionally it may become slightly harder to hit the SAR limit, allowing leeway in your scanning protocol for more slices, echoes, etc.

At registration some scanners may ask you which mode you wish to scan in, or they may even default to the First Level Controlled Mode. For maximum patient safety, you should opt for the Normal Mode and allow the scanner to determine the need for First Level scanning on a per sequence basis.

What happens if you enter the wrong patient weight?

Whatever patient weight (and height for some scanners) you enter, the scanner will adjust the RF transmit power to get the appropriate B_1 that produces the desired flip angle. This depends upon the "coil loading" – itself highly dependent upon body and coil geometry. The patient weight you enter will affect the scanner's estimation of SAR (not the actual SAR). Too high a value entered will allow the RF transmitter to operate at higher power, giving the possibility of exceeding the actual SAR limit. Entering a patient weight that is too low may result in limitations to your scanning because the scanner thinks it is exceeding the SAR limit. As SAR is a key patient safety parameter, you should always enter the correct patient weight.

Example 5.10   Wrong patient weight

You accidently entered the patient weight as 100 kg when they are actually 80 kg. The scanner informs you that the SAR for a particular sequence is 3.9 W kg^{-1} in the First Level Mode. What is the actual SAR?
   The scanner determines the RF transmit power P then divides this by the user entered patient weight.

$$RF\ power\ P = 3.9 \times 100 = 390\ W$$

Therefore, the actual SAR is 390/80 = 4.875 W kg^{-1} and exceeds the First Level limit. You may be legally compromised if the patient receives a burn.

SAR prediction and measurement

The scanner is required to have software to enable the prediction of SAR from each sequence. This is displayed prior to the commencement of the acquisition. During scanning the current SAR will be measured by the scanner every 10 seconds to ensure the 10 second limit is not exceeded. The current SAR value will also be displayed. The SAR monitor will also show head SAR, partial body SAR, SED, B_{1+}RMS, plus appropriate limit values. Be aware that the predicted SAR may differ significantly from the measured or current value. For more detailed information relevant to your particular scanner model consult your applications specialist or MRI service engineer.

CONCLUSIONS

In this chapter we have seen that:

- The physical consequence of RF exposure in MRI is tissue heating.
- RF interactions with the body are complex.
- The principal risk to patients is RF burns.
- The IEC limits are given in terms of temperature and SAR.
- SAR depends upon patient size, B_0^2, B_1^2 (α^2), the number and type of RF pulses and TR.

Provided projectile incidents are avoided and excluding implants, the RF exposure remains the most significant source of electromagnetic hazard from MRI.

Revision questions

1. "For uniform rectangular RF pulses, SAR increases approximately with the square of the flip angle."
   True or false?
2. What are the IEC 60601-2-33 core temperature increase limits?
   A. 0.5 °C is normal mode and 1.0 °C in first-level controlled
   B. 0.7 °C is normal mode and 1.0 °C in first-level controlled
   C. 1.0 °C is normal mode and 2.0 °C in first-level controlled
   D. 2.0 °C is normal mode and 4.0 °C in first-level controlled.

3. To reduce SAR:
   A. Decrease TR
   B. Reduce flip angle
   C. Increase the number of echoes
   D. Increase echo time
   E. Decrease the number of averages.
4. Which of the following is the most effective way to reduce SAR?
   A. Increase TR
   B. Reduce flip angle
   C. Reduce the number of echoes
   D. Use low SAR RF pulses
   E. Use parallel imaging.
5. An 80 kg patient has undergone a 2-minute scan with a SAR of 2 W kg^{-1}. The total RF energy absorbed is:
   A. 240 J
   B. 320 J
   C. 9600 J
   D. 14 400 J
   E. 19 200 J.
6. A patient is unwilling to have their MRI scan because they read an article in a newspaper saying that mobile phones cause cancer. Do you:
   A. Tell them to stop complaining and just get in the scanner?
   B. Say the article is probably rubbish?
   C. Reassure them that MR involves only short-term exposure to carefully controlled electromagnetic fields?
   D. Refer them to a MR Safety Expert if they need further information?
   E. Send them away?
7. In MRI entering a higher patient weight than the actual patient weight:
   A. Prevents the exceeding of a SAR limit
   B. Reduces the SAR limit, making the scan safer
   C. Allows you to scan faster
   D. Has no consequence
   E. Is not good practice.
8. In the absence of perfusion or other cooling mechanisms and for the same induced electric fields which tissue is most likely to heat up the most?

		Conductivity (S m^{-1})	Specific Heat Capacity (kJ kg^{-1} °C^{-1})
A	Brain	0.29	3.58
B	Bone	0.06	2.27
C	Lens	0.29	3.13
D	Muscle	0.69	3.42
E	Fat	0.04	2.35

References

1. Payne, D., Klingenböck, A., and Kuster, N. (2018). IT'IS Database for thermal and electromagnetic parameters of biological tissues, Version 4.0, May 15, 2018. DOI: 10.13099/VIP21000-04-0.

2. Schaefer, D.J. (2014) Bioeffects of radiofrequency power deposition. In: *MRI bioeffects, safety, and patient management* (Ed. F.D. Shellock and J.V. Crues III) pp. 131–154. Los Angeles, C: Biomedical Research Publishing Group.

3. Hand, J.W. (2008). Modeling the interaction of electromagnetic fields (10 MHz–10 GHz) with the human body: methods and applications. *Physics in Medicine and Biology* 53(16):R243–286.

4. Murbach, M, Neufeld, E, Kainz, W. et al. (2014). Whole-body and local RF absorption in human models as a function of anatomy and position within 1.5T MR body coil. *Magnetic Resonance in Medicine* 71:839–845.

5. Nagy, Z., Oliver-Taylor, A., Kuehne, A. et al. (2017). Tx/Rx head coil induces less RF transmit-related heating than body coil in conductive metallic objects outside the active area of the head coil. *Frontiers in Neuroscience* 26 January 2017. https://www.frontiersin.org/articles/10.3389/fnins.2017.00015/full

6. Athey, T.W. (1989). A model of the temperature rise in the head due to magnetic resonance imaging procedures. *Magnetic Resonance in Medicine* 9:177–184.

7. Mosteller, R.D. (1987). Simplified calculation of body-surface area. *New England Medical Journal* 317:1098.

8. El Edelbi, R., Lindemalm, S., and Eksborg, S. (2012). Estimation of body surface area in various childhood ages – validation of the Mosteller formula. *Acta Paediatricia* 101:540–544.

9. Adair, E.R. and Berglund, L.G. (1986). On the thermoregulatory consequences of NMR imaging. *Magnetic Resonance Imaging* 4:321–333.

10. National Radiological Protection Board (1992). Electromagnetic fields and the risk of cancer. Report of an Advisory Group on Non-Ionising Radiation. Chilton, UK: *Documents of the NRPB* 3(1).

11. International Commission on Non-ionizing Radiation Protection (1998). Guidelines for limiting exposure to time-varying electric, magnetic, and electromagnetic fields (up to 300 GHz). *Health Physics* 74:494–522.

12. Michaelson, S.M. and Lin, J.C. (1996). *Biological Effects and Health Implications of Radiofrequency Radiation*. New York: Plenum.

13. Elder, J.A. (2003). Ocular effects of radiofrequency energy. *Bioelectromagnetics Supplement* 6:S148–S161.

14. Hand, J.W. (1986). *Physical Techniques in Clinical Hyperthermia*. Letchwork, UK: Research Studies Press.

15. Van Rhoon, G.C., Samaras, T., Yarmolenko, P.S. et al. (2013). CEM43 °C thermal dose thresholds: a potential guide for magnetic resonance radiofrequency exposure levels? *European Radiology* 23:2215–2227.

16. National Toxicology Program (2018a). Toxicology and carcinogenesis studies on B6C3F1/N mice exposed to whole-body radio frequency radiation at frequency (1,900 MHz) and modulations (GSN and CDMA) used by cell phones. *Report NTP TR 596*. Available from https://ntp.niehs.nih.gov/ntp/htdocs/lt_rpts/tr596_508.pdf (accessed 13 March 2019).

17. National Toxicology Program. (2018b). *Toxicology and Carcinogenesis Studies in Hsd:Sprague Dawley SD Rats Exposed to Whole-Body Radio Frequency Radiation at a Frequency (900 Mhz) and Modulations (GSM and CDMA) Used by Cell Phones. Report TR-595*. Available from https://ntp.niehs.nih.gov/ntp/htdocs/lt_rpts/tr595_508.pdf (accessed 13 March 2019).

18. Milham, S.M. (1985). Mortality in workers exposed to electromagnetic fields. *Environmental Health Perspectives* 62:297–300.

19. Baan, R., Grosse, Y., Lauby-Secretan, B. et al. (2011). Carcinogenicity of radiofrequency electromagnetic fields. *Lancet Oncology* 12:624–626.

20. Cardis, E., Deltour, I., Vrijheid, M. et al. (2010). Brain tumour risk in relation to mobile telephone use: results of the INTERPHONE international case-control study. *International Journal of Epidemiology* 39:675–694.

21. Frei, P., Poulsen, A.H, Johansen, C. et al. (2011). Use of mobile phones and risk of brain tumours: update of Danish cohort study. *British Medical Journal* 343:d6387 doi: https://doi.org/10.1136/bmj.d6387

22. Benson, V.S., Pirie, K., Schüz, J. et al. (2013). Mobile phone use and risk of brain neoplasms and other cancers: prospective study. *International Journal of Epidemiology* 42:792–802.

23. Food and Drug Administration (2008). www.fda.gov/NewsEvents/Newsroom/PressAnnouncements/ucm624809.htm (accessed 19 December 2019)

24. Guy, A.W., Chou, C.K., Lin, J.C. et al. (1975). Microwave-induced acoustic effects in mammalian auditory systems and physical materials. *Annals of the New York Academy of Sciences* 247:194–218.

25. Röschmann, P. (1991). Human auditory system response to pulsed radiofrequency energy in RF coils for magnetic resonance at 2.4 to 170 MHz. *Magnetic Resonance in Medicine* 21:197–215.

26. Hudson, D. and Jones, A.P. (2018). A 3-year review of MRI safety incidents within a UK independent sector provider of diagnostic services. *British Journal of Radiology Open* 1: bjro. 20180006 https://doi.org/10.1259/bjro.20180006

27. Delfino, J.G., Krainak, D.M., Flesher, S.A. et al. (2019). MRI-related FDA adverse event reports: a 10-year review. *Medical Physics* doi: 10.1002/mp. 13768.

28. Martin, N.A. and Falder, S. (2017). A review of the evidence for threshold of burn injury. *Burns* 43:1624–1639.

29. Brix, L., Isaksen, C., Kristensen, B.H. et al. (2016). Third degree skin burns caused by a MRI conditional electrocardiographic monitoring system. *Journal of Radiology and Imaging* 1:29–32.

30. International Electrotechnical Commission (2015). *Medical Electrical Equipment – Part 2–33: Particular Requirements for the Safety of Magnetic Resonance Equipment for Medical Diagnosis. IEC 60601-2-33 3.3 edn.* Geneva: IEC.

31. Food and Drug Administration. (2014). *Criteria for significant risk investigations of magnetic resonance diagnostic devices.* Rockville, MD: Center for Devices and Radiological Health, FDA.

32. International Commission on Non-ionizing Radiation Protection (2004). Medical magnetic resonance (MR) procedures: protection of patients. *Health Physics* 87:197–216.

33. Health Protection Agency (2008). *Protection of patients and volunteers undergoing MRI procedures, Documents of the Health Protection Agency RCE-7.* Chilton: HPA.

Further reading and resources

https://it is.swiss/virtual–population/tissue–properties/database *Database of tissue properties.* (Accessed 17 August 2019).

Panych, L.P. and Madore B. (2018). The physics of MRI safety *Journal of Magnetic Resonance Imaging* 47:28–43.

Schaefer, D.J. (2014). Bioeffects of radiofrequency power deposition. In: *MRI bioeffects, safety, and patient management* (Ed. F.D. Shellock FD and J.V. Crues JV III) pp.131–154. Los Angeles, CA: Biomedical Research Publishing Group.

Shellock, F.G. (2014). Radiofrequency–energy induced heating during MRI: laboratory and clincal experiences. In: *MRI bioeffects, safety, and patient management* (Ed. F.D. Shellock and J.V. Crues III) pp. 155–170. Los Angeles, C: Biomedical Research Publishing Group.

www.drdonaldmcrobbie.com (Accessed 17 August 2019).

6

Acoustic noise

INTRODUCTION

One of the principal bugbears of patients undergoing MRI, along with being squeezed into a narrow tunnel, claustrophobia, and general anxiety about their health, is the noise. A survey of reportable MR incidents in the UK from 1990–2006 revealed eight related to acoustic noise out of a total of 163 [1]. UK Department of Health figures indicate nine noise-related incidents reported from 21 million scans between 1994 and 2011 – a rate of 0.00004%. Hudson and Jones [2] reported noise complaints as 0.89% of all MRI incidents, although with only six from 1.3 million patients (0.00045% incidence). In the USA FDA figures show acoustic noise as being responsible for 6% of MRI-related incidents reported [3]. With such a small number relating to so great a nuisance, it appears everyone accepts that MRI is loud. However, we must not become complacent as acoustic noise is a potential source of injury as well as discomfort. This chapter considers the generation and measurement of acoustic noise, human hearing function and damage, the range of noise from scanners and sequences, hearing protection, and regulatory limits. The implications of acoustic noise exposure for the fetus are considered in Chapter 7.

GENERATION OF ACOUSTIC NOISE IN MRI

The scanner's knocking sound is a consequence of the Lorentz force exerted on a wire (a gradient coil) from the movement of charge (i.e. current, I) within the static field. The maximum force is produced when the coil section is perpendicular to B_0. Figure 6.1 shows idealized gradient coil geometries. According to Equation 2.19, the arc sections contribute most to the force, and hence the vibration and acoustic noise.

If we consider a "Maxwell pair" z-gradient coil (Figure 6.1a), i.e. a loop concentric with the bore, then we can calculate the force as

$$F = 2\pi r I B_0 \tag{6.1}$$

This tells us that the force is proportional to:

- the current through the coil
- the radius
- B_0.

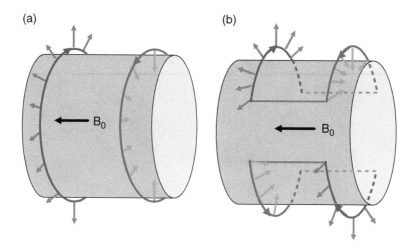

Figure 6.1 Forces on gradient coils. (a) a Maxwell pair G_z coil; the 'rearward' current results in an expansion force whilst the 'forwards' current causes a contraction. (b) One half of a Golay G_y or G_x coil; opposite forces apply at either end of each segment.

In the simplest terms we can compare an MRI system with a loudspeaker; both involve driving audio frequency current through a coil placed within a magnet. Real gradient coils have more complex geometries than are shown in the figure.

Example 6.1   Force on a gradient coil

What is the maximum force per unit radial length on a 70 cm diameter z-gradient coil with 100 A flowing through it in a 2.5 T field and how will it respond to a bipolar gradient pulse?
   Radial length is $2\pi r$

$$\frac{F}{2\pi r} = 100 \times 2.5 = 250 \ N$$

If the z-gradient coil is in a Maxwell pair configuration, then equal forces will be exerted around the ring, causing the coil to expand or contract depending upon the polarity of the pulse. The overall force is equivalent to 550 N – or half a tonne! (1 metric tonne = 1000 kg).

MEASURING NOISE: dB(A), dB(C), dB(Z)

The science of acoustics is complex and is not something you learn in radiography school, so we will discuss some of the basic concepts and measurements here.

Sound intensity and pressure level

What we call "acoustic noise", physically is a pressure wave transmitted through the air. Sound intensity (SI) is defined in a logarithmic scale in decibels (dB) as:

$$SI = 10 \log_{10}\left(\frac{S_1}{S_0}\right) \tag{6.2}$$

where S_0 is 1 pW m^{-2} (pico-watt per square meter) or 1×10^{-9} W m^{-2}.

Sound pressure level (SPL) is defined as:

$$SPL = 20\log_{10}\left(\frac{p}{p_0}\right) \tag{6.3}$$

where p_0=20 μPa (micro-pascal). Both p_0 and S_0 correspond to the threshold of hearing (for a healthy young adult).

The use of a logarithmic scale can cause confusion. Firstly, why is the multiplier 10 in Equation 6.2 and 20 in Equation 6.3? This is because one expression is in terms of power, whilst the other is in terms of pressure (force divided by area). In base-10 logarithms taking the square of a number results in a doubling, hence the factor 20 in Equation 6.3.

Secondly, when the SPL is doubled, the dB value increases by 6 (=$20\times\log_{10}2$) and the sound intensity quadruples, also 6 dB (=$10\times\log_{10}4$). Whether you use sound intensity or SPL to characterize acoustic noise, the answer always comes out the same in dB. This is convenient for practical measurements of noise.

MYTHBUSTER:

Acoustic noise measurements in deciBels are not additive. Two sound sources of 50 dB do not result in 100 dB, but in 56 dB. Halving an SPL of 100 dB does not result in 50 dB but in 94 dB.

Thirdly, decibels are multiplicative, not additive. For example, if the background noise of the cold head is 60 dB, and the sequence produces 100 dB, the total noise is not 160 dB (that would deafen the patient, literally), rather the total SPL is 100.086. Ear protection *attenuates* sound. In normal numbers attenuation is equivalent to multiplication by a number less than one, but in logarithms this becomes *subtraction*. So, if ear protection offers 30 dB attenuation, then (in theory at least) the noise exposure at the patient's ears reduces to 70 dB.

Example 6.2   Combined noise sources

The ambient noise in the scan room (from the cold head) is 60 dB, and the sequence is 100 dB. What is the combined noise?

A base-10 logarithm is the power of 10 to which a number must be raised, e.g. the logarithm of 100 is 2, i.e. $\log_{10}(100) = 2$ because $100 =10^2$. We have to invert Equation 6.3 to calculate p_1/p_0.

$$\frac{p_{ambient}}{p_0} = 10^{60/20} = 1000$$

$$\frac{p_{sequence}}{p_0} = 10^{100/20} = 100\,000$$

The total SPL =20 $\log_{10}$101 000 = 100.086 dB
DeciBels are not additive.

Figure 6.2 shows the relative SPL of various sources of noise in both dB and in pascals. Each 20-dB step represents an order of magnitude (factor of 10) in air pressure. This illustrates the amazing dynamic range of human hearing over seven orders of magnitude.

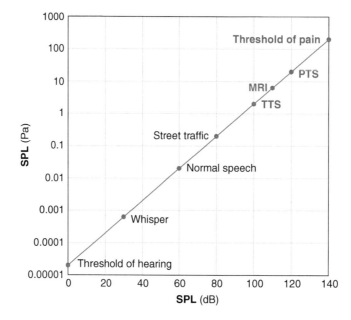

Figure 6.2   SPL in pascals (linear scale) and dB (logarithmic scale) showing the "loudness" of various sounds and thresholds for hearing damage.

SPL weightings

When measuring or specifying acoustic noise, various *weightings* are used, depending upon the purpose. These take the form of frequency responses or spectra over the audio range from 20–20 000 Hz (Figure 6.3).

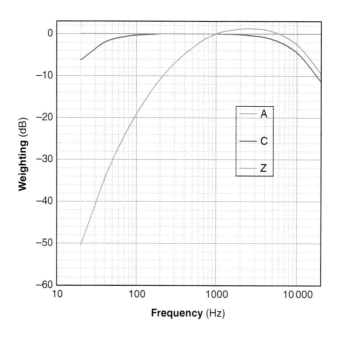

Figure 6.3   A, C and Z weightings.

dB(Z)-weighting

This is the simplest, being a flat or unweighted response. dB(Z) is related to the absolute pressure. It is defined by international standard *IEC 61672A* [4]. Z-weighting is useful for measuring peak sound level, L_{pk}.

dB(A)-weighting

The A-weighting, defined by *IEC 61672* [4], is adjusted to more closely match the response of the human ear. It is therefore most related to the perception of loudness. A-weighting (and human response) peaks in the range 1–8 kHz, dropping off sharply with lower frequencies below 500 Hz. For example, a 200 Hz tone with the same pressure as one at 1kHz will be 10 dB(A) less. Subjectively, this corresponds to "about half as loud" (human hearing doesn't exactly follow the base-10 logarithmic scale). A-weighting is based upon the hearing of a healthy young adult. Figure 6.4 shows how the hearing response varies with age, with a loss of high frequency response. This is why your granny can't hear dialogue on the TV at normal volume but still complains about the loud bass from your sound system!

dB(C)-weighting

The C-weighting is most suited to situations of high SPL, and is more linear than the A-weighting. The frequency response of human hearing flattens out at high SPL (Figure 6.4). Because ear protection devices are used in high SPL situations (MRI scanners, pneumatic drills, airplanes, firearms), their attenuation is specified in dB(C).

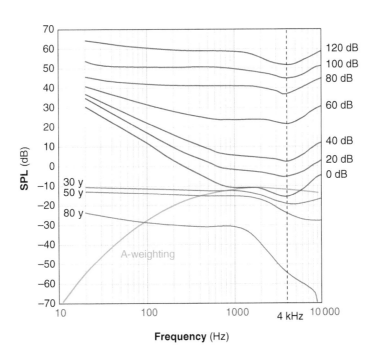

Figure 6.4 Equal loudness curves for different levels of noise (red lines), hearing response (loss) with age (blue lines).

Time-varying noise measurement

The level of sound produced by a MRI scanner varies in time throughout the sequence. For example, the change in amplitude of phase-encode gradient pulses can often be detected by ear. To measure acoustic noise over a time interval the parameter L_{eq} is used. This is the equivalent level of constant SPL that contains the same sound energy within the measurement period. L_{max} is the maximum SPL recorded over the measurement duration. For occupational exposure a daily noise level $L_{eq,d}$ is used (page 157).

Frequency specific noise measurement

Rather than stating the overall SPL over the whole audio range, sometimes frequency specific or "octave" measurements are given. An octave is a doubling in frequency. In musical terms the note "A" above middle C on the piano has a frequency of 440 Hz. A frequency of 880 Hz will also be an "A", but an octave higher. The higher "A" is also called the second harmonic; the third harmonic would be 1.32 kHz – a different note. Figure 6.5 shows a 125 Hz trapezoidal waveform and its spectrum. Note the absence of the even harmonics (2nd, 4th, etc.) and that the third harmonic at 375 Hz contains 11% of the amplitude of the first harmonic or 125 Hz fundamental frequency.

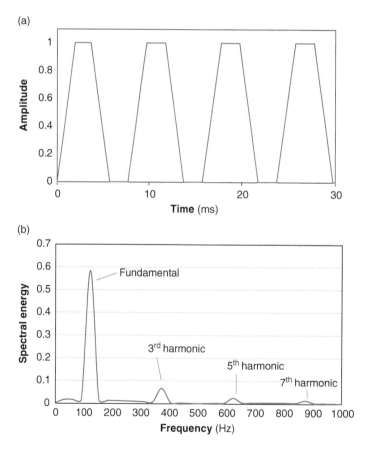

Figure 6.5   (a) 125 Hz trapezoidal waveform and (b) its frequency spectrum.

Table 6.1   Octave bands used in acoustics.

Lower Band Limit (Hz)	Center Frequency (Hz)	Upper Band Limit (Hz)
11	16	22
22	31.5	44
44	63	88
88	125	177
177	250	355
355	500	710
710	1000	1420
1420	2000	2840
2840	4000	5680
5680	8000	11 360
11 360	16 000	22 720

The audio spectrum can be divided into eleven octave bands (Table 6.1). Sometimes noise sources and protective equipment performance are specified according to octave bands. The fundamental frequency of human speech lies in the range 85–180 Hz for males and 165–225 Hz for females. Most humans have a vocal range of three octaves.

Measuring scanner noise

Measuring noise from a range of pulse sequences is a task that the MRSE may wish to undertake, for example, during scanner acceptance testing. It is important that the measurement device's performance is unaffected by the scanner. Prior to scanning, the device should be calibrated. For general purposes a meter offering at least $L_{A,eq}$ and $L_{A,pk}$ (A-weighted) measurements should suffice. Ensure the sequences lasts for at least as long as the measurement period. Subject to magnet safety and compatibility, place the microphone in the desired position. The most accurate measurements would entail having a patient or volunteer in the scanner, but it is more convenient (and ethical) to use a phantom. If evaluating different sequences, a constant microphone position should be maintained as the noise level varies along the bore [5]. The National Electrical Manufacturers Association (NEMA) has published a standard for acoustic noise measurement in MRI [6].

ANATOMY AND PHYSIOLOGY OF HUMAN HEARING

The anatomy and physiology of the human auditory system is complex and a full description is beyond the scope of this book. The purpose of the auditory system is to detect sound pressure waves, convert them to neural impulses and send those to the auditory cortex of the brain.

The auditory system

The *external ear* consists of the auricles (what we would call "ears") connected by the external auditory meatus via the tympanic membrane (ear drum) to the middle ear (Figure 6.6).

The *middle ear* lies within the temporal bone and contains the pharyngo-tympanic (or Eustacian) tube which equalizes pressure (think "head cold", air travel or SCUBA diving). Three small bones, the auditory ossciles: the malleus (hammer), the incus (anvil), and the stapes (stirrup) form a chain to transmit and amplify the vibrations through another membrane, the oval window, leading to the vestibule. Small muscles connected to the malleus and stapes provide a measure of sound damping as a response to high sound pressures, offering a degree of protection. A second membranous window, the round window, connects with the stapes. The vestibule is filled with perilymph fluid which is similar to cerebrospinal fluid (CSF).

The *inner ear* lies behind the petrous portion of the temporal bone and includes the labyrinthine system. This has three parts: the vestibule is the entrance chamber. Off this lie the three semi-circular canals responsible for detecting head movement, and the cochlea. The cochlea has the shape of a spiral, like a snail shell, narrowing towards the apex. The floor surface of the cochlea contains the organ of Corti in which the hair cells are situated, in contact with the endolymph fluid (also like CSF), their roots connected to nerve endings. There are only around 15 000 hair cells in the organ of Corti.

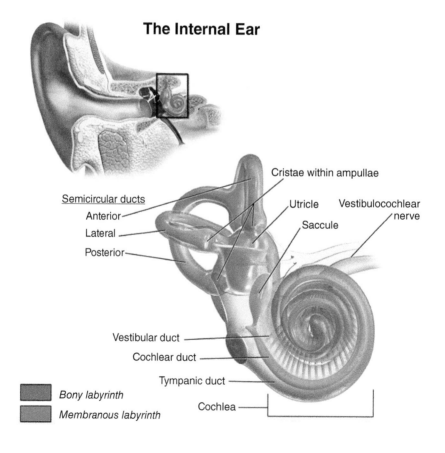

Figure 6.6 Internal ear anatomy. Source: Getty images.

Hearing damage

Damage to hearing arising from excessive noise exposure can take two forms. In a temporary threshold shift (TTS), caused by exposures in excess of 100 dB(A), a short-term hearing loss is experienced. You may have suffered from this following a rock concert or a visit to a nightclub. Temporary threshold shifts have been experienced in MRI patients who did not have hearing protection. The US Occupational Safety and Health Administration (OSHA) defines a standard threshold shift (STS) as a 10 dB increase in hearing threshold at 2, 3, and 4 kHz in the same ear [7]. A TTS of up to 50 dB may recover completely over of a few hours or weeks [8].

A permanent threshold shift (PTS) may result from a single large noise exposure of around 120 dB(A) or from repeated or continuous exposures causing temporary shifts. A PTS is a permanent hearing defect caused by irreparable damage to the hair cells. The likelihood of damage is related to the exposure time. In most countries an SPL greater than 85 dB(A) continuously over eight hours is considered unsafe. Figure 6.4 shows that the greatest sensitivity to damage is around 4 kHz at all SPL. The range 4–6 kHz is most likely to cause hearing impairment. Figure 6.7 shows examples of threshold shifts: one temporary, one permanent. The pain threshold of 140 dB(A) exceeds both the levels for TTS and PTS – by the time it hurts, it's too late. Small PTS (1–5 dB) have been shown to have an association with the number of volunteer scans experienced by MRI factory workers (Figure 6.8) [9].

The mechanisms of hearing loss are damage to the hair cells, synapses, or primary afferent neurones to which they are attached. Noise trauma can result in the loss of a large number of synapses and neurones even after hearing has returned to normal. Once damaged the hair cells do not regenerate.

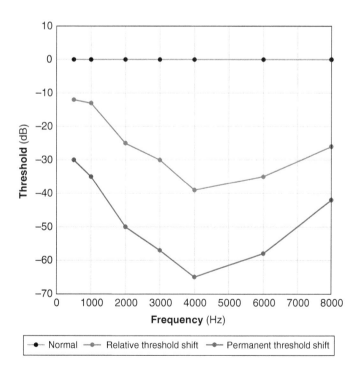

Figure 6.7   Example of audiometric determination of threshold shifts showing detrimental change in dB. The gray line shows no change from a normal audiogram. The red line indicates a shift which may be permanent.

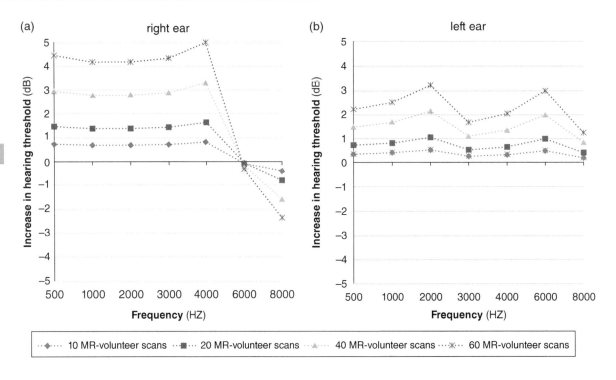

Figure 6.8 Increase in hearing threshold for MRI factory workers who have undergone multiple volunteer scans. Source: [9]. Reproduced with permission of BMJ Publishing Group Ltd.

Some patients may be more susceptible to hearing damage: tinnitus suffers, the very young (and unborn). Others may have reduced tolerance to excessive noise: psychiatric patients, the anxious, and those on certain medications.

MRI NOISE EXPOSURE

Field strength and gradient dependence

Acoustic noise has long been recognized as a source of annoyance and potential hazard. Figure 6.9 shows some early measurements of SPL from gradient echo sequences in a range of systems from 0.2 T to 1.5 T, clearly showing an upward trend with field strength [5].

MYTHBUSTER:

Acoustic noise is not simply dependent upon field strength and gradient specifications.

Pulse sequence dependence

Figure 6.10 shows noise measurements for various sequences (spin echo (SE), turbo spin echo (TSE), gradient echo (GRE), and echo planar (EPI)) at different B_0 with consistent scanning parameters [10–12]. Whilst there is much inter-system variability EPI and 3D-GRE sequences are generally among the loudest

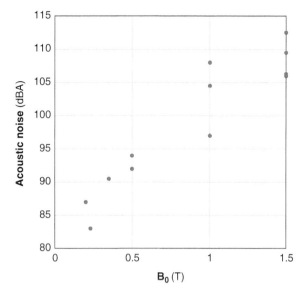

Figure 6.9   Field dependence of SPL using gradient echo sequences. Data from [5].

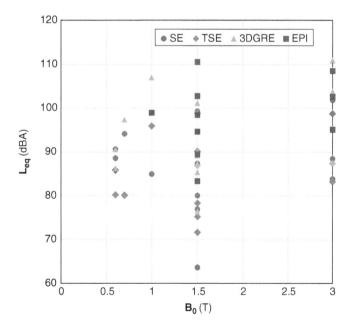

Figure 6.10   Sequence and field dependence of acoustic noise. Data from [10-12].

Peak frequencies

Knowledge of the peak frequencies for particular sequences can help to distinguish the most hazardous, e.g. 4–6 kHz. Figure 6.11 shows a representative sample of the frequency components for a TSE, MP-RAGE (3D gradient echo), EPI (used for BOLD fMRI) and FLAIR recorded from a 1.5 T scanner using recording studio software. Whilst EPI has the loudest single frequency

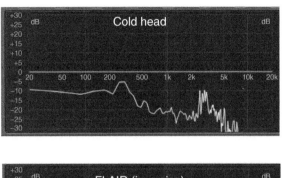

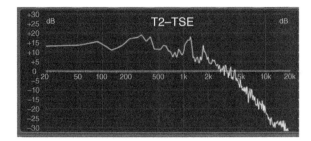

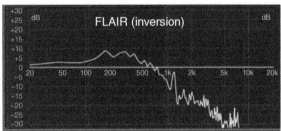

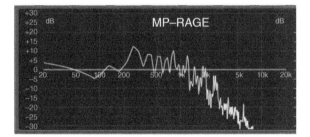

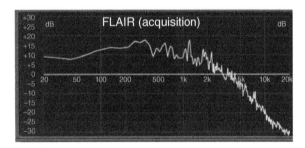

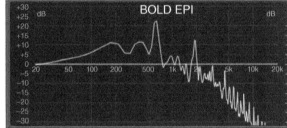

Figure 6.11   Audio frequency spectra for various sequences. dB values are relative to the dBm scale where its reference point of 0 dBm is defined as 1 milliwatt of AC signal power dissipated by a 600 Ω load.

component (630 Hz) and is subjectively the most annoying, the total noise level is slightly less than the T_2-TSE and the acquisition segment of FLAIR (by roughly 1–2 dB). However, EPI also has significant acoustic energy at 1.9 kHz (the third harmonic) arising from the dominance of the bipolar frequency encode gradient. Additionally, TSE has an overall greater intensity in the 1–3 kHz range, where human hearing is more sensitive.

Scanner design

The reason that simplistic assumptions based upon scanner specifications do not hold true is down to differences between how pulse sequences are programmed in different scanners, the geometry and construction of gradient coils, and methods of damping and sound attenuation built into the scanner. In addition to the sound or spectral components of the gradient waveforms, elements of the scanner structure will have mechanical resonances which may amplify particular frequencies.

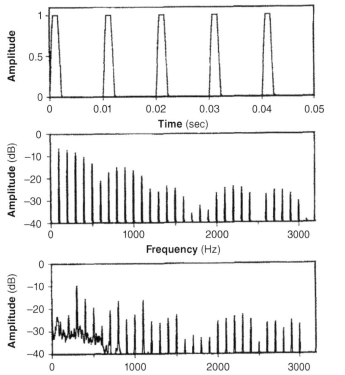

Figure 6.12   Transfer function measurement with a trapezoid pulse. Source [13]. Used with permission of Wiley.

By examining acoustic noise in the frequency domain, it is possible to make predictions about the level of noise from detailed knowledge of the pulse sequence programming [13]. Taking a "transfer function" approach, we can calculate the SPL output S(f) as

$$S(f) = H(f) \cdot G(f) \tag{6.4}$$

where G(f) is the input to the gradient amplifiers in terms of frequencies or the Fourier transform of the gradient pulse train, and H(f) is the acoustic transfer function of the scanner. H(f) can be experimentally determined by feeding white noise into the gradient coils or by using a pulse with known frequency components e.g. a trapezoid (Figure 6.12), an impulse or a sinc[1] function [14] which will have an approximately uniform range of intensities over a particular frequency range. The scanner acoustic transfer function can then be calculated from Equation 6.4 and then applied prospectively to estimate acoustic noise from real sequences.

Various methods have been implemented to reduce acoustic noise in the design of the scanner. These include optimized gradient coil design [15], mounting the coils in a vacuum [16], specialist sequence or gradient pulse design [17], and the deployment of active noise cancelation [18].

---

[1] Sinc function is defined as $\text{sinc}(x) = \dfrac{\sin(x)}{x}$. It has a value of 1 for x=0.

Scanner noise in the MR room

SPL follows an inverse square law with distance from the source; double the distance and the sound intensity will be a quarter, equal to a 6 dB reduction. The acoustic properties of the room, shape, and wall materials affect the spatial noise distribution. An approximate reduction of 10 dB in SPL with respect to the iso-center has been measured at the 0.5 mT line [19].

REDUCING ACOUSTIC NOISE IN PRACTICE

Whilst specific makes and models of scanners have various levels of acoustic noise for different sequences, we can – for a given sequence and scanner- make choices that will help to reduce the overall acoustic noise. Any parameter change that reduces gradient amplitude, dB/dt or the number of gradient pulses per second will reduce acoustic noise.

Slice width

For a given RF pulse waveform the slice width is inversely proportional to the slice select gradient G_{ss}. Increasing slice width in 2D acquisitions will reduce the acoustic noise.

Low SAR RF pulses

Low SAR RF pulses are longer than standard RF pulses and consequently have a narrower bandwidth. For a given slice thickness, a lower slice select gradient will be required. The selection of low SAR RF pulses may reduce the noise.

Field of view

Field-of-view (FOV) also depends upon the gradient amplitude. Increasing FOV without changing the receive bandwidth will decrease the gradient amplitude and noise (Figure 6.13a).

Pixel size

An increase in in-plane resolution or smaller pixel size will result in higher gradient amplitude and more acoustic noise.

TE and receive bandwidth

Increasing TE may allow a reduction in receive bandwidth (and vice-versa), resulting in a reduction in FE-gradient amplitude and lower noise (Figure 6.13b). For TSE (FSE) sequences noise reduction may be achieved by increasing the inter-echo spacing (IES) or reducing the turbo factor (echo train length), whilst minimizing the receive bandwidth. These changes increase the overall scan time.

TR

Increasing TR without any other parameter changes reduces the noise level (Figure 6.13c).

Number of slices, echoes

Reducing the number of slices or echoes will mean there is less gradient activity per TR period and will reduce the overall noise.

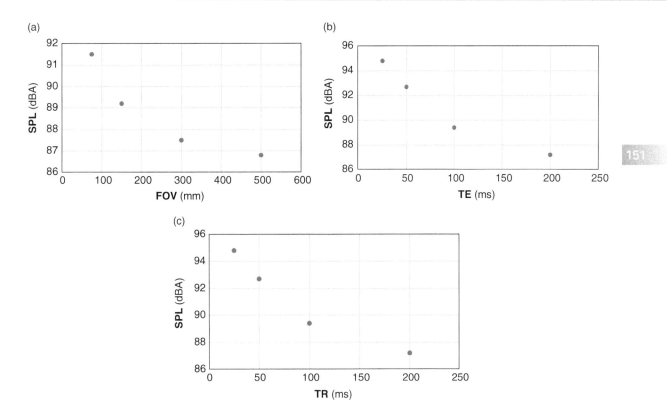

Figure 6.13   The influence of parameter changes on acoustic noise (a) FOV (b) TE (c) TR. Data from [5].

b-value

In diffusion-weighted imaging (DWI) or diffusion tensor imaging (DTI), the use of lower diffusion weighting or b-value will reduce the acoustic noise.

Sequence choice

We have seen above that the choice of a particular sequence over another does not guarantee less acoustic noise. Nevertheless, you should be aware of the relative noise levels of the major sequence types for your particular scanner. Those with the most gradient activity per unit time will tend to be the loudest. Consult your applications specialist or MRSE for more information. Some scanners offer specialist low-noise sequences (e.g. "zero-TE", "silent scan") or low noise gradient pulses ("whisper" or "softone").

HEARING PROTECTION

Hearing protection should be provided for all patients. This can take the form of ear plugs, ear defenders ("headphones" or "earmuffs") or both. Ear plugs and defenders can provide 10–30 dB of protection depending upon frequency and proper fitting. However, the specification of their attenuation characteristics is complicated by various different methodologies used in different parts of the world.

Specification of acoustic attenuation devices

In the USA, the performance of hearing protection is legally mandated using the Noise Reduction Rating (NRR) method. In Europe and the UK three methods are used: Single Number Rating (SNR), HML, and octave band. In Australasia the Sound Level Conversion valid for 80% of wearers (SLC$_{80}$) is used. They are all fundamentally different, producing different results.

The NRR method

The NRR method results in a single number, but the methodology is fairly complex. The NRR is defined as:

$$NRR = 107.9\,dB(C) - 3 - 10\log_{10} \sum_{f=125}^{8k} 10^{0.1(L_{Af}-A-2\sigma_A)} \qquad (6.5)$$

where L_{Af} is the A-weighted SPL at the center frequency of each octave band from 125 Hz to 8 kHz and each octave band has 100 dB of "pink" noise with the overall C-weighted SPL equal to 107.9 dB(C). Pink noise is random noise which has equal energy per octave. A is the mean real ear attenuation at threshold (REAT) and σ_A is the standard deviation of the attenuation measurements.

In practice, real life use of ear protection never works as well as it does under laboratory conditions. For this reason, OSHA in the US deregulates the specified NRR of a device by 50% [7]. Furthermore, if only A-weighted measurements are available 7 dB must be subtracted from the NRR. The actual attenuation is likely to be:

$$A = \frac{NRR-7}{2} dB \qquad (6.6)$$

MYTHBUSTER:

The actual acoustic attenuation offered by a piece of hearing protective equipment is not what it says on the device.

The NRR may be specified as two numbers. The first represents the protection afforded to a minimally trained person, assumed to be 80% of users; the second is appropriate for proficient users, assumed to be 20%. MR staff would be expected to be in the latter category, but patients might be in the former.

Example 6.3   NRR and earplugs

A pair of earplugs have a NRR of 39 dB. The scanner noise is 103 dB(A). What is the patient's noise exposure?
From Equation 6.6

$$A = \frac{NRR-7}{2} = \frac{39-7}{2} = 16\,dB$$

The noise exposure at ear is expected to be 87 dB.

The SNR method

This is the easiest method to apply. To use it you need the C-weighted average L_{Ceq} from the noise source (scanner). The acoustic noise at the ear is then

$$N_{ear} = L_{Ceq} - SNR + 4 \tag{6.7}$$

The additional 4 dB allows for real world factors. Although similar in concept, the SNR is not the same as NRR, as it uses different octave weightings.

The H-M-L method

The HML (high-medium-low) method offers a level of sophistication above both NRR and SNR. Attenuation values are specified for high frequencies (2–8 kHz), medium frequencies (1–2 kHz) and low frequencies (63–1000 Hz). The method requires both C- and A-weighted measurements of the noise source.

$$\text{If} \left| L_C - L_A \right| > 2$$

$$A = M - \left[\frac{M - L}{8}\right](L_C - L_A - 2) \tag{6.8a}$$

otherwise

$$A = M - \left[\frac{H - M}{4}\right](L_C - L_A - 2) \tag{6.8b}$$

As for SNR, a further 4 dB reduction is applied to account for real world factors.

Example 6.4   Protection using HML

An ear protection device has a HML rating of 34, 26, 20 and the sound levels are $L_A = 101$ dB and $L_C = 102.5$ dB. What sound level will be experienced at the ear?

$$L_C - L_A = 1.5\,dB$$

Use Equation 6.8b,

$$A = M - \left[\frac{H - M}{4}\right](L_C - L_A - 2) = 26 - \left[\frac{34 - 26}{4}\right](1.5 - 2) = 27\,dB$$

Allow 4 dB for the real world so the noise at ear is

$$N_{ear} = 101 - 27 + 4 = 78\,dB$$

The Octave band method

This is the most detailed method, but it requires measurement of the noise over eight octave bands: 63, 125, 250, 500, 1000, 2000, 4000 and 8000 Hz. It also needs the device attenuation figures for each band. An example is shown in Table 6.2.

Table 6.2   Octave band calculation example. See http://www.hse.gov.uk/noise/calculator.htm

Frequency (Hz)	63	125	250	500	1000	2000	4000	8000
NOISE (dB)	95	103	105	100	105	95	70	50
ATTENUATION (dB)	25	29	27	28	29	36	45	47
A-WEIGHTED NOISE						106.6 dB		
CALCULATED NOISE AT EAR						78 dB		
REAL WORLD NOISE AT EAR						82 dB		

SLC_{80} method

The SLC_{80} method is designed to be valid for 80% of wearers. It is defined as the C-weighted level of noise minus the in-ear noise measured using the A-weighting:

$$SLC_{80} = L_{Ceq,source} - L_{Aeq,ear} \tag{6.9}$$

Australia/New Zealand standard AS/NZS 1269.3 specifies 5 levels of protection, shown in Table 6.3. $LA_{eq,8\ hr}$ is the equivalent noise exposure averaged over an eight-hour shift.

Hearing protection in practice

It is standard practice that hearing protection is provided for all patients, usually as ear plugs or ear defenders (headphones/earmuffs).

Ear plugs

Formable ear plugs constituted from polyurethane foam are likely to offer 10–30 dB protection, dependent upon frequency and the effectiveness of the fit. The USA's National Institute for Occupational Safety and Health (NIOSH) summarizes the correct fitting procedure as "roll, pull, hold." Firstly, *roll* the ear plug between your fingers to compress it. Then *pull* the top of your ear with your other hand; this straightens the auditory canal and allows full insertion of the plug. Finally, *hold* the plug in place with your finger for 20–30 seconds as it expands. A good fit will result in muffled sounds. Cup your hands over your ears and if the sounds are much more

Table 6.3   Hearing protection class and SLC values used in Australia and New Zealand.

Class of protection	$L_{Aeq,8\ hr}$ (dB)	SLC (dB)
1	< 90	10–13
2	90–95	14–17
3	95–100	18–21
4	100–105	22–25
5	105–110	≥26

muffled in this configuration, then the plugs may not be fitted properly. A class 4 or 5 (in Australasia) ear plug is recommended. For example, the 3M E-A-Rsoft FX earplug (3M, St Paul, MN, USA) has an SLC80 of 26 dB, a NRR or 33 dB and a SNR of 38 dB. For babies, external disposable earmuffs or ear putty may be used.

Ear defenders

Ear defenders are probably easier to use as they will fit snuggly over most patient's ears. They offer approximately the same level of protection as ear plugs (properly fitted). NIOSH suggests a derating of the NRR of ear defenders ("earmuffs") by 25%. Ear defenders/headphones provided by the MR manufacturer often have plastic tubing attached for pneumatic sound transmission so that the patient can hear operator instructions or listen to music. This compromises the performance of the protection significantly. Contact between the ear defender and the scanner may result in noise transmission through vibration or though the ear defender material.

Limitations of hearing protection

The use of double protection: ear plugs and defenders does not result in the summation of their attenuations, but rather gives 5–10 dB additional protection over that of the most attenuating device. It may be worth doing this for very long, loud acquisitions, e.g. diffusion imaging or fMRI in research where the examination can last over an hour.

Remember too that just because you can't hear it, it can still do damage. The unconscious, sedated, or anaesthetized patient requires protection too, especially as they cannot warn you of discomfort. We will consider hearing effects on the fetus in the next chapter, but it has been estimated that *in utero* the noise exposure is about 30 dB less than the mother's [20].

Even with properly fitted multiple protective devices there will be a limit on the maximum attenuation possible set by noise conduction through tissue, particularly bone. The limit is thought to be in the range of 48–50 dB [21].

ACOUSTIC NOISE LIMITS

Workplace noise levels are usually mandated by law. They apply to staff working in MRI but not to patients, although the legal limits may inform patient limits.

Patient limits

The *IEC-60601-2-33* standard sets an absolute limit of 140 dB(Z) on scanner noise [22]. This is above the pain and damage thresholds, so initially it may seem unhelpful. However, this is a physical limit on the noise the scanner is technically capable of producing, and the IEC recognizes that no clinical scanner achieves this. *IEC-60601-2-33* also requires the use of hearing protection and instructions for its use if the scanner noise exceeds 99 dB(A). This has been derived from occupational limits. Using a baseline limit of 80 dB(A) over 16 hours, a "3 dB rule" is used to give the equivalent SPL for a one-hour duration of 94 dB (see Table 6.4). A further 5 dB is added to account for there being (usually) only one exposure a day.

The FDA *Criteria for Significant Risk Investigations of Magnetic Resonance Diagnostic Devices* [23] also has the 140 dB unweighted and 99 dB(A) limits.

Table 6.4   Times to reach occupational noise limits.

$L_{Aeq,d}$ (dB (A))	Time to reach limit				
	USA (OSHA)	ANZ[1]/Canada[2]	EU–EEA–UK		
			Lower Action Value 80 dB(A)	Upper Action Value 85 dB(A)	Limit 87 dB(A)
80	32 hours	16 hours	8 hours		
82	24.3	12	5		
85	16	8	2.5	8 hours	
88	10.6	4	1.3	4	6.4 hours
90	8		48 min	2.5	4.0
91	7	2			
92	6.1		30.2	1.6	2.5
94	4.6	1	19.1	1	1.6
95	4		15.2	48 min	1.3
96	3.5		12.1	38.1	1.0
97	3	30 min	9.6	30.3	48 min
98	2.6		7.6	24.1	38.1
100	2	15	4.8	15.2	24.1
102	1.5		3.0	9.6	15.2
103	1.3	7.5			
104	1.1		1.9	6.0	9.6
105	1		1.5	4.8	7.6
106	52 min	3.8	1.2	3.8	6.0
109	34	1.9			
110	30		28.8 s	1.5	2.4
112	22.8	57 s	18.2	57 s	1.5
115	15	28.8	9.1	28.8	45.6 s

[1] Australian values from https://www.safeworkaustralia.gov.au/noise (accessed 14 March 2019)
[2] Canadian values by Province. Available at Https://Www.Ccohs.Ca/Oshanswers/Phys_Agents/Exposure_Can.Html (accessed 14 March 2019).

In the UK the Medicines and Healthcare products Regulatory Agency [24] recommends hearing protection for all patients even when exposure is less than 99 dB(A). It relaxes this recommendation if the noise is significantly less than 85 dB(A).

The International Commission on Non-ionizing Radiation Protection (ICNIRP) [25] recommends that hearing protection is offered for exposures above 80 dB(A) and must be used for exposures above 85 dB(A).

The Royal Australian and New Zealand College of Radiologists (RANZCR) MRI Safety Guidelines [26] state that ear protection is mandatory for all patients.

There's a very simple rule of thumb: no ear protection, no scan.

Occupational exposure limits

Excessive acoustic noise is a major cause of industrial injury and is highly regulated in most countries. Limits are applied in the USA by the OSHA [7], in Europe by the Noise at Work Directive [27], in the UK by the Health and Safety Executive [28]. An absolute C-weighted limit is commonly set as 140 dB. Other exposures are established in terms of their equivalence to an eight hour or daily exposure- $L_{Aeq,8hr}$. Table 6.4 shows relevant values for the USA, Canada, the EU, UK, and Australasia (ANZ). The US, ANZ and Canadian limits use a "3 dB rule", i.e. a halving of the exposure time increases the limit by 3 dB. The EU-UK time limits can be calculated (in seconds) from

$$t_{limit} = T_0 \times 10^{0.1(L_{lim} - L_{exp})} \tag{6.10}$$

Where L_{lim} is the limit in dB(A) and L_{exp} is the exposure level. T_0 is 28 800 seconds (8 hours). Where there are multiple exposures during the day, the daily limit $L_{eq,d}$ is calculated from:

$$L_{eq,d} = 10\log_{10}\left[\frac{1}{T_0}\sum_{i=1}^{n}T_i 10^{0.1(L_{Aeq,T})_i}\right] \tag{6.11}$$

where n is the number of individual periods in the working day, T_i is the duration of period i, $(L_{Aeq},T)_i$ is the equivalent continuous A-weighted SPL that represents the sound the person is exposed to during period i, and the sum of all T_i is equal to duration of the person's working day, in seconds.

Example 6.5   Interventional MRI

A radiologist carries out 3 interventional procedures in the MR scanner in one day. The noise exposures are 103 dB(A) for 30 minutes, 115 dB(A) for 20 minutes and 110 dB(A) for 10 minutes. What is the daily equivalent noise limit?
   Use Equation 6.11 with T_0 = 480 mins

$$L_{eq,d} = 10\log_{10}\left[\frac{1}{480}(30\times 10^{10.3} + 20\times 10^{11.5} + 10\times 10^{11}\right]$$

$$= 10\log_{10}\left[16.5\times 10^9\right]$$

$$= 102.2\ dB$$

The total exposure time is 1 hour. This is less than the limit time for 102 dB in the USA (1.5 hours). An American radiologist would not be legally required to wear ear protection. They would not have to provide protection for other staff! A European radiologist would need ear protection rated with an SNR of at least 10 dB. Despite this example, all staff should wear hearing protection within the MR room during acquisition.

Each country has its own regulations regarding the measures that are required should the unprotected noise level exceed a limit. Usually this will involve the provision of hearing protection, signage, training, and, in some instances, audiometric monitoring or health surveillance. In the EU and UK hearing protection must be provided if the lower action level is exceeded, and its use becomes mandatory when the upper action level is exceeded. As good practice, MRI staff or other carers who remain in the MR examination room should always use hearing protection.

CONCLUSIONS

MR scanners are capable of producing sound pressure levels which may cause acoustic injury. Hearing protection for both patients and staff within the MR examination room is required. The actual effectiveness of hearing protection devices may be less than stated in their specifications. Different methods, limits, and laws apply in different countries.

Revision questions

1. In *IEC 60601-2-33* the maximum unweighted peak sound pressure level may not be greater than
   A. 85 dB
   B. 99 dB
   C. 99 dBA
   D. 120 dB
   E. 140 dB
2. Ear defenders are rated to 20 decibels sound attenuation using the SNR method. If the scanner noise is 100 dB(A), then the patient's ears will be exposed to about
   A. 5 dB(A)
   B. 50 dB(A)
   C. 80 dB(A)
   D. 84 dB(A)
   E. 94 dB(A)
3. A similar pulse sequence on a 3 T scanner will always be louder than on a 1.5 T scanner by
   A. 3 dB
   B. 5 dB
   C. 6 dB
   D. 10 dB
   E. We cannot say.
4. A temporary threshold shift TTS can be caused by exposure to
   A. 80 dB(A)
   B. 85 dB(A)
   C. 99 dB(A)
   D. Over 100 dB(A)
   E. 140 dB(Z)
5. Which of the following parameter changes will increase the acoustic noise?
   A. Reducing TR
   B. Increasing field of view
   C. Reducing the number of slices
   D. Reducing the turbo factor (echo train length)
   E. Increasing the flip angle.
6. If the noise from pulse sequence is 100 dB and the ambient noise in the MR room is 50 dB then the total sound pressure level (SPL) will be about:
   A. 50 dB
   B. 100 dB
   C. 106 dB
   D. 110 dB
   E. 150 dB

References

1. De Wilde, J.P., Grainger, D., Price D.L. et al. (2007). Magnetic resonance imaging safety issues including an analysis of recorded incidents within the UK. *Progress in Nuclear Magnetic Resonance Spectroscopy* 51:37–48.

2. Hudson, D. and Jones, A.P. (2018). A 3-year review of MRI safety incidents within a UK independent sector provider of diagnostic services. *British Journal of Radiology Open* 1: bjro. 20180006 https://doi.org/10.1259/bjro.20180006

3. Delfino, J.G., Krainak, D.M., Flesher, S.A. et al. (2019). MRI-related FDA adverse event reports: a 10-year review. *Medical Physics* doi: 10.1002/mp. 13768.

4. International Electrotechnical Commission (2013). *Electroacoustics – Sound level meters – Part 1: Specifications. 61672-1:2013*. Geneva: IEC.

5. Price, D.L., De Wilde, J.P., Papadaki, A.M. et al. (2001). Investigation of acoustic noise on 15 MRI scanners from 0.2 T to 3 T. *Journal of Magnetic Resonance Imaging* 13:288–293.

6. National Electrical Manufacturers Association (2010). *MS 4 – Acoustic Noise Measurement Procedure for Diagnostic Magnetic Resonance Imaging Devices*. Rosslyn, VA: NEMA.

7. Occupational Safety and Health Administration (1981). *Standard 1910.95 Occupational noise exposure*. Washington, DC: OHSA. https://www.osha.gov/laws-regs/regulations/standardnumber/1910/1910.95 (accessed 14 March 2019)

8. Ryan, A.F., Kujawa, S.G., Hammill, T. et al. (2016). Temporary and permanent noise-induced threshold shifts: A review of basic and clinical observations. *Otology & Neurotology* 37:e271–e275.

9. Bongers, S., Slottje, P., and Kromhout, H. (2017). Hearing loss associated with repeated MRI acquisition procedure-related acoustic noise exposure: an occupational cohort study. *Occupational and Environmental Medicine* 74:776–784.

10. Price, D., Delakis, I., Renaud C. et al. (2007). *3T MRI systems Issue 4. NHS CEP Report 06006*. NHS Purchasing and Supply Agency: London.

11. Price, D., Delakis, I., Renaud, C. et al. (2007). *1.5T MRI systems Issue 7. NHS CEP Report 06005*. NHS Purchasing and Supply Agency: London.

12. Price, D., Delakis, I., Renaud, C. et al. (2007). *0.6T – 1.0T open MRI systems Issue 6. NHS CEP Report 06030*. NHS Purchasing and Supply Agency: London.

13. Hedeen, R.A. and Edelstein, W.A. (1997). Characterization and prediction of gradient acoustic noise in MR imagers. *Magnetic Resonance in Medicine* 37:7–10.

14. Price, D.L., De Wilde, J.P., and McRobbie, D.W. (2004). A non-invasive method for obtaining the acoustic frequency response function for noise reduction. *Proceedings of the European Society of Magnetic Resonance in Medicine and Biology* 9–12 Sept. 2004, Copenhagen, Denmark, p. 426.

15. Mansfield, P., Glover, P.M., and Beaumont, J. (1998). Sound generation in gradient coil structures for MRI. *Magnetic Resonance in Medicine* 39:539–550.

16. Edelstein, W.A., Hedeen, R.A., Mallozzi, R.P. et al. (2002). Making MRI quieter. *Magnetic Resonance Imaging* 20:155–163.

17. Heismann, B., Ott, M., and Grodzki, D. (2015). Sequence-based acoustic noise reduction of clinical MRI scans. *Magnetic Resonance in Medicine* 73:1104–1109.

18. McJury, M. and Shellock, F.G. (2000). Auditory noise associated with MR procedures: a review. *Journal of Magnetic Resonance Imaging* 12:37–45.

19. Moelker, A.M., Maas, R.A.J.J., Lethimonnier, F. et al. (2002). Interventional MR imaging at 1.5T: quantification of sound exposure. *Radiology* 224:889–895.

20. Glover, P., Hykin, J., Gowland, P. et al. (1995). An assessment of the intrauterine sound intensity level during obstetric echo-planar magnetic resonance imaging. *British Journal of Radiology* 68: 1090–1094.

21. Berger, E.H., Word, W.D., Morrill, J.C. et al. (1996). *Noise & Hearing Conservation Manual, Fourth Edition*. Falls Church, VA: American Industrial Hygiene Association. https://blogs.cdc.gov/niosh-science-blog/2016/02/08/noise/ (accessed 14 March 2019).

22. International Electrotechnical Commission (2105). *Medical Electrical Equipment – Part 2–33: Particular Requirements for the Safety of Magnetic Resonance Equipment for Medical Diagnosis 60601-2-33 3.3 edn*. Geneva: IEC.

23. Food and Drugs Administration (2014). *Criteria for Significant Risk Investigations of Magnetic Resonance Diagnostic Devices - Guidance for Industry and Food and Drug Administration Staff.* Silver Spring, MD: FDA. https://www.fda.gov/RegulatoryInformation/Guidances/ucm072686.htm (accessed 14 March 2019).

24. Medicines and Healthcare Products Regulatory Agency (2015). *Safety Guidelines for Magnetic Resonance Imaging Equipment in Clinical Use.* London: MHRA. Available from https://assets.publishing.service.gov.uk/government/uploads/system/uploads/attachment_data/file/476931/MRI_guidance_2015_-_4-02d1.pdf (accessed 14 March 2019)

25. International Commission on Non-ionizing Radiation Protection (2004). Medical magnetic resonance (MR) procedures: protection of patients. *Health Physics* 87:197–216.

26. Royal Australian and New Zealand College of Radiologists (2017). *MR safety guidelines.* Sydney: RANZCR. https://www.ranzcr.com/college/document-library/ranzcr-mri-safety-guidelines (accessed 14 March 2019).

27. Directive 2003/10/EC (2003). *Noise.* Brussels: European Agency for Safety and Health at Work. https://osha.europa.eu/en/legislation/directives/82 (accessed 14 March 2019).

28. The Control of Noise at Work Regulations 2005. Statutory Instruments 2005 No. 1643. Schedule 1. London: The Stationery Office Limited. http://www.legislation.gov.uk/uksi/2005/1643/pdfs/uksi_20051643_en.pdf (accessed 4 March 2019).

Further reading and resources

McJury, M. (2014). Acoustic noise and MRI procedures. In: *MRI bioeffects, safety, and patient management* (Ed. F.D. Shellock and J.V. Crues III) pp. 88–130. Los Angeles, CA: Biomedical Research Publishing Group.

http://www.hse.gov.uk/noise/calculator.htm *Octave band calculator* (accessed 10 January 2019).

7

Pregnancy

INTRODUCTION

Despite the absence of ionizing radiation, the early deployment of MRI saw a cautious approach to the scanning of pregnant patients. Many departments implemented policies designed for the protection of the fetus from X-ray exposures to the new modality. A survey of 207 MR sites in the UK [1] revealed that almost half utilized a "ten day" or "twenty-eight day rule"[1] in MRI for females of reproductive age with 93% of sites restricting MR to the second or third trimester. Similarly, restrictive practices were common amongst pregnant MR staff: 51% of sites gave pregnant staff the option to opt out of magnet room duties at any stage of pregnancy, with 9% prohibiting access during the first trimester. Even today, such "folkloric" practices remain. What was driving this level of caution? We shall review the evidence for reproductive harm in cellular and animal models, before considering human epidemiological and MRI-based studies. Three potential sources of hazard: RF heating, acoustic noise, and gadolinium contrast administration are examined in greater detail.

CELLULAR EFFECTS AND ANIMAL STUDIES

Static field

Chapter 3 outlined the range of cell-level effects (and non-effects) attributed to static magnetic field exposure reported in the literature. There is very little evidence that these promulgate into the living animal.

A recent study of pregnant mice exposed daily for 75 minutes at the bore entrances of 1.5 and 7 T MRI magnets showed no effect on the duration of pregnancy, litter size, sex distribution, incidence of still births, malformations, or postpartum (the period immediately after birth) death of offspring. A slight delay in weight gain and in the time until eye opening (a developmental marker) was observed for the exposed group compared with controls [2]. Similar exposures did

---

[1] The 10 day and 28 day rules sought to restrict medical radiation exposures to within either 10 or 28 days from the last menstrual period in order to exclude or reduce the possibility of patient pregnancy and fetal exposure.

Essentials of MRI Safety, First Edition. Donald W. McRobbie.
© 2020 John Wiley & Sons Ltd. Published 2020 by John Wiley & Sons Ltd.

not affect mouse fertility but showed a reduced placental weight of offspring of intrauterine exposed female mice that correlated with a decrease in embryonic weight in those animals exposed at the strongest magnetic field [3]. In-utero exposure of mice at 7 T had no effect on their behavioral or learning capabilities [4].

In a 2009 review the International Commission on Non-Ionizing Radiation Protection (ICNIRP) concluded [5]:

> Exposure to static fields of up to 1 T has not been demonstrated to have an effect on fetal growth or postnatal development in mice [6,7].

> Other studies report a lack of effect on mouse fetal development following brief (2–7 d) exposure during organogenesis to fields of 4.7 T [8] and 6.3 T [9].

Time-varying magnetic fields

Pregnant mice exposed to MR fields with B_0 of 0.35 T, 23 mT m^{-1} gradients, and 61.2 mW RF power at 15 MHz showed no evidence of increased placental resorptions, still births, or teratogenicity (congenital abnormalities) [10]. There was a small reduction in crown-rump length (by 0.6 of a millimetre). Exposures of up to 12 000 Ts^{-1} at 2-3 kHz, resulting in massive muscular contractions, had no effect on the course of the pregnancy, litter numbers, or postnatal growth rate [11]. ICNIRP concluded that there was no clear evidence that exposure to low frequency or RF time-varying magnetic fields can adversely affect pregnancy outcome [5].

The National Toxicology Project into cell phone safety discovered no difference in littering, numbers or survival of pups, or sex distribution following continuous exposure of rats for the duration of their pregnancy to 0, 1.5, 3 or 6 W kg^{-1} at mobile telephony frequencies (900 and 1800 MHz). A lower birth weight was observed in the exposed group, but this returned to normal after a few weeks [12].

However, it is recognized that raised maternal temperature can result in developmental abnormalities in animals [13]. Critical thermal exposures are identified as:

- An extended core temperature increase of 2 °C
- A 2–2.5 °C increase for 30–60 minutes
- Greater than 4 °C increase for 15 minutes.

Additionally, fetal temperature may be 0.5 °C above maternal core temperature [14]. Normal Mode human scanning is designed to limit the core temperature rise to not more than 0.5 °C.

HUMAN STUDIES AND EPIDEMIOLOGY

Although animal models of pregnancy generally show no or marginal effects from magnetic field exposure, translation to humans remains problematical. Table 7.1 summarizes some of the results of early human exposure studies.

Like animal and cell studies, these are often limited by a lack of or incomplete dosimetry, often being undertaken as retrospective surveys. The slightly higher miscarriage and early birth rates reported by Kanal et al. [15] can be interpreted in terms of the MR technologist group being older than the control group. The other studies relate to clinical MRI exposures with various outcomes. For example, a lower gestation age in the exposed group, but similar birth weights when adjusted for gestation age [17], or increased length and improved gross motor function for the exposed babies [18].

Table 7.1   Summary of human MR and epidemiological studies into EMF and pregnancy.

Ref.	Subjects	Trimester	Exposure Conditions	Result	Comment
[15]	287 MR technologists, 964 others	All	10 mT–2 T	Slightly higher miscarriage and early birth rate	Age of non-MR subjects lower
[16]	20 children	2nd, 3rd	EPI 0.5 T	No hearing deficit	No controls
[17]	74 in utero	2nd, 3rd	EPI 0.5 T Up to 5 scans	No difference: gestation age-adjusted birth weight	Exposed: lower gestation age
[18]	20 in utero 35 controls		4 MRI scans	Increase in length/ gross motor function	Selection/ statistical issues
[19]	41 with history of prenatal death/perinatal hypoxia	3rd	1.5 T MRI	37 normal, 1 eye function, 1 hearing deficit	Abnormalities 'considered unrelated to MRI'
[20]	72 in utero	2nd, 3rd	1.5 T MRI	No effect on hearing, communication, socialization, or motor skills	2-year follow-up
[21]	15 exposures, 2 with GBCA	1st	1.5 T MRI	No adverse outcomes attributed to MRI	No controls

How do we interpret these conflicting data?

Fortunately, "Big Data" comes to our rescue. The problems with the studies summarized in Table 7.1 lie not just in their small sample sizes, lack of control groups, and inadequate dosimetry, but also in their attempt to detect very subtle or rare effects. A seminal study by Ray et al. [22] accessed the complete retrospective health records of the Canadian Province of Ontario providing 1742 first trimester MRI examinations compared to 1.4 million non-MRI pregnancies. They examined the incidence of stillbirth or neonatal death within 28 days, congenital anomalies, neoplasms, and hearing or vision loss from birth to four years. Table 7.2 shows the number, percentage, and incidence for each outcome, a crude and adjusted hazard ratio (HR) or ratio of incidence, and the absolute number difference per 1000 person–days[2] (or per 1000 pregnancies in the case of stillbirth or neonatal death). In the last column the 95% confidence intervals are also shown (Figure 7.1). Whilst there appears to be a small association with, e.g. vision loss, the absolute incidence difference is not significantly different from zero. The authors concluded that MRI during the first trimester was not harmful to the fetus with regard to stillbirth, neonatal death, congenital anomalies, hearing loss, or neoplasms. A smaller study [23] showed no effect on birth weight and growth between 751 1.5 T in-utero exposures and 10 042 non-exposed neonates.

Acoustic noise

Concern about the effect of high levels of acoustic noise on the fetus has existed since the 1990s [24]. Reeves et al. [25] is often cited as evidence of a lack of adverse effect. In this study 93 babies exposed to 1.5 T MRI during the second or third trimester were compared with over 1600 controls. Hearing function was assessed using oto-acoustic emission (OAE). These are sounds

---

[2] The use of "person-days" is a standard metric for determining disease prevalence in clinical trials.

Table 7.2   1st trimester MRI and pregnancy outcomes from Ray et al. [22].

Outcome	Number, (%), [Incidence per 1000 person-years]		Hazard Ratio (HR)		Adjusted risk difference per 1000 person-days (range 95% CI)
	MRI (n=1737)	Non-MRI (n=1 418 541)	Crude	Adjusted	
Still birth or neonatal death[1]	19 (1.1) [10.9]	9844 (0.7) [6.9]	1.57	1.68	4.7 (−1.6 to 11)
Congenital anomaly	165 (9.5) [33.8]	1 09 053 (7.7) [24.0]	1.29	1.16	3.8 (−1 to 9.6)
Vision loss	21 (1.2) [4.0]	10 124 (0.7) [2.1]	1.98	1.50	1.1 (−0.1 to 2.9)
Hearing Loss	50 (2.9) [9.6]	38 978 (2.8) [8.1]	1.24	1.04	0.3 (−0.5 to 3.7)
Any neoplasm	≤ 5 (0.3) [0.2]	4831 (0.3) [1.0]	0.19	0.53	−0.5 (−1.0 to 0.3)

The 5th column is the statistically adjusted risk ratio (MRI incidence/non-MRI incidence). The final column is the absolute incidence difference per 1000 person-days with the 95% confidence interval (CI) range in brackets.[1] This data is per 1000 pregnancies. The data are also shown in Figure 7.1.

generated by the cochlear hair cells at 1.5, 2, 3, and 4 kHz in response to an external auditory stimulus. The test requires minimal cooperation from the baby, is objective, and highly sensitive. The results showed that the 1.5, 2, and 3 kHz OAE were not significantly different (P>0.05) between exposed and control babies. The 4 kHz results showed a significant (P=0.02) 2.4 dB reduction for the exposed babies (Figure 7.2). However, when the 34 neonatal intensive care babies were removed from the analysis significance was not achieved for the 4 kHz OAE. This paper is often cited to attest to a lack of adverse effect on neonatal auditory function arising from in-utero MRI. This is not exactly the case. Peak hearing sensitivity occurs around 4 kHz, so are we detecting a subtle, but real, effect, masked by the low numbers of subjects?

Strizek et al. [23] also measured OAE and an auditory brain stem response. Their results are less equivocal: a smaller proportion (0.67%) of MR exposed babies had abnormal OAE than in the control group (1.4%). A slightly higher percentage of the MR group had abnormal brain stem response (5.2% vs 3.2%) near birth, but this reversed after three months (0% vs 0.34%). This is supported by Ray et al. [22] who calculated an inverse probability weight adjusted risk of hearing loss of 1.04, equivalent to no effect.

GADOLINIUM-BASED CONTRAST AGENTS

The situation is more complex for gadolinium-based contrast agents (GBCA) administered during pregnancy. A gadolinium concentration of 0.028×10^{-7} of administered dose per gram of fluid was detected in the amniotic fluid in macaques 50 days after administration of gadoteridol (ProHance, Bracco Diagnostics Inc. Monroe Township, NJ) [26]. Gadolinium was also detected in the femur (2.5×10^{-7}) and liver (0.15×10^{-7}) of all offspring, and also at lower levels in the skin, spleen, brain, and kidney of one out of eight animals.

In the large Canadian study [22], 397 of the patients had GBCA administration at any time during pregnancy. It is not known which particular agent was used for any given patient. The control group was 1.4 million non-MRI exposed women. The results (Table 7.3 and Figure 7.1) showed that gadolinium given any time during pregnancy was associated with an increased

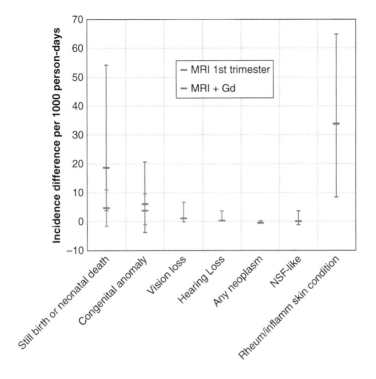

Figure 7.1   Incidence of adverse events from first trimester MRI during pregnancy and MRI with contrast at any time during pregnancy. Data from Ray et al. [22].

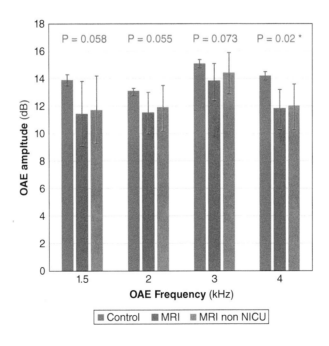

Figure 7.2   Neonatal cochlear function after MRI exposures assessed by oto-acoustic emission (OAE). If neonatal intensive care (NICU) babies are excluded there is no significant difference between MRI-exposed and controls. Data from Reeves et al. [25].

Table 7.3   MRI with gadolinium and pregnancy outcomes from Ray et al. [22].

Outcome	Number, (%) [incidence per 1000 person-years]		Hazard ratio		Adjusted risk difference per 1000 person-days (range 95% CI)
	Gd-MRI (n=397)	Non-MRI (n= 1 418 541)	Crude	Adjusted	
Still birth or neonatal death[1]	7 (1.8) [17.6]	9844 (0.7) [6.9]	2.60	3.70	18.6 (3.8 to 54.2)
Connective tissue or skin disease resembling NSF	≤5 (≤1.3) [3.3]	8705 (0.6) [1.8]	1.76	1.0	0.0 (−1.2 to 3.6)
Broad rheumatological or inflammatory infiltrative skin condition	123 (31.0) [125.8]	3 84 180 (27.1) [93.7]	1.33	1.36	33.7 (8.4 to 64.7)
Congenital anomaly	39 (10.3) [34.8]	1 09 053 (7.7) [24.0]	1.33	1.25	6.0 (−3.8 to 20.6)

The 5th column is the statistically adjusted risk ratio (Gd incidence/non-MRI incidence). The final column is the absolute incidence difference per 1000 person hours with the 95% confidence interval (CI) range in brackets.
The data are also shown in Figure 7.1.
[1] This data is per 1000 pregnancies.

incidence of rheumatological or inflammatory infiltrative skin conditions (31% GBCA vs 27% non-MRI), and stillbirth or neonatal death (1.8% GBCA vs 0.7% controls). The conclusion was that "gadolinium-enhanced MRI at any time of pregnancy was associated with rare adverse outcomes in childhood." The incidence of Gd-related stillbirth or neonatal death was estimated to be 1.9%, around 1 in 50. This corresponds of the risk of a fatal cancer from over 200 mSv of ionizing radiation- or more than 10 CT scans. We would not dream (even in our worst nightmares) of giving this much radiation to a pregnant patient.

MYTHBUSTER:

Gadolinium administered any time during pregnancy may be more harmful to the fetus than several CT scans of the abdomen or pelvis.

EXPOSURE LIMITS AND GUIDANCE

Most national practice guidelines follow the *IEC 60601-2-33* [27] recommendation that the RF exposure of pregnant patients should be restricted to the Normal Mode:

> "The instructions for use shall describe that scanning of pregnant PATIENTS with the WHOLE BODY RF TRANSMIT COIL should be limited to the NORMAL OPERATING MODE with respect to the SAR level."

That is, a maximum 0.5 °C maternal core temperature increase, or 2 W kg^{-1} whole body SAR. Additionally, steps to limit acoustic noise should be taken. Most significantly, MR is not contraindicated during the first trimester.

MYTHBUSTER:

MRI is not contraindicated during the first trimester, although a positive benefit vs risk analysis must have been carried out by the radiologist and referring clinican.

Fetal SAR and temperature

The whole-body SAR limit should restrict core maternal temperature increase to a maximum of 0.5 °C, but the possibility exists of local hotspots occurring within fetal tissue. Moreover, amniotic fluid lacks the cooling mechanism of perfused tissues. RF modeling has estimated fetal SAR and temperature for exposures of 2 W kg^{-1} from a quadrature body transmit coil operating at 64 MHz (1.5 T) and 128 MHz (3 T) [28]. The results (Figure 7.3) showed that peak SAR in any 10 g of fetal tissue was 40–60% of the peak maternal SAR at 64 MHz, and 50–70% at 128 MHz. First Level exposures at 1.5 T can result in peak fetal SAR hotspots reaching 14 W kg^{-1} [29]. However, this is significantly less than for adults (60 W kg^{-1}) or children (43 W kg^{-1}). Further work showed that temperatures in fetal tissue could exceed 38 °C if the maternal SAR is 2 W kg^{-1} over 7.5 minutes [30]. These results encourage a conservative approach to scanning during pregnancy.

RF exposures from parallel transmission ("RF shimming") may result in significantly higher SAR than for quadrature (circularly polarized) RF transmission. Estimated temperatures reached 40.8 °C for both fetus and mother in a 3 T system with RF optimized for uniform B$_1$ [29]. RF exposure during pregnancy should be restricted to the quadrature mode only.

MYTHBUSTER:

Parallel transmission for B$_1$ shimming does not reduce fetal SAR and should not be used on pregnant patients.

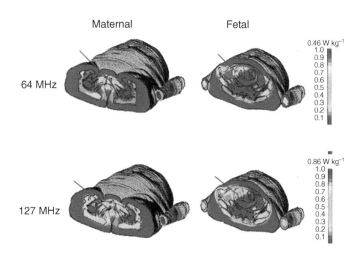

Figure 7.3   Fetal SAR predictions: top row 64 MHz maternal (L), fetal (R); bottom row 127 MHz maternal (L), fetal (R). The position of maximum local SAR (10 g) is indicated. Source [28]. Reproduced with permission of Wiley.

Minimizing SAR

Methods to control and limit SAR were considered in Chapter 5, page 127. These include using:

- Low SAR RF pulses
- Hyperechoes where available
- Reduced flip angles
- Reduced number of echoes and slices
- Longer TR.

Consider also that the body model used by the scanner for SAR estimation may not be based upon a heavily pregnant patient, that their thermal regulation may be less effective, and exercise a cautious approach.

Acoustic noise

In an attempt to estimate the acoustic attenuation offered to the fetus by the maternal tissues and amniotic fluid, a (male) subject swallowed a microphone to simulate the position of the fetus in the scanner [31]! An attenuation of around 30 dB was measured, but the limitations of this experiment are obvious. There may actually be an *increase* in sound intensity of around 4 dB for low frequencies (125 Hz), but with attenuation of only 10 dB at 4 kHz, the most damage sensitive frequency [32].

The limitation of acoustic noise was considering in Chapter 6. This includes the use of:

- Acoustically optimized gradient pulses
- Low SAR RF pulses (because smaller slice selection gradient pulses can be used)
- Larger fields-of-view or pixel dimensions
- Lower or fewer b-values and diffusion directions
- Fewer slices or echoes
- Longer TE or smaller receive bandwidths.

In addition to the potential effect on fetal hearing, take into consideration the effect of excessive acoustic noise on the mother's anxiety or stress level.

Professional guidance

Whilst the contraindication of MRI during the first trimester has largely been abandoned, there are various conditions to be observed. These generally include the need for consent, risk–benefit considerations (including delaying the scan), the use of alternative imaging, cautious use of contrast agents, restriction to the Normal Mode, and minimizing acoustic noise. It is important to be aware of the professional guidance that exists in your country, as subtle differences may occur. Guidance is available from the American College of Radiology [33], the Health Protection Agency (now Public Health England) [34], the International Commission on Non-Ionizing Radiation Protection [35], the Medicines and Healthcare Products Regulatory Agency [36], and the Royal Australian and New Zealand College of Radiologists (RANZCR) [37].

The ICNIRP guidance [35] contains a robust and forward-looking warning about gadolinium:

There is at present insufficient knowledge to establish unequivocal guidance for the use of MRI procedures on pregnant patients. In these circumstances, it is advised that MR procedures may be used for pregnant patients only after critical risk/benefit analysis, in particular in the first trimester, to investigate important clinical problems or to manage potential complications for the patient or fetus. The procedure should be conducted using a verbal and written informed consent procedure. The pregnant patient should be informed on the potential risks, also compared with those of other alternatives. Excessive heating is a potential teratogen; because of uncertainties in the RF dosimetry during pregnancy, it is recommended that exposure duration should be reduced to the minimum and that only the normal operation level is used. In addition, large doses of MRI gadolinium-based contrast agents have been shown to cause post-implantation fetal loss, retarded development, increased locomotive activity, and skeletal and visceral abnormalities in experimental animals. Such agents should only be used during pregnancy if the potential benefit justifies the risk to the fetus.

Staff exposure

Just as for patients, limitations on MR staff activities during pregnancy have been relaxed recently. It is expected that MR staff may continue to work normally in MRI at any time during pregnancy [33,36–38]. This includes positioning the patient, scanner operation, injecting, and entering the scanner room in response to an emergency. However, on account of precautions relating to acoustic noise, they should not enter the MR examination room *during* an acquisition, i.e. whilst there is gradient activity. Other concerns, e.g. the need to lift patients or coils, should also be considered. RANZCR recommends that pregnant persons who are neither patients nor MRI staff be excluded from the MRI scanner room at all times [37]. Different work health and safety regulations may apply in different countries; for example, the UK and EU countries require specific risk assessments with regard to staff pregnancy and work practice. Also, different countries may have particular definitions as to whether the fetus is legally designated as "a member of the public" [27], or whether the exposure of an accompanying parent or domestic carer is considered as a "medical exposure" or that of a member of the public. In such instances overarching legal requirements may apply. Not all countries are the same; whilst physics and physiology are the same everywhere, regulation and practice may not be.

CONCLUSIONS

MRI can be performed safety during pregnancy with significant benefit to both mother and, where appropriate, the fetus. Scanning should be restricted to the Normal Mode and acoustic noise minimized. Until more information is available parallel transmission should not be used. Care (and restraint, preferably avoidance) should be exercised regarding the use of gadolinium contrast, which may turn out to be a significant source of risk and harm to the unborn child. Controversially, in cases where gadolinium contrast may be required, CT *may* prove a safer option. Pregnant staff should avoid the MRI scanner room (zone IV) during actual scanning.

Revision questions

1. A member of the MR team is pregnant. To manage the risk to the unborn child they should:
   A. Work in CT instead because the risks are well known and easier to control
   B. Avoid MRI during the first trimester in accordance with guidance
   C. Only work on 1.5 T scanners
   D. Only work in reception
   E. Avoid being in the magnet room during scanning.

2. When scanning a pregnant MR patient, you should:
   A. Restrict RF to the Normal Mode
   B. Restrict RF exposure to 1 W kg^{-1}
   C. Use parallel transmission to reduce SAR
   D. Minimize acoustic noise
   E. Administer gadolinium contrast agents as routinely.
3. To scan a patient during the first trimester:
   A. A positive benefit vs risk analysis is required
   B. Patient consent is required
   C. Scanner noise should be limited to 80 dB(A)
   D. Do not scan. MR is contraindicated
   E. Only scan if CT results are inconclusive.
4. Concerning the effects of MRI examinations on pregnancy:
   A. MRI has been shown to affect neonatal hearing and vision
   B. MRI has been shown to be a cause of stillbirth
   C. MRI has no effect on birth weight
   D. Administration of gadolinium contrast is safe as it does not cross the placenta
   E. Administration of gadolinium contrast has resulted in rare but serious adverse events including inflammatory and infiltrative skin conditions.

References

1. De Wilde, J., Rivers, A., and Price, D. (2005). A review of the current use of magnetic resonance imaging in pregnancy and safety implications for the fetus. *Progress in Biophysics and Molecular Biology* 87:335–353.
2. Zahedi, Y., Zaun, G., Maderwald, S. et al. (2014). Impact of repetitive exposure to strong static magnetic fields on pregnancy and embryonic development of mice. *Journal of Magnetic Resonance Imaging* 39:691–699.
3. Zaun, G., Zahedi, Y. Maderwald, S. et al. (2014). Repetitive exposure of mice to strong static magnetic fields in utero does not impair fertility in adulthood but may affect placental weight on offspring. *Journal of Magnetic Resonance Imaging* 39:683–690.
4. Hoyer, C., Vogt, M.A., Richter, S.H. et al. (2012). Repetitive exposure to a 7 Tesla static magnetic field of mice in utero does not cause alterations in basal emotional and cognitive behavior in adulthood. *Reproductive Toxicology* 34:86–92.
5. International Commission on Non-ionizing Radiation Protection (2009). ICNIRP guidelines on limits of exposure to static magnetic fields. *Health Physics* 96:504–514.
6. Sikov, M.R., Mahlum, D.D., Montgomery, L.D. et al. (1979). Development of mice after intrauterine exposure to direct-current magnetic fields. In: (Eds. R.D. Phillips, M.F. Gillis, W.T. Kaune et al.) *Biological effects of extremely low frequency electromagnetic fields, Proceedings of the 18th Hanford Life Sciences Symposium*. Springfield, VA: National Technical Information Service, pp. 462–473.
7. Konermann, G. and Monig, H. (1986). Studies on the influence of static magnetic fields on prenatal development of mice. *Radiologe* 26:490–497 (in German).
8. Okazaki, R., Ootsuyama, A., Uchida S. et al. (2001). Effects of a 4.7 T static magnetic field on fetal development in ICR mice. *Journal of Radiation Research (Tokyo)* 42:273–283.
9. Murikami, J., Toril Y., and Masuda, K. (1992). Fetal development of mice following intrauterine exposure to a static magnetic field of 6.3T. *Magnetic Resonance Imaging* 10:433–437.
10. Heinrichs, W.L., Fong, P., Flannery, M. et al. (1988). Midgestational exposure of pregnant BALB/c mice to magnetic resonance imaging conditions. *Magnetic Resonance Imaging* 6:305–313.
11. McRobbie, D. and Foster, M.A. (1985). Pulsed magnetic field exposure during pregnancy and implications for NMR fetal imaging: a study with mice. *Magnetic Resonance Imaging* 3:231–234.
12. National Toxicology Program (2018). Toxicology and Carcinogenesis Studies in Hsd:Sprague Dawley SD Rats Exposed to Whole-Body Radio Frequency Radiation at a Frequency (900 MHz) and Modulations

(GSM and CDMA) Used by Cell Phones. Report TR-595. Available from https://ntp.niehs.nih.gov/ntp/htdocs/lt_rpts/tr595_508.pdf (accessed 13 March 2019).

13. Ziskin, M.C. and Morrissey, J. (2011). Thermal thresholds for teratogenicity, reproduction, and development. *International Journal of Hyperthermia* 27:374–387.

14. Schröder, H.J. and Power, G.G. (1997). Engine and radiator: fetal and placental interactions for heat dissipation. *Experimental Physiology* 82:403–414.

15. Kanal, E., Gillen, J., Evans, J.A. et al. (1993). Survey on reproductive health among female MR workers. *Radiology* 187:395–399.

16. Baker, P.N., Johnson, I.R., Harvey, P. et al. (1994). A three-year follow-up of children imaged in utero with echo-planar magnetic resonance imaging. *American Journal of Obstetrics and Gynecology* 170:32–33.

17. Myers, C., Duncan, K.R., Gowland, P.A. et al. (1998). Failure to detect intrauterine growth restriction following in utero exposure to MRI. *British Journal of Radiology* 71: 549–551.

18. Clements, H., Duncan, K.R., Fielding, K. et al (2000). Infants exposed to MRI in utero have a normal paediatric assessment at 9 months of age. *British Journal of Radiology* 73:190–194.

19. Kok, R.D., De Vries, M. M., Heerschap, A. et al. (2004). Absence of harmful effects of magnetic resonance exposure at 1.5 T in utero during the third trimester of pregnancy: a follow-up study. *Magnetic Resonance Imaging* 22:851–854.

20. Bouyssi-Kobar, M., du Plessis, A.J., Robertson, R.L. et al. (2015). Fetal magnetic resonance imaging: exposure times and functional outcomes at preschool age. *Pediatric Radiology* 45:1823–1830.

21. Choi, J.S., Ahn, H.K., Han, J.Y. et al. (2015). A case series of 15 women inadvertently exposed to magnetic resonance imaging in the first trimester of pregnancy. *Journal of Obstetrics and Gynecology* 35:871–872.

22. Ray, J.G., Vermeulen, M.J., Bharatha, A. et al. (2016). Association between MRI exposure during pregnancy and fetal and childhood outcomes. *Journal of the American Medical Association* 316:952–961.

23. Strizek, B., Jani, J.C., Mucyo, E., et al. (2015). Safety of MR imaging at 1.5 T in fetuses: a retrospective case-control study of birth weights and the effects of acoustic noise. *Radiology* 275:530–537.

24. American Academy of Pediatrics (1997). Noise: a hazard for the fetus and newborn. *Pediatrics* 100:724–727.

25. Reeves, M.J., Brandreth, M., Whitby, E.H. et al. (2000). Neonatal cochlear function: measurement after exposure to acoustic noise during in utero MR imaging. *Radiology* 257:802–809.

26. Prola-Netto, J., Woods, M., Roberts, V.H.J. et al. (2018). Gadolinium chelate safety in pregnancy: barely detectable gadolinium levels in the juvenile nonhuman primate after in utero exposure. *Radiology* 286:122–128.

27. International Electrotechnical Commission (2105). *Medical Electrical Equipment – Part 2-33: Particular Requirements for the Safety of Magnetic Resonance Equipment for Medical Diagnosis 60601-2-33 3.3 edn*. Geneva: IEC.

28. Hand, J.W., Li, Y, Thomas, E.L. et al. (2006). Prediction of specific absorption rate in mother and fetus associated with MRI examinations during pregnancy. *Magnetic Resonance in Medicine* 55:883–893.

29. Murbach, M., Neufeld, E., Samaras, T. et al. (2017). Pregnant women models analyzed for RF exposure and temperature increase in 3T RF shimmed birdcages. *Magnetic Resonance in Medicine* 77:2048–2056.

30. Hand, J.W., Li, Y., and Hajnal, J.V. (2010). Numerical study of RF exposure and the resulting temperature rise in the fetus during a magnetic resonance procedure. *Physics in Medicine and Biology* 55:913–930.

31. Glover, P., Hykin, J., Gowland, P. et al. (1995). An assessment of the intrauterine sound intensity level during obstetric echo-planar magnetic resonance imaging. *British Journal of Radiology* 68: 1090–1094.

32. Richards, D.S., Frentzen, B., Gerhardt, K.J. et al. (1992). Sound levels in the human uterus. *Obstetrics and Gynecology* 80: 186–190.

33. Kanal, E., Barkovich, A.J., Bell, C. et al. (2013). Expert Panel on MR Safety: ACR guidance document on MR safe practices: 2013. *Journal of Magnetic Resonance Imaging* 37:501–530.

34. Health Protection Agency (2008). *Protection of patients and volunteers undergoing MRI procedures, Documents of the Health Protection Agency RCE-7*. Chilton, UK: HPA.

35. International Commission on Non-ionizing Radiation Protection (2004). Medical magnetic resonance (MR) procedures: protection of patients. *Health Physics* 87:197–216.
36. Medicines and Healthcare Products Regulatory Agency (2015). *Safety Guidelines for Magnetic Resonance Imaging Equipment in Clinical Use*. London: MHRA. Available from https://assets. publishing.service.gov.uk/government/uploads/system/uploads/attachment_data/file/476931/MRI_guidance_2015_–_4-02d1.pdf (accessed 14 March 2019)
37. Royal Australian and New Zealand College of Radiologists (2017). *RANZCR MRI Safety Guidelines*. Sydney: RANZCR. https://www.ranzcr.com/college/document-library/ranzcr-mri-safety-guidelines (accessed 15 March 2019).
38. Temperton, D.H. (2009). Pregnancy and work in diagnostic imaging departments, 2nd edn. London: British Institute of Radiology.

Further reading and resources

American College of Obstetricians and Gynecologists (2017). Guidelines for diagnostic imaging during pregnancy and lactation. *Obstetrics & Gynecology* 130:e210–e216.

Colletti, P.M. (2014). MRI procedures and pregnancy. In: *MRI bioeffects, safety, and patient management* (Ed. F.D. Shellock FD and J.V. Crues III). Los Angeles, CA: Biomedical Research Publishing Group, pp. 217–241.

Health Protection Agency (2008). *Protection of patients and volunteers undergoing MRI procedures, Documents of the Health Protection Agency RCE-7*. Chilton, UK: HPA.

International Commission on Non-ionizing Radiation Protection (2004). Medical magnetic resonance (MR) procedures: protection of patients. *Health Physics* 87:197–216.

Medicines and Healthcare Products Regulatory Agency (2015). *Safety Guidelines for Magnetic Resonance Imaging Equipment in Clinical Use*. London:MHRA. Available from https://assets.publishing.service.gov.uk/government/uploads/system/uploads/attachment_data/file/476931/MRI_guidance_2015_–_4-02d1.pdf (accessed 14 March 2019).

Royal Australian and New Zealand College of Radiologists (2017). *RANZCR MRI Safety Guidelines*. Sydney: RANZCR. https://www.ranzcr.com/college/document-library/ranzcr-mri-safety-guidelines (accessed 15 March 2019).

Temperton D.H. (2009). *Pregnancy and work in diagnostic imaging departments, 2nd edn*. London: British Institute of Radiology.

8

Contrast agents

INTRODUCTION

The use of gadolinium-based contrast agents (GBCA) to modify relaxation times was first proposed very early in the history of MRI [1]. Gadolinium Gd^{3+} ions were incorporated (or chelated) onto larger macromolecules, also known as "ligands" (from the Greek word "to bind"), to increase safety- free gadolinium is toxic; and to increase the tendency of the agent to accumulate in lesions. Chelation, deriving from the Greek "chela" for claw, is a chemical process whereby a metal ion is bonded to two or more *coordination points* of attachment on the ligand. The first agents were designed for use in the central nervous system (CNS), specifically for brain tumors where the agent crosses the blood brain barrier. Owing to the large magnetic susceptibility of the gadolinium ions, enhanced relaxation occurs within their microscopic vicinity (<1 nm) as water molecules associate with the Gd^{3+} through an exchange process.

Since the introduction of the first commercially approved agent (Magnevist; Schering AB, Berlin, now Bayer HealthCare) in 1988, GBCAs have been used for the detection and diagnosis of non-CNS lesions, tumor staging, MR angiography, arthrography, perfusion, and permeability imaging. It is estimated that GBCA is used in up to 40% of MR examinations, with around 30 million administrations per year [2]. Table 8.1 lists currently available agents. In this chapter we will use the trade names, as most readers will be familiar with these rather than the chemical or formula names and acronyms.

Recently, there has been significant media attention on the side effects of gadolinium agents and the issue is considered as controversial. This chapter outlines the physical and chemical properties of the agents as related to their stability and incidence of adverse reactions. Those responsible for the administration of MR contrast should consult the Further Reading and References sections at the end of this chapter. Readers should also be aware that this is a current and ongoing area of research.

PHYSICAL AND CHEMICAL PROPERTIES

Gadolinium (Gd) is a "rare earth" transition metal belonging to the lanthanides group of the periodic table. It was discovered in 1880 by Jean Charles de Marignac, but is named after Johan Gadelin, who discovered the mineral gadolinite. It has atomic number 64 (with 64 protons), existing in six stable isotopes with mass numbers 154, 155, 156, 157, 158, and 160, 158 being the most abundant.

Essentials of MRI Safety, First Edition. Donald W. McRobbie.
© 2020 John Wiley & Sons Ltd. Published 2020 by John Wiley & Sons Ltd.

Table 8.1 Gadolinium-based contrast agents.

Trade name	Generic name	Acronym	Chemical formula	Structure
Omniscan[1]	Gadodiamide	Gd-DTPA-BMA	$C_{16}H_{28}GdN_5O_9$	Linear, non-ionic
OptiMark[2]	Gadoversetamide	Gd-DTPA-BMEA	$C_{20}H_{34}GdN_5O_{10}$	Linear, non-ionic
Magnevist[3]	Gadopentetate dimeglumine	Gd-DTPA	$C_{28}H_{54}GdN_5O_{20}$	Linear, ionic
Eovist/Primovist[3]	Gadoxetate disodium	Gd-EOB-DTPA	$C_{23}H_{33}GdN_3O_{11}^{+3}$	Linear, ionic
MultiHance[4]	Gadobenate dimeglumine	Gd-BOPTA	$C_{36}H_{62}GdN_5O_{21}$	Linear, ionic
ProHance[4]	Gadoteridol	Gd-HP-DO3A	$C_{17}H_{29}GdN_4O_7$	Macro-cyclic, non-ionic
Gadovist/Gadavist[3]	Gadobutrol	Gd-DO3A-Butrol	$C_{18}H_{31}GdN_4O_9$	Macro-cyclic, non-ionic
Dotarem[2]	Gadoterate meglumine	Gd-DOTA	$C_{23}H_{42}GdN_5O_{13}$	Macro-cyclic, ionic

Manufacturers: [1] GE Healthcare; [2] Guebert Group; [3] Bayer HealthCare marketed as Gadavist (USA) and Gadovist (Europe); [4] Bracco Imaging. Production of Ablavar formerly Vasovist (Lantheus Imaging) ceased in 2017.

174

Gadolinium-152 is radioactive by alpha decay with a half-life of 10^{14} years. Gd-157 is highly efficient at capturing neutrons and is used as a shielding material in nuclear reactors. Gadolinium exhibits fluorescence and is widely used in screens and detectors for X-ray imaging. Gadolinium is used in MR for its paramagnetic properties but has a Curie temperature of around 17°C (compare with Table 2.3); at just below room temperature it becomes ferromagnetic.

Gadolinium does not occur naturally in biology. A dose of 100–200 mg kg^{-1} is lethal in 50% of administrations (the "LD50") to rodents. Gadolinium's toxicity is associated with its competition with other ions, particularly calcium (Ca^{2+}) to occupy protein binding sites. Gadolinium's atomic radius is 180 pm (180×10^{-12} m), similar to calcium (194 pm). When bonded to a ligand molecule by chelation, its toxicity is reduced significantly; the LD50 for the agents listed in Table 8.1 range from 6–30 mmol kg^{-1} in mice. The stability of chelation increases with the number of coordination points. When the bonds break, the metal ion is said to dissociate from the ligand. *Transmetallation* occurs when the Gd is replaced by another metal ion. For a primer on moles and molar solutions see Example 8.1 below.

Example 8.1 Moles and mass

What is the mass of 1 mmol of gadolinium chloride (Gd Cl$_3$) and how many Gd ions are there?

One mole is defined as the atomic weight in grams (g mol^{-1}). The atomic weight of gadolinium is 157 and chlorine 35. The total molecular weight is 157 + (3 × 35) = 262. A mole of Gd Cl$_3$ weighs 262 g, so a milli-mole is 0.262 g. A molar solution is one mole dissolved in 1 liter of solvent. The number of molecules or atoms in a mole is given by Avogadro's number (N_A): 6.022×10^{23}. 1 mmol of Gd Cl$_3$ contains around 6×10^{20} (six hundred quintillion) gadolinium ions.

Relaxation properties

GBCAs work by reducing the relaxation time T_1 in regions where the agent accumulates, e.g. within a tumor, or in transit within blood vessels in an angiographic acquisition. T_2 is also affected, but at the doses encountered in tissue, the main effect of GBCAs is seen as hyper-intense signal on T_1-weighted images (Figure 8.1). The agent's relaxivities, r_1 and r_2, are specified in liters per milli-mole per second (L mmol^{-1} s^{-1}). Values for specific agents are shown in Table 8.2. The effect on the tissue relaxation rate R_i can be calculated from

$$R_i = R_0 + r_i C_A \tag{8.1}$$

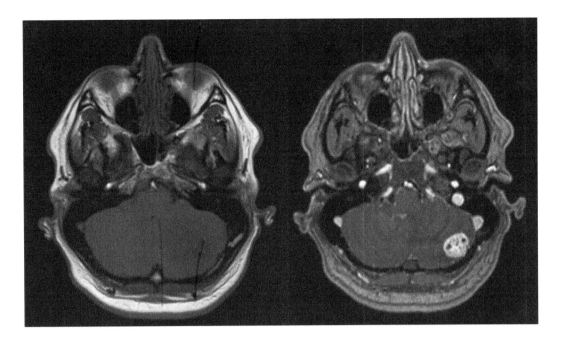

Figure 8.1 T$_1$-weighted brain pre- (L) and post (R) contrast showing enhancement of a hemangioblastoma. Source: Flinders Medical Centre, Adelaide, Australia. Reproduced with permission.

Table 8.2 Typical relaxivities of commercial GBCAs at 1.5 and 3T [3].

Agent	r$_1$ (L mmol^{-1} s^{-1})		r$_2$ (L mmol^{-1} s^{-1})		Concentration (mmol ml^{-1})
	1.5T	3T	1.5T	3T	
Omniscan (gadodiamide)	4.3	4.0	5.2	5.6	0.5
OptiMark (gadoversetamide)	4.7	4.5	5.2	5.9	0.5
Magnevist (gadopentetate dimeglumine)	4.1	3.7	4.6	5.2	0.5
Eovist/Primovist (gadoxetate disodium)	6.9	6.2	8.7	11.0	0.25
MultiHance (gadobenate dimeglumine)	6.3	5.5	8.7	11.0	0.5
ProHance (gadoteridol)	4.1	3.7	5.0	5.7	0.5
Gadovist/Gadavist (gadobutrol)	5.2	5.0	6.1	7.1	1.0
Dotarem (gadoterate meglumine)	3.6	3.5	4.3	4.9	0.5

where R_i is the relaxation rate R_1 or R_2 (s^{-1}), R_0 is the unenhanced relaxation rate (without Gd), and C_A is the concentration of the agent. The relaxation times are:

$$T_1 = \frac{1}{R_1} \qquad (8.2a)$$

$$T_2 = \frac{1}{R_2} \qquad (8.2b)$$

Example 8.2   Relaxation times

If a gadolinium-based contrast agent with $r_1 = 4$ and $r_2 = 5$ L $mmol^{-1}$ s^{-1} accumulates in a tissue with a T_1 of 800 ms and T_2 of 100 ms at a concentration of 0.1 mmol kg^{-1}, what will the observed relaxation times be?

From Equations 8.1 and 8.2,

$$R_1 = \frac{1}{0.8} + 4 \times 0.1 = 1.65 \ s^{-1}$$

therefore

$$T_1 = \frac{1}{1.65} = 0.606 \ s \ or \ 606 \ ms.$$

$$R_2 = \frac{1}{0.1} + 5 \times 0.1 = 10.5 \ s^{-1}$$

and

$$T_2 = \frac{1}{10.5} = 0.095 \ s \ or \ 95 \ ms$$

Both T_1 and T_2 are reduced, but the greater reduction is in T_1, resulting in hyper-intense or bright appearance on a T_1-weighted image.

Most agents are provided in half molar concentration (0.5 $mmol^{-1}ml^{-1}$) and the standard patient dose is 0.1 $mmol^{-1}kg^{-1}$, corresponding to a total mass of chelated Gd of about one gram (see Example 8.3 below); this compares with a typical body content of around 2 g of zinc and 4 g of iron. A dose of *one* molar concentration Gadovist requires half the volume of the half-molar agents. The maximum dose is generally 0.2 $mmol^{-1}kg^{-1}$, 30–150 times less than the mouse LD50. Administered GBCAs have a smaller volume compared to iodinated contrast used in CT and X-ray angiography; a CT contrast injection may contain 150 ml of fluid with 120 mmol of the agent.

Another class of MR contrast agents based upon super-paramagnetic iron oxide (SPIO), so-called negative agents, work by reducing T_2 and signal intensity. These are not currently in clinical use and will not be considered further.

Physical properties of CGCAs

The host molecules, chelating agents or ligands can be divided into four categories according to their chemical structure:

- Linear, non-ionic: Omniscan, OptiMark
- Linear, ionic: Magnevist, Eovist/Primovist, MultiHance, (Ablavar)
- Macro-cyclic, non-ionic: ProHance, Gadovist/Gadavist
- Macro-cyclic, ionic: Dotarem.

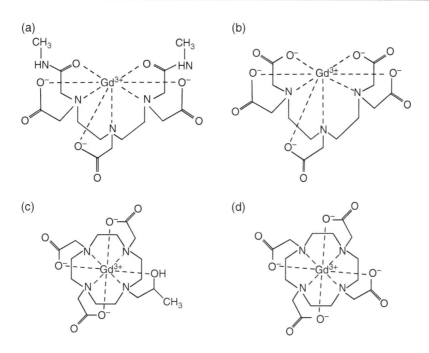

Figure 8.2   Structure of gadolinium-based contrast agents (a) linear non-ionic- Gadodiamide (Omniscan); (b) linear ionic- Gadopentetate dimeglumine (Magnevist); (c) macrocyclic non-ionic- Gadoteridol (ProHance); (d) macrocyclic ionic- Gadoterate meglumine (Dotarem). The coordination bonds are shown as dashed lines. The ionic agents have a net negative charge.

Figure 8.2 shows the chemical structural representation of an example of each type of ligand. The eight coordination bonds, the "claws" of the ligand, are shown as dashed lines. The non-ionic chelates have zero net charge, the +3 charge of the Gd being balanced by the three O^- ions. The ionic agents have an additional O^- making their overall charge negative. This further prevents the Gd ion dissociating from its ligand. In the macrocyclic molecules the Gd ion is embedded in the center of a cyclic structure, rendering it more secure.

The agents can also be categorized by their route of excretion: all via glomerular filtration through the kidneys. Eovist and MultiHance bind to proteins and are also cleared through the hepatobiliary system. The times for 50% clearance in a patient with healthy renal function, or biological half-lives, are shown in Table 8.3. Figure 8.3 shows the estimated concentration versus time for an agent with a biological half-life of 1.5 hours in a patient with normal renal function; after 12 hours only 0.4% remains, and almost complete clearance has occurred by 24 hours. A patient with reduced renal function with an estimated glomerular filtration rate (eGFR[1]) of 30–60 will have a significantly lower clearance rate, with around 6% remaining after 24 hours, and much more remaining in cases of severe renal failure (eGFR < 30).

Table 8.3 also shows the osmolality of the agents. Blood osmolality is around 275–297 mosm kg^{-1} (milli-osmoles per kilogram). Osmolality relates to the tendency of concentrations

---

[1] eGFR is derived from a measurement of blood creatinine in mL min^{-1} 1.73 m^{-2} (mL per minute per 1.73 meters squared – equivalent to body surface area). It is an indicator of kidney function; a normal eGFR in a young adult will be greater than 90 mL min^{-1} 1.73 m^{-2}.

Table 8.3 Physical properties of GBCAs [3].

Type	Agent	Molecular weight (g mol^{-1})	Osmolality[1] (mosm kg^{-1})	Viscosity[1] (mPa-s)	Clearance $t_{1/2}$ (hr)
Linear, non-ionic	**Omniscan** (gadodiamide)	591.7	789	1.4	1.3
	OptiMark (gadoversetamide)	661.8	1110	2.0	
Linear, ionic	**Magnevist** (gadopentetate dimeglumine)	938.0	1960	2.9	1.6
	Eovist/Primovist (gadoxetate disodium)	684.8	688	1.2	0.93
	MultiHance (gadobenate dimeglumine)	1058.1	1970	5.3	1.6
Macro-cyclic, non-ionic	**ProHance** (gadoteridol)	558.7	630	1.3	1.57
	Gadovist/Gadavist (gadobutrol)	604.7	1603	5.0	1.81
Macro-cyclic, ionic	**Dotarem** (gadoterate meglumine)	753.9	1350	2.0	1.6

[1] At 37°C.

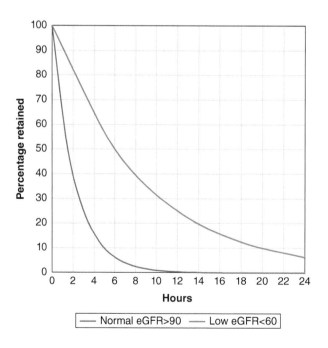

Figure 8.3 Typical clearance for a patient with normal renal function and low eGFR (< 60 mL min^{-1}1.73 m^{-2}).

Table 8.4   Stability of CBCAs: laboratory test results [3].

Type	Agent	Stability Log K_{therm}	Stability (in-vivo conditions) Log K_{cond}	Dissociation half-life[1]	Excess ligand (%)
Linear, non-ionic	**Omniscan** (gadodiamide)	16.9	14.9	<5s	5
	OptiMark (gadoversetamide)	16.6	15.0	<5s	10
Linear, ionic	**Magnevist** (gadopentetate dimeglumine)	22.1	17.7	<5s	0.1
	Eovist/Primovist (gadoxetate disodium)	23.5	18.7	<5s	0.5
	MultiHance (gadobenate dimeglumine)	22.6	18.4	<5s	0.0
Macro-cyclic, non-ionic	**ProHance** (gadoteridol)	23.8	17.1	3.9 hr	0.1
	Gadovist/Gadavist (gadobutrol)	21.8	14.7	43 hr	0.1
Macro-cyclic, ionic	**Dotarem** (gadoterate meglutamine)	25.6	19.3	338 hr	0.0

[1] pH 1, 25° C

of solutions to equalize across a semi-permeable membrane by the redistribution of the solvent. The overall osmotic pressure of a dose of GBCA is small compared to that of blood. A low osmolality is desirable in a contrast agent, particularly if extra-vasation occurs. Similarly, a low viscosity is desirable as it renders the agent less "sticky." Blood viscosity is around 2.8 mPa-s (milli-pascal-seconds) at 37 °C.

From a safety perspective, the most important aspect of contrast agents is their stability. There are two main metrics to describe this: *thermodynamic* stability and *kinetic* stability. Thermodynamic stability relates to the amount of energy required to break the bonding of the Gd ion to the ligand. Thermodynamic stability is quantified by the constant K_{therm} which expresses the ratio of bound chelate to free chelate once thermal equilibrium has been achieved. It is independent of pH. The *conditional stability constant* K_{cond}, estimated for the in-vivo pH of 7.4, is more clinically relevant. These values are shown in Table 8.4 as base-10 logarithms; a difference of one therefore represents a tenfold difference in concentration; a value of 15 indicates that there may be one free Gd ion per 10^{15} chelated ions.

MYTHBUSTER:

Not all GBCAs have similar chemical stability. The difference in stability between two CBCAs with log K_{cond} of 15 and 18 is 1000 times. Gadolinium ions are one thousand times more likely to dissociate from the ligand with the lower value of log K_{cond}.

Example 8.3 Number of Gd ions

How many gadolinium ions are in a 0.1 mmol kg^{-1} dose of a contrast agent with atomic weight 600 administered to an 83 kg patient? What mass of gadolinium is this?

1 mole of contrast agent = 600 g per kg;

Total dose is 83 × 0.1 × 10^{-3} = 0.0083 mol. 1 mole contains 6.02 × 10^{23} molecules, so the dose will contain 5 × 10^{21} Gd ions.

1 mole of Gd weighs 157 g, the concentration is 8.3 mmol, so the total chelated Gd content is

$$8.3 \times 157 \times 10^{-3} = 1.3 \, g.$$

The entire human body contains around 2 g of zinc and 4 g of iron.

Example 8.4 Free Gd ions

If the agent in Example 8.3 has a conditional stability constant log K_{cond} equal to 15, how many free Gd ions will be present?

The ratio of bound to free ions is 10^{15}, so the number of free ions is 5 × 10^{21} ÷ 10^{15} = 5 × 10^6. There will be about 5 million free gadolinium ions. These can recombine with the ligand, but in-vivo there will be competition from other ions such as calcium, zinc, and iron.

How many free Gd ions would be present if the log K_{cond} was 19?

The dose contains 5 × 10^{21} Gd ions and the ratio of bound to free ions will be 10^{19}, so the number of free ions is 5 × 10^{21} ÷ 10^{19} = 5 × 10^2. There will only be 500 free gadolinium ions, compared to 5 million for the other agent.

Also shown in Table 8.4 are the dissociation half-lives, giving an indication of the speed of dissociation or the kinetic stability. These are measured at 20 °C with pH = 1 so are not directly relevant to the clinical situation. Nevertheless, they indicate the greater intrinsic stability of the three macro-cyclic agents. Some of the agents contain extra ligand in the vial, as much as 10% in the case of OptiMark. It has been shown in animal studies that this improves their safety profile.

The stability data in Table 8.4 does not tell the whole story. In-vivo there will be competition for the ligands' metal binding sites from other ions. For example, ProHance exhibits less transmetallation of Gd with zinc at physiological pH than the ionic linear agent Magnevist, which transmetallizes less than a linear non-ionic agent Omniscan [4]. A significant increase in gadolinium toxicity resulting from transmetallation with zinc (Zn^{2+}), calcium (Ca^{2+}), and copper (Cu^{2+}) has been observed in rodents subjected to large doses of linear agents [5]. Transmetallation with Zn^{2+} has also been observed in the blood and urine of humans after a single dose of the linear Omniscan, but not for the macrocyclic ProHance [6].

CONTRAST REACTIONS AND ADVERSE EVENTS

Any medicinal product will have a range of possible side effects, some of which may be adverse. An adverse reaction is a noxious and unintended response to a medicinal product. For GBCAs these may take the form of acute reactions of an allergic nature, or, rarely, in the form of nephrogenic systemic fibrosis (NSF). Recent research has demonstrated that evidence for long-term retention of Gd in human tissues, particularly the brain and bone can be observed in T_1-weighted images. The clinical consequences of this are, as yet unknown.

General reactions

General reactions to GBCA are acute and transitory in nature ranging from nausea (1.5%), hives (0.2%), to more severe reactions (0.001%) [2]. These can be compared with iodinated CT contrast

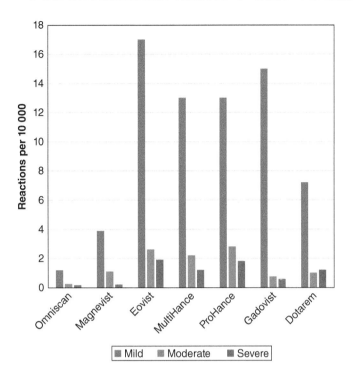

Figure 8.4 Incidence of allergic reactions. Data from [10].

reactions: 0.2–0.7% acute; 0.04% severe; 0.0006% fatal [7]. Most GBCA reactions are allergy-like: headache, nausea with or without vomiting, injection site reactions, rash, dizziness, and itchiness (pruritus). Three quarters of incidences are transient, requiring no further treatment. The ACR Manual on Contrast Media [8] categorized adverse reactions and appropriate responses and treatment. MR medical practitioners should be aware of these, or other available national or international advice on contrast reactions, e.g. from the European Society of Urogenital Radiology [9]. The ACR Manual also advises practitioners to be cognisant of their patients' previous reactions and any history of asthma or allergies to food, chemicals, or medication. In each case, a positive benefit versus risk analysis should be undertaken. Preventative measures may include premedication with antihistamines or corticosteroids. Further monitoring of the patient is required where reactions have occurred.

Figure 8.4 shows the results of a meta-analysis of the published incidences of allergic-like reactions (according to the ACR classifications) from various agents [10]. The overall prevalence was stated as 9.2 per 10 000 administrations (0.092%). Note that this *excludes* physiological reactions such as the potentially fatal NSF. The NSF storm which had been brewing since the late 1990s broke in 2006 [11].

NSF

Fifteen renal dialysis patients identified from March 1997 onwards presented an unusual condition characterized by thickening and hardening of the skin of the extremities with an increase in dermal fibroblast-like cells, closely resembling scleromyxoedema [12]. Initially, it was named "nephrogenic fibrosing dermopathy" [13], until its systemic nature affecting other organs was noticed [14]; we now know it as Nephrogenic Systemic Fibrosis or NSF. Its link to gadolinium was made by Thomas Grobner, an Austrian nephrologist, in 2006 [15]; initially Gd-DTPA (Magnevist) was implicated, but a published correction [16] identified the agent as Gd-DTPA-BMA or Omniscan.

In the USA over 1600 NSF cases were reported to the FDA with only 60 US hospitals accounting for 93% of these [17]. The overall prevalence of NSF from Omniscan was 3.4 per 10 000 (0.034%) and 0.23 per 10 000 from Magnevist for patients with renal insufficiency. There was a greater risk for both high dose one-off administrations and for repeated injections within six months of each other. Figure 8.5 plots the percentage of 815 confirmed and unconfounded (by the administration of more than one agent) incidences for various GBCAs: 78.7% from Ominscan, 19.3% from Magnevist, and 1.3% from OptiMark. The very low reported incidences for Gadovist (0.4%) and Dotarem (0.2%) did not meet the clinical criteria for NSF [18]. 75% of cases occurred in the USA with others reported in Denmark (5.6%), Germany (4.9%), the United Kingdom (4.7%), and Japan (2.3%). 99% of incidences were for patients with acute renal failure with 81% suffering from chronic kidney disease (CKD): 79% stage 5 with an estimated glomerular filtration rate (eGFR) of less than 15 mL min^{-1}1.73 m^{-2} and 1.8% stage 4 (eGFR >15 but <30 mL min^{-1}1.73 m^{-2}); and 75.6% on dialysis. 97.7% of incidence occurred within two years of the Gd administration, about one third occurring within one month of injection.

NSF is characterized by thickening and tightening of the skin resulting in a "woody" feel and an appearance similar to orange peel, with subcutaneous edema (Figure 8.6, [19]); it can result in joint stiffness or immobility, or difficulty in bending. Skin changes can also extend from the extremities to the trunk. The systemic nature of the disease may involve the lungs, heart, liver, kidneys, skeletal muscles, diaphragm, and other organs, and can prove fatal. It is a very serious adverse reaction and has led to many lawsuits in the USA.

In response most regulatory agencies placed restrictions upon the use of higher risk linear agents. In the EU the European Pharmacovigilance Working Party introduced new product labeling stating that Omniscan was contraindicated in patients with severe renal impairment (GFR < 30 mL min^{-1}1.73 m^{-2}), and those with or undergoing liver transplantation. In 2010 the European Medicines Agency introduced a risk rating for GBCA as high, medium or low risk (Table 8.5). High risk agents were contraindicated for patients with severe renal failure (GFR < 30 mL min^{-1}1.73 m^{-2}), for transplantation patients during the perioperative liver-transplantation period,

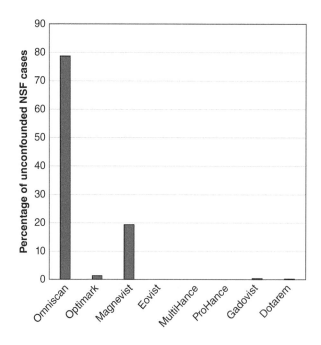

Figure 8.5   Incidence of unconfounded cases of NSF. Data from [18].

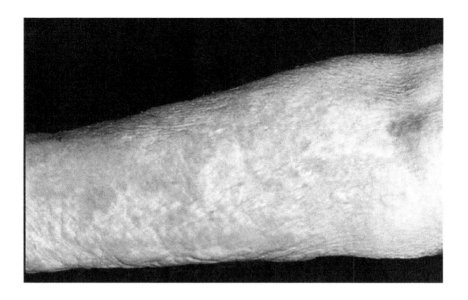

Figure 8.6   Skin thickening and 'orange peel' appearance in a patient with NSF. Source [19] Used with permission of Elsevier.

Table 8.5   Classification of agents by NSF risk and observed long term retention in tissue [2,20,35].

Agent	Structure	NSF reported?	EMA Risk rating	ACR NSF safety group	Long term Gd retention?	EMA position (European Union and UK only)
Omniscan (gadodiamide)	Linear, non-ionic	Yes	High	1	Yes	License suspended
OptiMark (gadoversetamide)	Linear, non-ionic	Yes	High	1	No	License suspended
Magnevist (gadopentetate dimeglumine)	Linear, ionic	Yes	High	1	Yes	License suspended except for intra-articular use
Eovist/Primovist (gadoxetate disodium)	Linear, ionic	No	Medium	3	No	Maintain
MultiHance (gadobenate dimeglumine)	Linear, ionic	No	Medium	2	Yes	Only licensed for liver scans
Ablavar (gadofosveset trisodium)[1]	Linear, ionic	No	NA	3	No	Not licensed in the EU
ProHance (gadoteridol)	Macro-cyclic, non-ionic	No	Low	2	No	Maintain
Gadovist/Gadavist (gadobutrol)	Macro-cyclic, non-ionic	No	Low	2	No	Maintain
Dotarem (gadoterate meglumine)	Macro-cyclic, ionic	No	Low	2	No	Maintain

[1] Ablavar (Vasovist) $C_{33}H_{40}GdN_3Na_3O_{15}P$ withdrawn from the US market for commercial reasons.

and for neonates. The American College of Radiology also defines NSF safety groups: group 1 agents are associated with the greatest number of NSF cases; group 2 agents are associated with few, if any, cases of NSF; group 3 agents have only recently been commercially available and therefore evidence on NSF is not yet available [20].

With restrictions upon the use of the high risk (ACR group 1) agents and more responsible dosing, there are few, if any, cases of NSF being reported currently. Gadolinium toxicity and controversy has not gone away however; it has intensified.

Retention

The long-term retention of gadolinium in tissues is well established by basic science. As long ago as 1992 deposition in brain tissue was reported [21]; retention in bone was reported in the early 2000s [22–24]. An interesting case report showed that zinc-gadolinium transmetallation does occur in humans [25]. In human serum non-ionic linear agents have shown levels of dissociated Gd in blood ten times the level from ionic linear agents, whilst macrocyclics remained stable [26]. Preclinical studies in rodents measured Gd retention in skin, liver, femur with the highest observed for Omniscan, Optimark, and Magnevist [27] (Figure 8.7).

The above evidence of the long-term retention of gadolinium made little impact until March 2014 when Kanda et al. [28] showed that unenhanced MR signal hyper-intensity in the brain, specifically the dentate nucleus and globus pallidus, correlated with the number of prior gadolinium contrast administrations. Whilst details of the specific agents used were unavailable subsequent research has shown that this effect mainly occurs with linear agents, and that macrocyclic agents appear to deposit with an order of magnitude less. Table 8.5 itemizes human brain retention study results [2]. Unsurprisingly, it is the agents mostly associated with NSF that exhibit retention: linear ionic Magnevist showing statistically significant signal intensity differences [29], whilst macrocylic Dotarem and Gadovist did not [30]. Signal changes in the dentate nucleus and globus pallidus of children have been observed following four Magnevist injections but not after similar Dotarem administrations [31]. Most significantly retention occurs regardless of renal function, unlike NSF [32]. The same study identified 0.1–58.8 μg of retained gadolinium per gram of tissue with a response dependent on the dose of Omniscan administered.

The sixty-four thousand (or multi-billion) dollar question is: does this matter? Are there any clinical consequences of long term gadolinium retention? As yet this remains unanswered, however gadolinium has been associated with: nephrotoxicity; apoptosis and necrosis in renal tubular cells in humans and in vitro; white blood cell reduction in mice; pancreatitis in humans; neurotoxicity in rats: tremours, seizures, ataxia (appearance of drunkenness), corpus callosum damage, and hemorrhage; and encephalopathy in humans [33]. Whilst the evidence is sketchy, the human data arising from individual case reports only, gadolinium is a known toxin. The most infamous case of alleged gadolinium toxicity was reported in the media on 7 November 2017 when news broke that Hollywood movie star Chuck Norris was suing several pharmaceutical companies over the alleged poisoning of his wife, Gena, by gadolinium. This caused a surge in public awareness of gadolinium toxicity [34].

Current advice

Most jurisdictions acknowledge the occurrence of both NSF and long term Gd retention, advising caution and constraint, noting a lack of observed (so far) health effects from retention, whilst reiterating the clinical benefits of MR contrast examinations to large numbers of patients. There are differences in regulatory and professional guidance, particularly between Europe and other regions. You should be aware of the guidance that applies in your country.

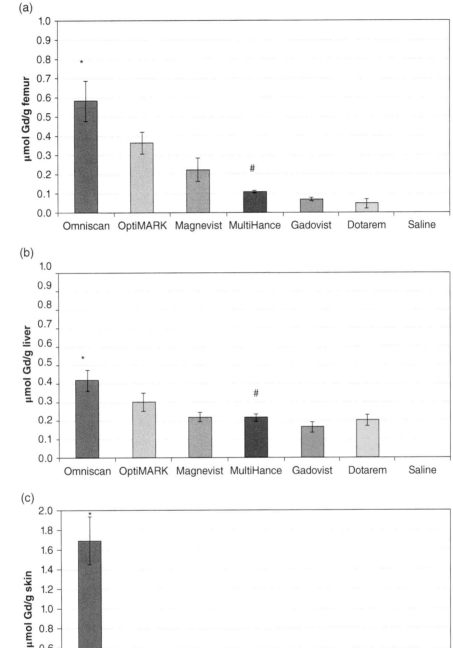

Figure 8.7 Gd retention in rats for (a) femur; (b) liver; (c) skin. Source [27]. Used with permission of Springer Nature.

Following the initial retention studies, in July 2017 the European Medicines Agency [35] revoked the licenses of Omniscan, Magnevist, and OptiMark. They are now unavailable in the 27 European Union countries plus the UK. Initial advice from the FDA regarding Gd retention in the brain was given in May 2017. The following year new Medication Guides for GBCAs were introduced to be given to patients receiving GBCA [36].

Links to guidance documents for the USA, Canada, Europe, UK, Australia, and New Zealand are given at the end of this chapter.

PREGNANCY AND LACTATION

Pregnancy

The association of a small risk of stillbirth or neonatal death following GBCA to the mother was noted in Chapter 7 [37]. GBCAs are known to cross the placenta and small amounts of a macrocylic agent (ProHance) have been detected in juvenile primates following maternal doses: 2.5×10^{-7} of the dose in the femur; 0.15×10^{-7} in the liver [38].

The administration of GBCA to pregnant patients is not absolutely contraindicated but caution is required. Lower risk agents should be used with the minimum dose. For example, the ACR Manual on Contrast Media [20] requires that:

- Clinicians and radiologists review each case, administering GBCA only if the potential benefit to the patient *and* fetus outweighs the risk from free Gd ions to the fetus
- The information cannot be gained without the use of contrast or by another modality
- The information is required during the pregnancy
- The above is documented.

Additionally, patient consent is recommended. Other guidance was highlighted in Chapter 7.

Breast-feeding

It is estimated that less than 0.04% of the dose of GBCA passes into the mother's milk and that uptake by the infant is 1% of that, so that the total ingested dose is less than 0.0004%. It is considered that cessation of breast feeding for 24 hours is not essential [39]. Recommendations on the use of GBCA during pregnancy and lactation vary by agent and jurisdiction, so check the labeling and any relevant national guidance. For example, the ACR Manual on Contrast Media [20] states that:

- The small amount of GBCA excreted into breast milk and absorbed by the child suggests that it is safe to continue breast-feeding after Gd administration
- If she is concerned the mother may make an informed decision to cease breast-feeding for 12–24 hours
- In such a case milk expressed in this period should be discarded.

CONCLUSIONS

As the controversy rages in the media and is discussed within the professions, what lessons can be learned? The most important is not to ignore the problem. NSF probably could not have been predicted as it is an entirely new disease. However, its appearance followed indiscriminate off-label use of medicinal products; it is an unnatural disease caused by human activity. Gadolinium retention, on the other hand, was reported in the scientific literature many years before the MR community recognized it; the data on chemical stability of GBCAs has been available for decades. Ultimately, the choice and dosage of a pharmaceutical is a clinical decision, but basic science and recent clinical and animal studies point to the higher stability, and hence, greater intrinsic safety of the macro-cyclic agents. All professional and regulatory bodies advise on restricting the uses of GBCAs where possible, limiting the dosage to recommended levels, and the use of the more stable agents. It is not known whether gadolinium retention in tissues may prove harmful in the future. The story of gadolinium contrast agents has taken dramatic turns in recent years and may not yet be finished. MR professionals need to keep abreast of the ongoing research in this area including the possible development of new agents using other paramagnetic ions.

187

Revision questions

1. The most commonly used gadolinium-based contrast agents:
    A. Reduce T_1 where they are accumulated, decreasing the MR signal intensity
    B. Increase T_1 where they are accumulated, increasing the MR signal intensity
    C. Reduce T_1 where they are accumulated, increasing the MR signal intensity
    D. Increase T_2 where they are accumulated, increasing the MR signal intensity
    E. Do not affect T_2 at all.
2. The most chemically stable MR contrast agents are:
    A. Linear, ionic
    B. Macro-cyclic
    C. Linear, non-ionic
    D. Iodine-based
    E. They are all the same.
3. A GBCA with a stability constant log K_{con} equal to 15 means that:
    A. 1 in 15 of the gadolinium ions may dissociate from the chelating agent
    B. There are 15 chelating ligands per gadolinium ion
    C. The number of free gadolinium ions is 10^{15}
    D. There may be 1 free gadolinium ion per 10^{15} chelated gadolinium ions
    E. The agent will be 25% more stable than an agent with K_{con} equal to 12.
4. The MR contrast agents most associated with nephrogenic systemic fibrosis are:
    A. Gadovist, MultiHance, and Dotarem
    B. Primovist, ProHance, and Ablavar
    C. Omniscan, OptiMark, and Magnevist.
5. In countries where they are available, high risk (for NSF) agents should not be administered to patients with a glomerular filtration rate (GFR) of
    A. Greater than 60 mL min^{-1}1.73m^{-2}
    B. 45–60 mL min^{-1}1.73m^{-2}
    C. 30–45 mL min^{-1}1.73m^{-2}
    D. Less than 30 mL min^{-1}1.73m^{-2}
    E. They can be given to any patient.
6. Gadolinium-based contrast agents can be given to a pregnant woman:
    A. At any time, because the agent does not cross the placenta
    B. Never, they are an absolute contraindication
    C. Only for fetal imaging
    D. Only after the first trimester
    E. Only after a positive benefit to risk assessment by the radiologist.

References

1. Weinmann, H.J., Brasch, R.C., Press, W.R. et al. (1984). Characteristics of gadolinium-DTPA complex: a potential NMR contrast agent. *American Journal of Roentgenology* 142:619–624.

2. Runge, V.M. (2016). Safety of the gadolinium-based contrast agents for magnetic resonance imaging, focusing in part on their accumulation in the brain and especially the dentate nucleus. *Investigative Radiology* 51:273–279.

3. Hao, D., Ai, T, Goerner, F. et al. (2012). MRI contrast agents: basic chemistry and safety. *Journal of Magnetic Resonance Imaging* 36:1060–1071.

4. Puttagunta, N.R., Gibby, W.A., and Puttagunta, V.L. (1996). Comparative transmetallation kinetics and thermodynamic stability of gadolinium-DTPA bis-glucosamide and other magnetic resonance imaging contrast media. *Investigative Radiology* 31:619–624.

5. Cacheris, W.P., Quay, S.C. and Rocklage, S.M. (1990). The relationship between thermodynamics and the toxicity of gadolinium complexes. *Magnetic Resonance Imaging* 8:467–481.

6. Puttagunta, N.R., Gibby, W.A., and Smith, G.T. (1996). Human in vivo comparative study of zinc and copper transmetallation after administration of magnetic resonance imaging contrast agents. *Investigative Radiology* 31:739–742.

7. Beckett, K.R., Moriarity, A.K., and Langer, J.M. (2015). Safe use of contrast media: what the radiologist needs to know. *RadioGraphics* 35:1738–1750.

8. ACR Committee on Drugs and Contrast Media (2013). *ACR Manual on Contrast Media Version 9.* Reston, VA: American College of Radiology.

9. European Society of Urogenital Radiology (2018). *ESUR Guidelines on Contrast Agents Version 10.0* http://www.esur.org/guidelines/ (Accessed 5 March 2019).

10. Behzadi, A.H., Zhao, Y., Farooq, Z. et al. (2018). Immediate allergic reactions to gadolinium-based contrast agents: A systematic review and meta-analysis. *Radiology* 286:471–482.

11. Colletti, P.M. (2009). Nephrogenic systemic fibrosis and gadolinium: a perfect storm. *American Journal of Roentgenology* 191:1150–1153.

12. Cowper, S.E., Robin, H.S., Steinberg, S.M. et al. (2000). Scleromyxoedema-like cutaneous diseases in renal-dialysis patients. *Lancet* 356:1000–1001.

13. Leboit, P.E. (2003). What nephrogenic fibrosing dermopathy might be. *Archives of Dermatology* 139:928–930.

14. Ting, W.W., Stone, M.S., Madison, K.C. et al. (2003). Nephrogenic fibrosing dermopathy with systemic involvement. *Archives of Dermatology* 139:903–906.

15. Grobner, T. (2006A). Gadolinium – a specific trigger for the development of nephrogenic fibrosing dermopathy and nephrogenic systemic fibrosis? *Nephrology Dialysis Transplantation* 21:1104–1108.

16. Grobner, T. (2006B). Erratum. *Nephrology Dialysis Transplantation* 21:1745.

17. Bennett, C.L., Qureshi, Z.P., Sartor, A.O. et al. (2012). Gadolinium-induced nephrogenic systemic fibrosis: the rise and fall of an iatrogenic disease. *Clinical Kidney Journal* 5:82–88.

18. Spinazzi, A. (2014). MRI contrast agents and nephrogenic systemic fibrosis. In: *MRI bioeffects, safety, and patient management* (Ed. F.D. Shellock and J.V. Crues III) pp 256–281. Los Angeles, CA: Biomedical Research Publishing Group.

19. Perazella, M.A. and Rodby, R.A. (2007). Gadolinium-induced Nephrogenic Systemic Fibrosis in patients with kidney disease. *American Journal of Medicine* 120:561–562.

20. ACR Committee on Drugs and Contrast Media (2018). *ACR Manual on Contrast Media Version 10.3.* Reston, VA: American College of Radiology.

21. Koeberl, C. and Bayer, P.M. (1992). Concentrations of rare earth elements in human brain tissue and kidney stones determined by neutron activation analysis. *Journal of Alloys and Compounds* 180:63–70.

22. Gibby, W.A. and Gibby, K.A. (2004). Comparison of Gd DTPA–BMA (Omniscan) versus Gd HP-DO3A (ProHance) retention in human bone tissue by inductively coupled plasma atomic emission spectroscopy. *Investigative Radiology* 39:138–142.

23. White, G.W., Gibby, W.A., and Tweedle, M.F. (2006). Comparison of Gd(DTPA–BMA) (Omniscan) versus Gd(HP-DO3A) (ProHance) relative to gadolinium retention in human bone tissue by inductively coupled plasma mass spectroscopy. *Investigative Radiology* 41:272–278.

24. Darrah, T.H., Prutsman-Pfeiffer, J.J., Poreda, R.J. et al. (2009). Incorporation of excess gadolinium into human bone from medical contrast agents. *Metallomics* 1:479–488.

25. Greenberg, S.A. (2010). Zinc transmetallation and gadolinium retention after MR imaging: case report. *Radiology* 257:670–673.
26. Frenzel, T., Lengsfeld, P., Schirmer, H. et al. (2008). Stability of gadolinium-based magnetic resonance imaging contrast agents in human serum at 37 degrees C. *Investigative Radiology* 43:817–828.
27. Sieber, M.A., Lengsfeld, P., Frenzel, T. et al. (2008). Preclinical investigation to compare different gadolinium-based contrast agents regarding their propensity to release gadolinium in vivo and to trigger nephrogenic systemic fibrosis-like lesions. *European Radiology* 18:2164–2173.
28. Kanda, T., Ishii, K., Kawaguchi, H. et al. (2014). High signal intensity in the dentate nucleus and globus pallidus on unenhanced T1-weighted MR Images: relationship with increasing cumulative dose of a gadolinium-based contrast material. *Radiology* 270:834–841.
29. Radbruch, A., Weberling, L.D., Kieslich, P.J. et al. (2015). Gadolinium retention in the dentate nucleus and globus pallidus is dependent on the class of contrast agent. *Radiology* 275:783–791.
30. Radbruch, A., Weberling, L.D., Kieslich, P.J. et al. (2015). High-signal intensity in the dentate nucleus and globus pallidus on unenhanced T1-weighted images: evaluation of the macrocyclic gadolinium-based contrast agent Gadobutrol. *Investigative Radiology* 50: 805–810.
31. Ryu, Y.J., Choi, Y.H., Cheon, J.E. et al (2018). Pediatric brain: gadolinium deposition in dentate nucleus and globus pallidus on unenhanced T1-weighted images is dependent on the type of contrast agent. *Investigative Radiology* 53:246–255.
32. McDonald, R.J., McDonald, J.S., Kallmes, D.F. et al. (2015). Intracranial gadolinium deposition after contrast-enhanced MR Imaging. *Radiology* 275:772–782.
33. Rogosnitzky, M. and Branch, S. (2016). Gadolinium-based contrast agent toxicity: a review of known and proposed mechanisms. *Biometals* 29:365–376.
34. McNamara, C. and Rahmani, G. (2018). Gena Norris and gadolinium deposition disease – the impact of celebrity health disclosure on public awareness. *Magnetic Resonance in Medicine* 80:1277–1278.
35. European Medicines Agency (2017). EMA's final opinion confirms restrictions on use of linear gadolinium agents in body scans. 21 July 2017, EMA/457616/2017.
36. Food and Drug Administration (2018). *FDA Drug Safety Communication: FDA warns that gadolinium-based contrast agents (GBCAs) are retained in the body; requires new class warnings*. https://www.fda.gov/Drugs/DrugSafety/ucm589213.htm (accessed 15 July 2019).
37. Ray, J.G., Vermeulen, M.J., Bharatha, A, et al. (2016). Association between MRI exposure during pregnancy and fetal and childhood outcomes. *Journal of the American Medical Association* 316:952–961.
38. Prola-Netto, J., Woods, M., Roberts, V.H.J. et al. (2018). Gadolinium chelate safety in pregnancy: barely detectable gadolinium levels in the juvenile nonhuman primate after in utero exposure. *Radiology* 286:122–128.
39. Wang, P.I., Chong, S.T., and Kielar, A.Z. (2012). Imaging of pregnant and lactating patients: Part 1. Evidence-based review and recommendations. *American Journal of Roentgenology* 198:778–784.

Further reading and resources

Beckett, K.R., Moriarity, A.K., and Langer, J.M. (2015). Safe use of contrast media: what the radiologist needs to know. *RadioGraphics* 35:1738–1750.
Thomsen, H.S. and Webb, J.A. (eds) (2014). *Contrast Media: Safety issues and ESUR guidelines*. Heidelberg: Springer.
US National Library of Medicine. *PubChem*. www.pubchem.ncbi.nlm.nih.gov (accessed 22 August 2019).

National guidance documents

Australia

Royal Australian and New Zealand College of Radiologists (2017). *RANZCR Statement on Gadolinium Retention*. https://www.ranzcr.com/whats-on/news-media/171-ranzcr-statement-on-gadolinium-retention (accessed 15 July 2019).
Therapeutic Goods Administration (2017). *Gadolinium-based contrast agents for MRI scans*. https://www.tga.gov.au/alert/gadolinium-based-contrast-agents-mri-scans (accessed 15 July 2019).

Canada

Canadian Association of Radiologists (2017). *New CAR guidelines on the use of gadolinium-based-contrast agents in kidney disease*. https://car.ca/news/new-car-guidelines-use-gadolinium-based-contrast-agents-kidney-disease/ (accessed 15 July 2017).

European Union

European Medicines Agency (2017). *Gadolinium-containing contrast agents*. https://www.ema.europa.eu/en/medicines/human/referrals/gadolinium-containing-contrast-agents (accessed 15 July 2019).
European Society of Urogential Radiology (2018). *ESUR Guidelines on Contrast Agents Version 10.0* http://www.esur.org/guidelines/ (accessed 15 July 2019).

New Zealand

MedSafe (2017). Gadolinium based contrast agents for MRI and retention of gadolinium in the brain. https://www.medsafe.govt.nz/safety/EWS/2017/GadoliniumContrastAgents.asp (accessed 15 July 2019).
Royal Australian and New Zealand College of Radiologists (2017). *RANZCR Statement on Gadolinium Retention*. https://www.ranzcr.com/whats-on/news-media/171-ranzcr-statement-on-gadolinium-retention (accessed 15 July 2019).

UK

Medicines and Healthcare Products Regulatory Agency (2018). *Gadolinium-containing contrast agents: Omniscan and iv Magnevist no longer authorised, MultiHance and Primovist for use only in liver imaging*. https://www.gov.uk/drug-safety-update/gadolinium-containing-contrast-agents-omniscan-and-iv-magnevist-no-longer-authorised-multihance-and-primovist-for-use-only-in-liver-imaging. (accessed 15 July 2019).
Royal College of Radiologists (2019). *Guidance on gadolinium-based contrast agent administration to adult patients*. https://www.rcr.ac.uk/system/files/publication/field_publication_files/bfcr193-gadolinium-based-contrast-agent-adult-patients.pdf (accessed 15 July 2019).

USA

American College of Radiology (2018). ACR Manual on Contrast Media Version 10.3. Reston, VA: ACR. https://www.acr.org/Clinical-Resources/Contrast-Manual (accessed 15 July 2019).
Food and Drug Administration (2018). FDA Drug Safety Communication: *FDA warns that gadolinium-based contrast agents (GBCAs) are retained in the body; requires new class warnings*. https://www.fda.gov/Drugs/DrugSafety/ucm589213.htm (accessed 15 July 2019).
Radiological Society of North America (2018). *RSNA statement on Gadolinium-based MR contrast agents*. https://www.rsna.org/uploadedfiles/rsna/content/role_based_pages/media/rsna-gadolinium-position-statement.pdf (accessed 15 July 2019).

9

Passive implants

INTRODUCTION

Having reviewed the technological and biological aspects of MR exposures we now come to what many would consider the heart of MR safety: the safe scanning of patients with implants. A passive device is one that is implanted within or affixed to the patient, but which does not use any electrical power. Its function is generally mechanical; for example, in orthopedics: joint replacements, spinal rods, external limb fixation devices; or in cardiovascular surgery: stents to repair an artery, artificial heart valves, or clips to isolate an aneurysm in the brain.

The chapter reviews the potential sources of hazard from passive devices, explains the testing methodologies used to ascertain the MR safety of implants, illustrated with some examples of devices. For the aspiring MRSO or MRMD this chapter should be read in conjunction with Chapter 2 for the underlying theoretical aspects. Those wishing to act as an MRSE should also engage deeply with the material in Appendix 1.

RISKS FROM PASSIVE IMPLANTS

Walk into your MRI department (if you are appropriately authorized to do so) and what do you see? Lots of signage such as shown in figure 9.1. The red circle with the red line through it is the international symbol for prohibition; the sign is telling us that patients with both passive and active implants are excluded! This does not accord with MR practice; patients with passive implants have long been scanned, but clearly the signs indicate that some risks do exist.

The potential sources of hazard from MRI for the patient with passive implants are:

- Movement of the device from translation or rotation due to magnetic forces
- Displacement of the device arising from Lenz's Law forces
- Heating from the RF or imaging gradient exposures
- Vibration from the imaging gradient exposure
- Induction of electrical currents.

It is logical and convenient to consider the nature of the risks arising from each of the electromagnetic field components: the B_0 static field; the RF transmission field B_1; and the time-varying imaging gradients G_x, G_y, G_z. It is arguably more scientific to categorize the risks

Essentials of MRI Safety, First Edition. Donald W. McRobbie.
© 2020 John Wiley & Sons Ltd. Published 2020 by John Wiley & Sons Ltd.

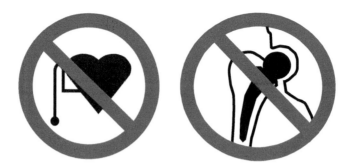

Figure 9.1   Signage on the MRI examination room prohibiting entry for persons with implants.

Table 9.1   Categorization of interactions of passive devices with magnetic fields in MRI.

Effect on the Device	Interaction		
	Static magnetic forces	Magnetic forces due to motion	Induction
Translation	Static field B_0 Spatial gradient dB/dz	Lenz's Law: static field gradient dB/dz, velocity v	-
Torque (twisting)	Static field B_0	Lenz's Law: static field gradient dB/dz, velocity v	-
Vibration	-	-	Gradient dB/dt
Electric currents	-	Static field gradient dB/dz Velocity v	Gradient dB/dt RF dB/dt (frequency, B_1)
Localized heating	-	-	Gradient dB/dt duty cycle; RF dB/dt frequency amplitude duty cycle

according to the underlying physical interactions. Table 9.1 shows that each potentially hazardous effect may have more than one physical cause, some resulting from the interaction of field components rather than from a single source. Other factors also play a decisive role in the strength of these interactions: the device material (dia-/paramagnetic or ferromagnetic), its magnetic susceptibility, saturation status, electrical conductivity, geometry (shape, size, angle with respect to the field, position), velocity, and anatomical location.

Static magnetic forces

Chapter 2 examined how the nature and strength of the forces of magnetic attraction and torque depend upon:

- The magnetic properties of the material (dia-/para-/ferromagnetic, its magnetic susceptibility χ) and its condition (hard/soft ferromagnetic, saturated/unsaturated)
- The shape of the object and its orientation to the static magnetic field B_0
- The fringe field B_0, its spatial gradient $\left(\dfrac{dB}{dz}\right)$ or the field-gradient product $\left(B \cdot \dfrac{dB}{dz}\right)$.

These are summarized in Table 9.2.

Table 9.2   Summary of static magnetic field forces.

Material type	Magnetic susceptibility χ	Translational force	Torque
Diamagnetic	Small, negative	$F = \dfrac{\chi}{\mu_0} VB_0 \dfrac{dB}{dz}$	$T = \dfrac{1}{\mu_0} \chi^2 VB_0^2 g_t$
Paramagnetic / weakly ferromagnetic	Small, positive	$F = \dfrac{\chi}{\mu_0} VB_0 \dfrac{dB}{dz}$	$T = \dfrac{1}{\mu_0} \chi^2 VB_0^2 g_t$
Strongly ferromagnetic	Unsaturated	$F_z = \dfrac{1}{\mu_0} VB_0 \dfrac{dB}{dz} g_d$	$T = \dfrac{1}{\mu_0} VB_0^2\ g_t{'}$
	Saturated	$F_z = \dfrac{1}{\mu_0} VB_{sat} \dfrac{dB}{dz}$	$T = \dfrac{1}{\mu_0} VB_{sat}^2 g_t$

μ_0 is the permeability of free space; V is the object's volume; g_d, g_t and $g_t{'}$ are shape factors that depend upon the demagnetizing factors (d_1, d_2, d_3), larger for long thin objects and dependent upon the angle of the object to B_0. The full expressions are given in Chapter 2 and Appendix 1.

Table 9.3 and Figure 9.2 show some χ values for common implant materials plus a few strongly ferromagnetic materials which may be present in devices. Figure 9.3 shows the theoretical ratio of translational to gravitational force on a spherical object with density 8000 kg m^{-3} as a function of magnetic susceptibility for a 1.5 T and 3 T static field with spatial gradients dB/dz of 5 and 7.5 T s^{-1}. The material saturates at 1T. Even objects with susceptibility as low as 0.01–0.1 can experience forces greater than gravity.

Diamagnetic materials

The forces and torques on diamagnetic materials are very small; χ is very small, and χ-squared even smaller. Devices made from these materials (e.g. gold, copper, polyethylene) do not present a translational or twisting hazard in the MR environment at any time. Plastics are inherently diamagnetic with χ around -10^{-5}.

Paramagnetic materials

For paramagnetic objects, e.g. a titanium or titanium alloy aneurysm clip, the translational force is proportional to the product B_0·dB/dz. Torque increases with the square of B_0, so will be four times greater at 3 T compared with 1.5 T. Fortunately, the torque also depends upon the susceptibility squared; e.g. for titanium $\chi^2 = 0.00018^2 = 0.0000000324$ or 3.24×10^{-8}, a very small number.

Example 9.1   Torque on a paramagnetic stent

What is the maximum torque on a 2 cm long Nitinol stent weighing 20 mg in a B_0 of 3 T?
The volume of stent material is

$$V = \frac{m}{\rho} = \frac{20 \times 10^{-6}}{6450} = 3.1 \times 10^{-9}\ m^3$$

The maximum torque occurs at an angle of 45° to B_0 (Equation 2.16):

$$T_{max} = \frac{1}{4\mu_0} \chi^2 V B_0^2 = \frac{1}{16\pi \times 10^{-7}} \times 0.000245^2 \times 3.1 \times 10^{-9} \times 3^2 = 3.3 \times 10^{-10}\ Nm$$

The maximum twisting force is

$$F = \frac{T}{0.5 \times d} = 3.3 \times 10^{-8} N$$

This is negligible compared (~6000 times smaller) with the gravitational force of 0.196×10^{-3}N.

Table 9.3 Magnetic and electrical properties of metals.

Material	Magnetic Susceptibility χ	Density ρ (kg m⁻³)	Saturation Field B_{sat} (T)	Electrical Conductivity σ ×10⁶ (S m⁻¹)	σ/ρ ×10³	Skin Depth at 100 MHz ×10⁻⁶ (m)	Specific Heat Capacity C (J kg⁻¹ °C⁻¹)
Diamagnetic							
Silver (Ag)[1]	−0.000024	10 490	-	62	5.9	6.4	235
Gold (Au)[1]	−0.000034	19 300	-	45	2.3	7.5	129
Copper (Cu)[1]	−0.0000096	8960	-	59	6.6	6.6	384
Polyethylene[2]	−0.0000096	923	-	~0	~0	~0	1550
Paramagnetic							
Aluminium (Al)[1]	0.000021	2700	-	38	14.1	8.2	904
Titanium (Ti)[1]	0.00018	4507	-	2.5	0.55	31.8	520
Nitinol[3] 50% Ni 50% Ti	0.000245	6450	-	1.2	0.19	45.9	837
Platinum (Pt)[1]	0.00026	21 450	-	9.4	0.44	16.4	133
Elgiloy[4]/ Phynox	0.0039	8300	-	1.1	1.3	47.2	450
Palladium (Pd)[1]	0.00079	12 023	-	10	0.96	15.9	240
Co-Cr-Mo [5] (ASTM 75)	0.00092	8400	-	14	1.7	13.4	450
Weakly ferromagnetic							
316 LVM[6,7] stainless steel (ASTM F 138)	0.0006	8000	< 0.001	1.3	0.16	44.1	502
316 L[7] stainless steel	0.0042	8000	< 0.01	1.3	0.16	44.0	502
316[8,9] stainless steel	0.003	8000	-	1.4	0.16	42.5	502
17-7 PH stainless steel	0.4–2.6	7810	-	1.3	0.16	31.2	450
Strongly ferromagnetic							
Cobalt (Co)[1]	250	8900	0.6	17	1.8	0.79	421
Nickel (Ni)[1]	600	8908	0.5	14	1.6	0.55	445
Martensitic SS[9]	400–1100	7800	1.4	1.8	0.23	1.33	450–510
Mumetal[9]	~10 0000	8760	0.7	17	1.9	0.039	460
Pure iron (Fe)[1]	~20 0000	7874	2.16	10	1.3	0.036	449

Sources: [1] [1]; [2] [2], [3] [3], [4] [4], [5] [5], [6] [6], [7] [7], [8] [8], [9] [9]. Values may vary depending upon heat treatment and processing.

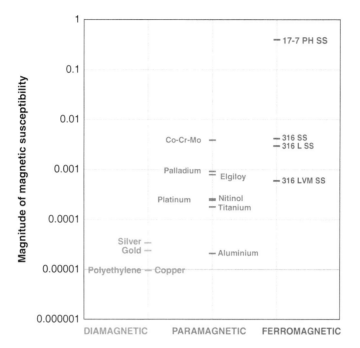

Figure 9.2   Magnitude of magnetic susceptibility for implant materials. Note that the susceptibility of diamagnetic materials is negative.

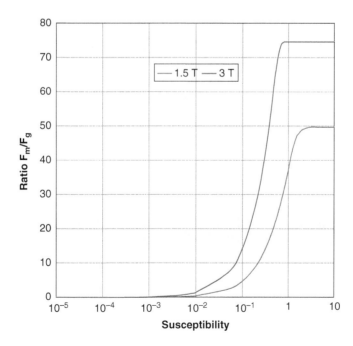

Figure 9.3   Ratio of the maximum magnetic translational force to gravitational force for a spherical object of density 8000 kg m^{-3} (similar to stainless steel) versus magnetic susceptibility for 1.5 and 3 T magnets with dB/dz of 5 and 7.5 T m^{-1}. The object saturates at 1 T. Simulation for illustration only.

Example 9.2   Translation force on a paramagnetic stent

If the patient above passes through a spatial gradient dB/dz of 5 Tm^{-1} where B = 2 T what is the maximum translational force on the stent?

From Equation 2.10

$$F = \frac{\chi}{\mu_0} V B_0 \frac{dB}{dz} = \frac{1}{4\pi \times 10^{-7}} \times 0.000245 \times 3.1 \times 10^{-9} \times 2 \times 5 = 6.0 \times 10^{-6} N.$$

This is still negligible compared to the force due to gravity but 180 times greater than the torque.

Ferromagnetic materials

For strongly ferromagnetic objects where $\chi \gg 1$ (e.g. nickel, 405 stainless steel), the value of magnetic susceptibility becomes irrelevant; the shape of the object is more important as the scanner bore is approached. If the metal is saturated, as is likely close to the bore entrance the forces become dependent simply upon the value of the fringe field gradient dB/dz. This is the field property used in the American Society for Testing and Materials (ASTM) device testing and conditions [10]. Once fully inside the bore, there is no further attractive force as dB/dz becomes zero- but there the torque from B_0 will be at its maximum value. The object is likely to become saturated before it enters the bore, so the maximum level of torque may even occur outside the magnet (see Figure 2.15).

MYTHBUSTER:

The translational or projectile magnetic force within the bore of the scanner is very low and is zero at the iso-center. A spatial gradient is required to produce the force. Conversely magnetic torque is at a maximum within the bore.

Example 9.3   Ferromagnetic aneurysm clip

A patient with a ferromagnetic aneurysm clip of length 10 mm is introduced into a 1.5 T MRI scanner passing through a 3 Tm^{-1} spatial gradient. Which force will be the stronger, the twisting force or the translational force?

For simplicity (this may not be true) assume that the clip is aligned at the at the worst-case angle and saturates at 1.5 T. The maximum force from the torque T about a central point of rotation is

$$F_{torque} = \frac{T}{l}$$

The ratio of the force from the torque to the translational force is (from Table 9.2)

$$F_{trans} / F_{torque} = 4l \frac{dB}{dz} \Big/ B_{sat} = 0.04 \times \frac{3}{1.5} = 0.08$$

The force from the torque will be 12 times that from translation. This is postulated as the cause in a case of an aneurysm clip related fatality [11].

"Weakly ferromagnetic" materials

Stainless steel (SS) deserves a special mention. It comes in two major types: austenitic and martensitic. Martensitic stainless steels are strongly ferromagnetic; devices or surgical instruments made from these are likely to be MR Unsafe. This includes the 400 series of steels and PH17-7 sometimes used in older implants. Austenitic stainless steels are usually considered to be "non-ferromagnetic". In reality they are weakly ferromagnetic. The degree of ferromagnetism depends upon the crystalline structure of the metal which is determined by the method of its formation and fabrication. Different heating, cooling and machining processes can result in different magnetic properties. For example, 316 (and its L and LVM versions) "surgical" SS is austenitic but may contain small amounts of martensite impurities which will exhibit ferromagnetic behavior, but with only a small effect in relation to the bulk susceptibility of the metal. The tiny domains of martensite can saturate, albeit with very low saturation fields. Saturation can also be partial, not covering the whole of the object. The values given in Table 9.3 for the steels are indicative only, and may vary by batch, supplier, and history.

Figure 9.4 shows the ratio of magnetic to gravitational force at 3 T and 7.5 T m^{-1} on spheres of equal mass composed from various materials commonly used in implants. With the exception of 316 SS the magnetic force on the objects is less than gravity. This is usually taken as an indication of safety in the MR environment, although elongated objects may exhibit greater force. 17-7 PH stainless steel has a minimum susceptibility of 0.4, enough under the conditions of Figure 9.4 to result in a force 30–40 times gravity depending upon its shape.

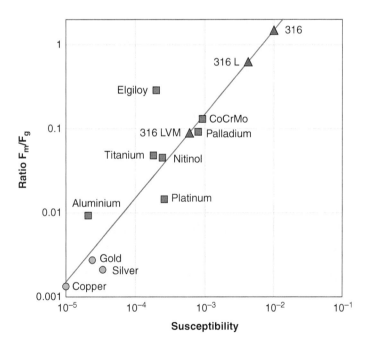

Figure 9.4   Ratio of the magnetic translational force to gravitational force for spherical objects composed of materials commonly used in implants for B_0 =3T with dB/dz=7.5T m^{-1}. The red line is for a spherical object of density 8000 kg m^{-3} as in Figure 9.3.

Example 9.4   Saturation of stainless steel

What value of external B_0 would be required to saturate a passive implant made from 316 LVM stainless steel?
  B within the device is given by

$$B_{int} = \chi B_0$$

Using $\chi = 0.0006$ and $B_{sat} = 0.001$ T

$$B_0 = \frac{B_s}{\chi} = \frac{0.001}{0.0006} = 1.67 \, T$$

The metal will not saturate in a 1.5 T scanner, but will saturate in a 3 T scanner. This is good for MR safety at 3 T as the maximum force will be limited above 1.67 T, depending only upon dB/dz.

Magnetic forces due to motion

Lenz's Law was considered in Chapter 2. This force produced in *any* metal originates from electromagnetic (Faraday) induction arising from motion within the static field spatial gradient which, in turn, generates eddy currents with a magnetic field that opposes the change in B_0. The strength of the opposing field is proportional to:

- The induced current density J
- Velocity v
- The material's electrical conductivity σ
- Object size
- The magnitude of dB/dz.

Table 9.3 shows values of electrical conductivity for various materials. Those with high conductivity will exhibit the greatest force: e.g. aluminium, copper, and gold. Titanium, Elgiloy, and Nitinol have lower conductivities and will be less affected.

  How big a problem is this? It has been evaluated for artificial heart valves [12,13] but the Lenz force on a moving valve is less than the typical force from a beating heart of around 7 N [14]. Examples 9.5 and 9.6 illustrate the forces with simple models of an orthopedic implant. As the examples show, it is unlikely to be problem. The very outcome of the tilting aluminium or copper sheet experiment informs us that the Lenz's forces from movement are likely to be significantly less than the gravitational force[1].

---

[1] You may ask why the tilting aluminium or copper plate experiment works at all when dB/dz within the bore is zero or negligible? The answer is that it is the rate of change of magnetic *flux* that induces the current. Flux is proportional to the area of the object which effectively changes as the angle to B_0 changes. This effect could also be present in a metallic heart valve as its orientation to B_0 changes in opening and closing.

Example 9.5   Lenz force on an orthopedic implant

What is the maximum current density induced the shaft of a Co-Cr-Mo hip joint replacement of diameter = 22 mm, length = 120 mm, and parallel to B_0 if the MR couch speed is 50 mm s^{-1} and the maximum spatial gradient is 5 Tm^{-1}? What is the equivalent magnetic dipole moment resulting from the motion and the repulsive force?

The conductivity of Co-Cr-Mo is 14×10^6 S m^{-1}. From Equation 2.25 the maximum current density will occur on the surface of the shaft as

$$J_{max} = v\sigma \frac{r}{2}\frac{dB}{dz}$$

$$= 0.5 \times 0.05 \times 14 \times 10^6 \times \frac{0.022}{2} \times 5 = 19{,}250 \, A m^{-2}$$

To estimate the magnetic moment we need to consider the electrical current around an equivalent circuit. This is obtained from the average current density divided by the cross-sectional area available for current flow.

The average J occurs for the average radius which is $\pi r/4$. The average current path will also occur at this radius and is $\pi^2 r/2$. The effective cross-sectional area is the volume divided by the current path

$$Area = \frac{\pi r^2 d}{\pi^2 r/2} = 2rd/\pi = 2 \times 0.011 \times 0.12/\pi = 0.00084 \, m^2$$

So the induced current will be

$$I = \pi/4 \times 19250 \times 0.00084 = 12.7 \, A$$

For simplicity assume I flows in a loop with radius $\pi r/4$ (an overestimation), the magnetic moment (Equation A1.8) will be

$$m = I\pi \left(\frac{\pi r}{4}\right)^2 = 12.7 \times \pi \times \left(\frac{\pi \times 0.011}{4}\right)^2 = 0.003 \, A m^2$$

and the force is

$$F_z = m\frac{dB}{dz} = 0.003 \times 5 = 0.015 \, N$$

The force due to gravity is
$$F_g = g\rho V = 9.8 \times 8400 \times \pi \times 0.011^2 \times 0.12 = 3.76 \, N$$
This is around 250 times greater than the Lenz's Law force.

Example 9.6   Torque from Lenz's effect

What is the force resulting from magnetic torque caused by motion on the implant in the previous example at angle of 30° to B_0?

The torque is (Equation 2.14):

$$T = mB\sin\theta$$

This has a maximum around the bore entrance as in Example 9.5. *Let us assume B = 1.5 T (from a 3 T scanner). The torque will be*

$$T = 0.003 \times 1.5 \times 0.5 = 0.0022 \, N\,m$$

With a twisting force of

$$F_{Lenz} = \frac{0.0022}{0.06} = 0.037 \, N$$

This is around one hundredth of the gravitational force (3.76 N).

MYTHBUSTER:

The forces due to Lenz's law on large metallic implants are generally negligible up to 3T at normal MR couch velocities.

Induction

Induction from movement of the implant through dB/dz can result in surprisingly large eddy currents of several amperes from a maximum dB/dt of the order of 0.25 T s^{-1} (see Example 9.5). Induced eddy currents from the gradients will be more than two orders of magnitude greater. This could have three consequences: electrical excitation or shock, vibration and heat generation.

Induced electric fields

As Example 9.7 shows the electric fields and hence induced voltages are relatively small. This result follows directly from Maxwell's equations (Chapter 2 and Appendix 1). For the RF B$_1$ field, the rate of change dB/dt is much greater (see Example 9.8) and Figure 9.5. However, the nervous system is electrically insensitive to stimulation from high frequency fields, and the only concern will be heating of the implant and adjacent tissue.

Example 9.7   Induced E in a hip implant

Estimate the peak induced electric field in the ball of a titanium hip replacement of radius 12 mm situated 15 cm from the iso-center experiencing a 50 mTm^{-1} gradient with rise time 0.3 ms.

Neglecting "concomitant gradients" (See Appendix 1) and the inductance of the object, the B$_z$ amplitude of the gradient is

$$B = 0.15 \times 50 \times 10^{-3} = 0.0075 \, T$$

$$dB / dt = 25 Ts^{-1}.$$

The maximum induced E-field is (Equation 2.23)

$$E = \frac{0.012}{2} \times 25 = 0.15 \, V m^{-1}$$

This is less that the peripheral nerve stimulation threshold of around 1 V m^{-1}. In practice the inductance of the metal object will reduce E further.

Example 9.8   dB/dt from the RF transmission

What dB/dt is produced by B$_1$ of amplitude 10 µT at 128 MHz (3 T)?

$$\left|\frac{dB_1}{dt}\right| = \left|\frac{d}{dt}(B_1 \cos \omega t)\right| = 2\pi f B_1$$

$$= 2 \times \pi \times 128 \times 10^6 \times 10 \times 10^{-6} = 8,042 \, Ts^{-1}.$$

Vibration

The dB/dt in an implant from the imaging gradients may be of the order of a hundred times that arising from movement within the static fringe field dB/dz. The Lenz's law twisting and translational forces will be significantly stronger – not as much as a hundred times because of the damping effect of the self-inductance of the device. The outcome of gradient activity on the

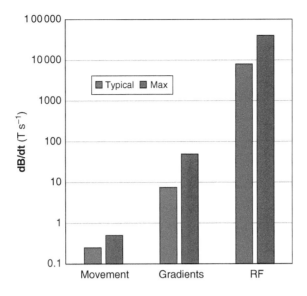

Figure 9.5   Typical and maximum values of dB/dt arising in MRI from movement within the fringe field spatial gradient, the imaging gradients, and the RF B_1 field.

implant is vibrational rather than translational motion. Mechanical factors: the strength of embedding of the implant within tissue, damping, and flexibility will also determine the amount of vibration. Significant vibration can occur for devices of greater than 10 cm in dimension, such as hip implants [13]. For higher conductivity materials the vibrational forces could equal or exceed those from gravity. Patient discomfort from induced vibration in cervical spine fixation devices has been reported [15].

MYTHBUSTER:

The greatest motion of non-ferromagnetic implants arises from vibration caused by Lenz's Law forces from induced eddy currents in the implant. This is enabled by its electrical conductivity. Low conducting materials: titanium, Nitinol, Elgiloy, will vibrate less than those with higher conductivity: Co-Cr-Mo, aluminium, copper.

Implant heating

Both the gradient activity and the RF transmission can result in the heating of implants. The physical mechanism is Faraday induction. Equation 2.27 gives the general expression which applies both to dB/dt arising from the gradients and the RF (Figure 9.5). Specific absorption rate (SAR) is proportional to:

- Electrical conductivity σ
- The inverse of density ρ
- The square of the induced electric field.

The ratio of σ/ρ is shown in Table 9.3. For the same mass, 316 series SS, Nitinol, and titanium implants will exhibit an order of magnitude less heating than other materials such as silver, gold, and cobalt-chromium-molybdenum (Co-Cr-Mo).

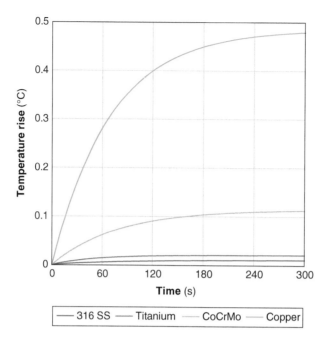

Figure 9.6 Estimated theoretical heating of metal spheres of radius 1 cm embedded in the ASTM RF heating phantom exposed to an imaging gradient dB/dt of 20 T s⁻¹ with duty cycle D of 0.1 (for the gradient rise/fall times). For illustration only.

The form of the temperature rise is shown in Figure 9.6 given mathematically by

$$\Delta T = \Delta T_f \left(1 - e^{-t/\tau}\right) \tag{9.1}$$

The temperature of the object (and the tissue in contact with it) rises rapidly at first and reaches thermal equilibrium with its surroundings when the heat generated equals the heat transferred to the surroundings. The time constant τ is determined by the mass $(=\rho V)$, specific heat capacity C of the object, its surface area A, and the heat transfer coefficient h (W m⁻² °C⁻¹). The final temperature increase ΔT_f reached is that which would occur within the time τ in the absence of cooling mechanisms:

$$\tau = \frac{\rho VC}{hA} \tag{9.2a}$$

$$\Delta T_f = \frac{\tau\, SAR}{C} \tag{9.2b}$$

Heating by the gradients

Heating of implants by the gradients is significantly less than from the RF, but not always negligible. Examples 9.9 & 9.10 and Figure 9.6, whilst limited in their scope and assumptions, illustrate the general behavior of various metals: the heating of implant materials is small or negligible with a typical gradient dB/dt of 20 T s⁻¹, but the higher conductivity metals: copper, silver, and gold, can heat up substantially in air (Figure 9.7)

In practice pulse sequences with significant gradient switching, such as echo planar imaging (EPI) and steady state free precession sequences (e.g., FIESTA, TRUFISP, B-FFE, etc.) may

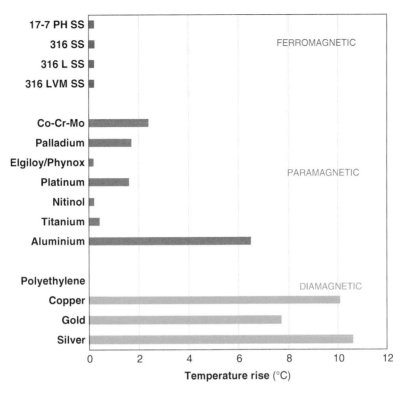

Figure 9.7 Equilibrium maximum temperature of 1 cm radius metal spheres exposed to an imaging gradient dB/dt of 20 T s⁻¹ m, duty cycle 0.1 in air. For illustration only.

contribute to implant heating. A 2 °C temperature rise in an aluminium replica of a hip implant in air has been measured, although the titanium original (with its lower electrical conductivity) did not heat up [16]. Copper objects which heated up by 10 °C in air, only achieved 1.2 °C when embedded in a saline-equivalent gel. Given the properties of metals used in the larger orthopedic implants, heating by the gradients is not expected to add a significant thermal burden.

Example 9.9   Power dissipation from the gradients

What power will be dissipated in the 10 mm radius ball of a hip implant made from Co-Cr-Mo at a location with peak dB/dt = 50 T s⁻¹ and a duty cycle D = 0.1? What if the implant was titanium?

The peak power density is

$$P_V = \sigma D \left(\frac{r}{2} \frac{dB}{dt} \right)^2$$

The average power density is 0.4 of the peak value (Equations 2.30, 2.31)

$$P_V = 0.4 \times 14 \times 10^6 \times 0.1 \times \left(\frac{0.01}{2} 50 \right)^2 = 35\,000\ W\,m^{-3}$$

To obtain the power multiply by the volume

$$P = 35\,000 \times \frac{4}{3} \times \pi \times 0.01^3 = 0.15\,W.$$

By contrast the same object made from titanium would only experience 0.026 W.

Example 9.10   Metal object suspended in air

What temperature will the Co-Cr-Mo object in Example 9.9 reach in air?
  Temperature rise is related to power per unit mass (the specific absorption rate). This is

$$SAR = \frac{P}{\frac{4}{3}\pi r^3 \rho}$$

$$= \frac{0.15}{\frac{4}{3}\pi \times 0.01^3 \times 8400} = 4.17 \ W kg^{-1}$$

The thermal conductivity κ of air is 0.026 (W m^{-1} °C^{-1}) so the heat transfer coefficient from convection will be (Equation A1.96)

$$h_{conv} = \frac{\kappa}{L} = \frac{0.026}{0.01} \times 3 = 7.8 \ W m^{-2} \ °C^{-1}$$

The final temperature increase is given by Equations 9.2a & b (the surface area of a sphere is $4\pi r^2$)

$$\Delta T_f = \frac{\rho V \ SAR}{hA} = \frac{8400 \times \frac{4}{3}\pi \times 0.01^3 \times 4.17}{7.8 \times 4 \times \pi \times 0.01^2} = 15 \ °C$$

Note that this analysis has ignored the influence of the object's inductance upon the rise time. For a full analysis see [16]. If the sphere is embedded in the ASTM RF heating phantom which has $\kappa = 0.54$ W m^{-1} °C^{-1}, the temperature increase is restricted to 0.7 °C.

RF heating

Heating of metallic implants mainly occurs from the dB_1/dt of the RF transmission pulses; the B_1 field is a rapidly time-varying magnetic field and so will induce electric fields and current densities in objects. For RF induction a number of complications arise. These include the skin effect, whereby the induced current flows mainly on the surface of the material (see Table 9.3 and section Skin depth, page 354) neglecting the influence of self-inductance, the effect of being embedded in tissue leading to local variations in B_1, the potential for the antenna effect, and the cooling mechanisms available (perfusion and thermal conduction). These make the calculation of RF heating on metallic implants extremely complex and only achievable with any degree of validity using sophisticated electromagnetic and thermal modeling.

Example 9.11   Power dissipation from B_1

What power will be dissipated in the 10 mm radius titanium ball of a hip implant in a 1.5 T scanner with peak $B_1 = 10$ µT and a duty cycle D = 0.1? This corresponds to a whole-body SAR of around 1 W kg^{-1} and a $B_{1,}$RMS of 3.2 µT.
  At 64 MHz the current is restricted to the surface by the skin effect, and the volume and mass of metal involved will be small. Assume all the current is contained within one skin depth = 40 µm (this is an approximation). This results in an average factor for power (as it is proportional to I^2 and intergrating Equation A1.85 squared) of 0.43. The power can be obtained from modifying Equation A1.80

$$P = \frac{1}{15}\pi\sigma\omega^2 B_1^2 \left\{ r^5 - (r-\delta)^5 \right\} D \times 0.43$$

$$= \frac{1}{15}\pi \times 2.5 \times 10^6 \times (2\pi \times 64 \times 10)^2 \left\{ 0.01^5 - (0.01 - 0.000040)^5 \right\} \times 0.1 \times 0.43 = 0.72 \ W$$

By way of contrast a similar device made from Co-Cr-Mo would dissipate 1.7 W. Changing the frequency to 128 MHz increases the power absorbed in the titanium to 2.0 W. Note that the simplistic assumption of a squared dependence of power (and SAR) on frequency does not hold. Full EM modeling is required to generate reliable numerical estimates.

Example 9.12   Implant heating from B_1

What final temperature is reached in Example 9.11?
  The average SAR is

$$SAR = \frac{P}{\frac{4}{3}\pi r^3 \rho} = \frac{0.72}{\frac{4}{3} \times \pi \times 0.01^3 \times 4507} = 38 \text{ W kg}^{-1}$$

The thermal conductivity κ of the phantom material is 0.54 (W m^{-1} °C^{-1}) so the heat transfer coefficient h_{conv} from convection is (Equation A1.96)

$$h_{conv} = \frac{\kappa}{L} = \frac{0.54}{0.01} \times 3 = 162 \text{ W m}^{-2} \text{ °C}^{-1}$$

The final temperature increase is given by Equation 9.2 (4πr^2 is the surface area of a sphere)

$$\Delta T_f = \frac{\rho V \, SAR}{hA} = \frac{4507 \times \frac{4}{3}\pi \times 0.01^3 \times 38}{162 \times 4 \times \pi \times 0.01^2} = 3.5 \text{ °C}$$

Without resorting to such computational heroics three general points can be made from simple "back of an envelope" estimations. Firstly, the choice of metal: those with lower conductivity will heat less. However due to the skin effect a more conductive metal will, conversely, have a higher RF resistance than for DC or low frequency currents, thus reducing the power dissipated. Why? Maxwell's equations state that the induction is of electric field, or in a wire, voltage; this will not change. Power is voltage squared, divided by resistance so the power and heating will be less than expected than when considering the DC resistance of the metal. Figure 9.8 shows the estimated maximum temperature rise for small spherical objects of various materials exposed to B_1 at 64 MHz in the ASTM phantom. A high conductivity, low permeability material will absorb more power and heat tissue more.

Once thermal equilibrium is achieved, the temperature ceases to increase even if the scan (and associated SAR) is maintained (Figure 9.9). The figure also shows the estimated (by a simplistic model) heating of a titanium object in air, with a notably higher maximum temperature rise – reaching over 40 °C *increase*. Metallic structures *not* embedded in tissue can experience very significant temperature rises. This is especially important for halo vests, external fixation devices, and stereotactic frames. The use of high conductivity, diamagnetic materials can result in extreme heating. For example, silver non-MR ECG electrodes are highly likely to result in serious RF burns (see Figure 5.11a). For fully embedded implants blood perfusion restricts the temperature increase.

MYTHBUSTER:

Low magnetic susceptibility, e.g. in diamagnetic metals, does not guarantee safety in the MR environment. Their high conductivity means they will experience more RF heating.

Secondly, the assumption that the RF field simply ends or attenuates rapidly at the edge of the coil may not be the case. Near field radiative or "virtual transmission line" effects can extend the RF fields: electric and magnetic, in tissue ([17] and Figure 2.30) significantly beyond the volume of the RF transmit coil. Whilst we can attest that neither the electrical induction nor the associated heating outside the transmitter coil volume will exceed that within the coil's volume, we cannot presume that either is negligible.

MYTHBUSTER:

The notion that the RF field attenuates rapidly beyond the extent of the transmit coil, whilst true in air, is *not* the case in tissue: the electric and magnetic fields can extend significantly beyond the volume of the transmit coil.

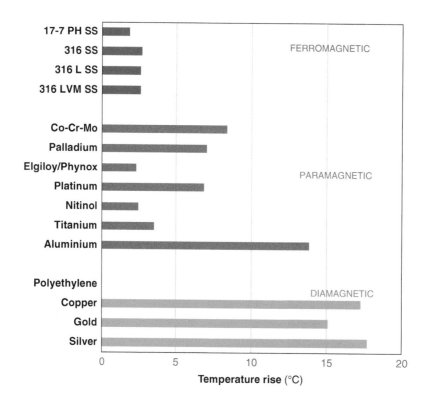

Figure 9.8 Maximum theoretical temperatures from a simplistic model of the heating of 1 cm radius sphere of various materials immersed in the ASTM RF heating phantom in a B_1 of 10 µT at 64 Hz with a duty cycle of 0.1. This is roughly equivalent to a whole-body SAR of 1 W kg^{-1}. For illustration only.

Thirdly, the antenna effect, whereby a metallic implant of around a half wavelength will greatly amplify the induction, leading to excess heating particularly at the vertices, i.e. pointed ends. We saw in Chapter 5 that half-wavelength values in tissue are not simply the oft-quoted 13 cm at 3 T and 26 cm at 1.5 T, but depend upon the dielectric constant of the surrounding tissue (Table 9.4).

MYTHBUSTER:

The use of "resonant lengths" of 13 and 26 cm at 3 T and 1.5 T may not be valid in most tissues as tissue dielectric constants differ significantly from that of water.

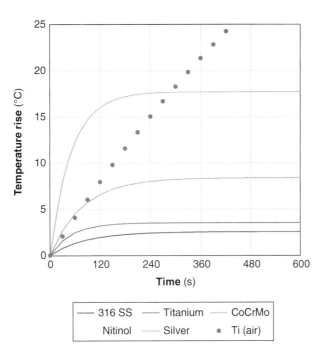

Figure 9.9 Estimated RF heating of objects made from various metals in the ASTM RF phantom for a B_1 of 10 μT at 64 Hz with a duty cycle of 0.1. An initial sharp rise is followed by a temperature plateau even although the RF remains active. For comparison, the estimated heating of the titanium object in air is shown (dotted line). For illustration only.

Table 9.4 Resonant half-wavelengths in some tissues.

Tissue	Dielectric constant ε_r		$\lambda/2$ (cm)	
	64 MHz	128 MHz	64 MHz	128 MHz
Water	84.6	84.6	25.5	12.7
Muscle	72.2	63.5	27.6	14.1
Bone (cancellous)	30.9	26.3	42.2	22.9
Bone (cortical)	16.7	14.7	57.4	30.6
Fat	13.6	12.4	63.6	32.3

Electromagnetic and thermal modeling

The only way to properly assess the heating risk of implants is either by full electromagnetic modeling or by measurement under carefully controlled conditions. Figure 9.10 shows the SAR of bilateral Co-Cr-Mo (ASTM 75) hip implants in female and male models at 64 and 128 MHz, at different locations within a birdcage body coil for a whole-body SAR of 2 W kg^{-1} [5]. Local SAR in 10 g of tissue at either the ball or shaft end of the implants ranged from 27–73 W kg^{-1} but was not necessarily greater at 128 MHz (3 T). Additionally, the maximum localized SAR was observed in the inner thigh (254 W kg^{-1}) at 64 MHz or the skin of the left arm (96.3 W kg^{-1}) at 128 MHz. These results emphasize the inherent limitations in making simplistic generalizations about RF interactions.

MYTHBUSTER:

A metallic implant will not necessarily exhibit more SAR and hence local tissue heating at 3T compared with 1.5 T.

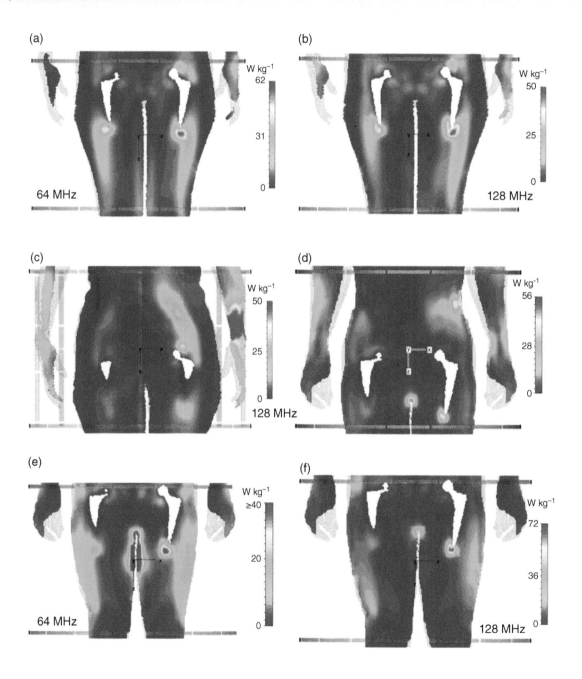

Figure 9.10   Computation of local SAR from bilateral Co-Cr-Mo hip implants at 1.5 and 3T in male and female model exposed to 2 W kg⁻¹ whole-body RF. Horizontal lines show the coil position. Top row: maximum SAR (a) female 64 MHz; (b) female 128 MHz. Middle row: SAR at joint ball (c) female 128 MHz; (d) male 128 MHz. Bottom row: SAR at tip of shaft (e) male 64 MHz; (f) male 128 MHz. Source [5]. Reproduced with permission of Wiley.

ASTM TESTING

ASTM International (formerly the American Society for Testing and Materials) has published methodologies for testing:

- The magnetic translational force: *ASTM F2052-15 for Measurement of Magnetically Induced Displacement Force on Medical Devices in the MR Environment* [10]
- The magnetic torque: *ASTM F2213-17 for Measurement of Magnetically Induced Torque on Medical Devices in the MR Environment* [18]
- RF-induced heating: *ASTM F2182-11a for Measurement of Radio Frequency Induced Heating Near Passive Implants During MRI* [19].

These are used to determine the MR conditions and labeling [20].

Translational force: ASTM F2502

The testing of a passive implant or medical device involves introducing it into the vicinity of a whole-body MRI magnet. The device is freely suspended from a fine string and is brought towards the center of the bore opening[2] to ensure that both B_0 and dB/dz act solely in the z-direction (Figure 9.11). A magnetic object will deflect from the vertical towards the bore axis. The magnetic force on the device can be calculated as

$$F_m = mg \tan \alpha \qquad\qquad (9.3)$$

A deflection angle α of less than 45° indicates that the magnetic force of attraction is less than the gravitational force. This is often taken as a criterion for MR safety, but ASTM F2052-15 does not strictly require this as an acceptance condition. The angle θ resulting from both the translational force and torque is ignored. The deflection test is simple to perform, requiring a non-magnetic jig, thread, and a protractor. Small, very light objects can be combined for greater precision; the result will be the same.

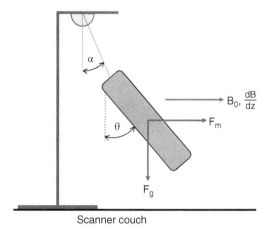

Scanner couch

Figure 9.11   ASTM 2052 deflection test [10]. The device is centred at the test position. The true deflection angle is α. Angle θ is also affected by magnetic torque.

---

[2] The test previously did not specify measurement on the bore axis.

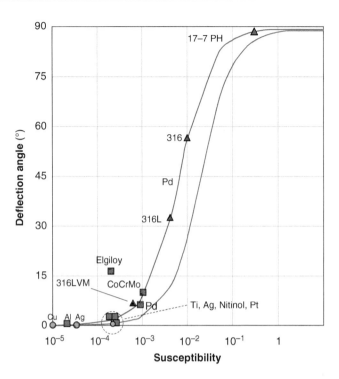

Figure 9.12 Calculated deflection angles for spheres composed of different implant materials for $B_0 = 3\,T$ and $dB/dt = 7.5\,T\,m^{-1}$ gradient. The red line corresponds to a metal with density of 8000 kg m^{-3}; the blue line is for $B_0 = 1.5\,T$, $dB/dz = 5\,T\,m^{-1}$.

Figure 9.12 shows the theoretical predictions for the deflection test conducted for two magnets: $B = 1.5\,T$, $dB/dz = 5\,T\,m^{-1}$; and $B_0 = 3\,T$, $dB/dz = 7.5\,T\,m^{-1}$. The curves are for ferromagnetic objects with a saturation field of 1 T and a density of 8000 kg m^{-1} (equivalent to steel). Also shown are the calculated deflection angles for spheres of various other metals. This is further illustrated diagrammatically in Figure 9.13 for spheres of various implant materials of equal mass for $B = 3\,T$ and $dB/dz = 10\,T\,m^{-1}$.

Limitations of the deflection test

One limitation is that no account is taken of the shape of the object. For unsaturated metals the force depends strongly upon the shape: elongated objects experiencing much greater forces when aligned with the B_z axis (Figures 2.15, 2.17). Another limitation relates to the reporting of the MR Conditions. A device can only be tested in fields up to the maximum value of B, dB/dz and the B·dB/dz product of the magnet used for testing. The new requirement that the measurements are performed on axis limits the peak values of these quantities. A mathematical extrapolation to higher field values can be applied if the deflection angle is less than 2°.

Torque: ASTM F2213

The ASTM standard for measuring magnetically induced torque is more complex, comprising five alternative methods:

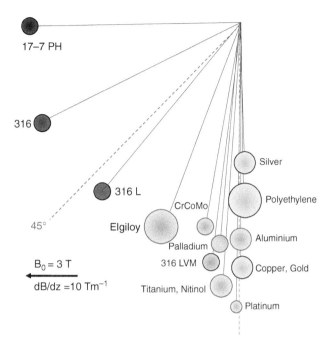

Figure 9.13   The deflection angles for spheres of various materials of equal mass in a B_0 of 3 T with dB/dz = 10 T m^{-1}. Red objects are ferromagnetic, blue – paramagnetic, and green diamagnetic (deflecting to the right).

- Suspension – suitable if the forces are less than the gravitational force
- Low friction surface – suitable if the forces are less than the gravitational force
- Torsional spring – using a torsion pendulum
- Pulley – using a low friction pulley attached to a rotating platform
- Calculation based upon the translational force test.

As the torsional spring and pulley methods require specialist apparatus they will not be described here. Typically they would only be used for objects which displayed significant rotation in simpler tests. Refer to the standard for details [18].

Suspension method

The suspension method set up is shown in Figure 9.14. The object is placed at the iso-center where the translational force is zero and the torque a maximum. Starting with the long axis of the device parallel to B_0, the object is twisted through 45° increments up to 360° noting any tendency for it to realign with the field. If none is observed the torque is negligible and no further testing is required. If there is some realignment, then the low friction surface method should be used.

Low friction surface method

In this method the device is first placed upon a low friction non-metallic surface. The surface is tilted with respect to the vertical until the object just begins to move, and the angle of elevation ϕ at which this occurs is recorded. The coefficient of friction η is calculated from

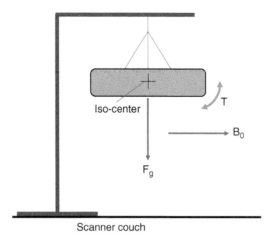

Figure 9.14   The 'suspension test' from ASTM-F2213 for magnetic torque [18]. The jig is placed as close as possible to the magnetic iso-center.

$$\eta = \tan\phi \tag{9.4}$$

The low surface plate is then placed at the magnet iso-center with the device on top, rotated in 45° increments up to 360° as before. If no realignment with B_0 is observed then the torque is less than

$$T < d\eta\,mg \tag{9.5}$$

d is the object length. If rotation within the field occurs, then one of the more sophisticated methods must be performed.

Calculation based upon measured displacement force

Using the results from the translation force test ASTM F2052 it is possible to calculate upper bounds for the magnetic torque on simple devices comprized of one material. If the saturation field B_{sat} of the device material is known the maximum torque can be estimated:

$$T_{max} = B_{sat}F_m\,/\,4\frac{dB}{dz} \tag{9.6}$$

F_m is the magnetic force calculated in Equation 9.3. If the saturation of the device material is unknown then the saturation field of iron (2.2T) is used:

$$T_{max} = 2.2F_m\,/\,4\frac{dB}{dz} \tag{9.7}$$

As for ASTM F2052 acceptance criteria are not defined, but must be included in the report along with the method used, and as appropriate: ϕ, η, B_{sat}, and the upper bound of the torque in N-m.

Radiofrequency heating of implants ASTM F2182

The ASTM standard for assessing the RF heating of passive implants is designed primarily for 1.5 and 3 T closed bore systems. The test methodology involves positioning the implant (using a non-conducting, non-metallic holder) in a realistic location within a tissue-equivalent phantom and subjecting it to RF transmission at around 2 W kg⁻¹ for 15 minutes. Fiber optic thermometer probes are positioned around the implant at locations where heating is anticipated. The temperature measurements are repeated for a further 15 minutes to ensure thermal equilibrium is reached. The measurements are repeated without the device in the phantom and the local SAR in 10g calculated from

$$SAR_{10g} = C\frac{\Delta T}{\Delta t} \tag{9.8}$$

where C is the specific heat capacity of the gel and ΔT the temperature rise over time Δt.

The dimensions of the phantom are shown in Figure 9.15. An optional "head and neck" section may be added. The standard provides detailed instructions for making the filler material: a gelled saline consisting of 1.32 g L⁻¹ sodium chloride (NaCl) and 10 g L⁻¹ polyacrylic acid (PAA) in water with a volume of 24.6 L (or 28.2 L with the optional extension). The gel has an electrical conductivity σ = 0.47 (± 10%) S m⁻¹, specific heat capacity C = 4,140 J kg⁻¹ °C, a relative permittivity ε_r = 80 (± 20), and a thermal diffusivity of 1.3×10^{-7} m² s⁻¹.

The report must contain the maximum temperature rise, the local background SAR at each probe position, the whole-body SAR, as well as the ambient conditions, scanner, and sequence details. The report must state whether SAR was calculated using calorimetry (Equation 9.8) or read out from the scanner console.

Limitations of the RF heating test

The most significant limitation of the test is the lack of perfusion cooling as occurs in the majority of tissues in the body. This means that the temperature rises measured are a worst case, unlikely to be exceeded in the body. The electrical and thermal properties of the phantom material represent an average and may not correspond exactly to the tissue in which the device is implanted. Finally, the B_1 and E distributions in the phantom may not adequately replicate those that occur in human anatomy.

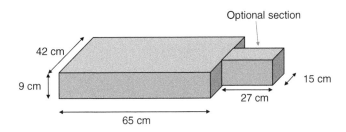

Figure 9.15   ASTM RF heating phantom as specified in ASTM F218 [19]. The 'head' section is optional.

EXAMPLES OF PASSIVE IMPLANTS

Aneurysm clips

In certain jurisdictions the scanning of patients with intracranial aneurysm clips is still considered as controversial. There have been at least two fatalities reported: one resulting from a ferromagnetic clip implanted in 1978 [11] and in 2016, a death related to a clip inserted in 1982. Example 9.3 considered the magnetic forces involved. In view of this it is essential to know the make and model of the aneurysm clip. For a clip that has been removed from its initial packaging magnetic testing is recommended prior to insertion.

Common materials used for their fabrication include the paramagnetic Elgiloy/Phynox, MP35 (nickel-chromium-cobalt alloy), titanium/titanium alloy, or weakly ferromagnetic 316 LVM stainless steel. A small minority still implanted may have 17-7 PH or 405 martensitic stainless steel which are ferromagnetic and unsafe. McFadden [21] attests that clips (McFadden Vari-Angle, Yasargil, Sundt Slim-Line, Spetzler, Surgica) made since 1980 do not contain stainless steel. Small deflection angles (<17°) have been measured for stainless steel, Elgiloy, and Phynox clips, but none for titanium or titanium alloy at 3 T [22]. At 8 T stainless steel clips deflected 50–53°, Phynox/Elgiloy 36–48°, MP35N 18–22°, and titanium-based only 5–6° [23].

The small size of the devices means that RF heating will be minimal under the specified conditions (Figure 9.16)

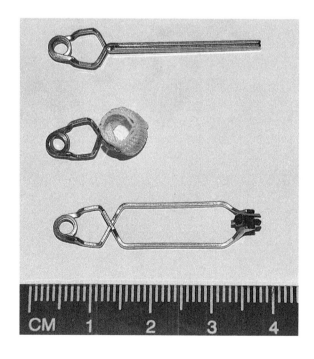

Figure 9.16 Examples of aneurysm clips (top, Codman Slim-Line Aneurysm Clip, straight, blade length 25 mm; middle, Codman Slim-Line Aneurysm Graft Clip, 5 mm diameter × 5 mm width; bottom, Codman Slim-Line Aneurysm Clip, reinforcing 30° angle, 6 mm × 18 mm. Source: Frank Shellock. Reproduced with permission.

Orthopedic implants

The vast majority of modern orthopedic devices present no significant risks during MRI. Materials used include 316 series stainless steels, Co-Cr-Mo, titanium and titanium alloys, and ceramics. Significant displacements (>45° in the deflection test) were only noted at 7 T for two devices in a ten-year review of the literature [23]. Heating was generally less than 2 °C, with only two instances of higher temperature increases: 9.2 and 5.3 °C for a Co-Cr-Mo and titanium alloy hip implant [24]. An investigation of the latest types of plates and screws made from 316 L SS (ISO 5832) and titanium alloys at 1.5 T showed deflection angles of up to 7.7° and 4.3° respectively, and heating of 0.74 and 0.43 °C [25].

Some older devices and components have been shown to be ferromagnetic, but analysis suggests that, with fixation into bone, rotation or translation is unlikely up to 3 T [27].

External fixation devices

One class of devices: frames, external fixation devices, and prosthetic limbs, is unsafe. These devices offer significant loops for induced current with the intervening tissue completing the loop (Figure 9.17). Additionally the portion of the device suspended in air can attain a higher temperature than if embedded in tissue (see Section: RF heating.). External fixation devices made from 316 L, titanium alloy, Elgiloy, and MP35N stainless steel displayed heating in a phantom of up to 2.1 and 1.1 °C for 2 W kg^{-1} at 1.5 and 3 T [28]. Figure 9.18 summarizes the results of simulations of the effect of the length of the connecting rods, the insertion depth of the fixation screws, and the type of connecting rod material used: carbon fiber, a perfect electrical conductor (PEC), and plastic glass. More heating is predicted for 64 MHz (1.5 T) and a shallow insertion depth. Carbon fiber (a very good electrical conductor with conductivity of 5.6×10^6 S m^{-1}) produced similar

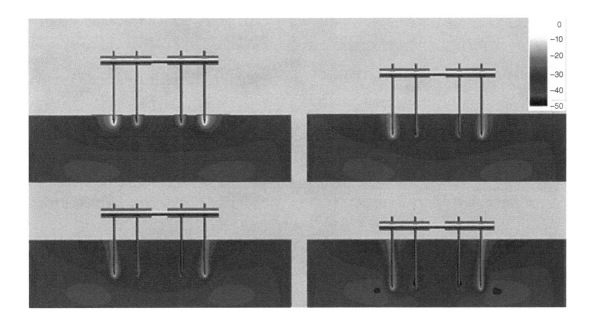

Figure 9.17   Power loss (equivalent to SAR) around external fixation device pins with different insertion depths at 1.5 T. Source [29], licensee BioMed Central Ltd.

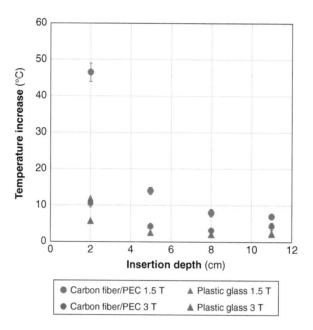

Figure 9.18   Maximum temperature increase around the external fixation device pins shown in Figure 9.17 with rods composed of different materials. PEC is 'perfect electrical conductor.' Data from [29].

heating to a pure metal; the plastic glass rods produced less heating, but still in the range 2–12 °C depending upon the insertion depth [29]. An example of an external fixation device is considered in Chapter 11.

Spinal rods and fixation devices

Spinal rods have been used since their introduction by Harrington in the 1960s to treat scoliosis in pediatric patients (Figure 9.19) [30]. Small deflection angles of less than 5° were measured at 3 T. Even at 7 T titanium-based devices deflected by less than 8°, with Co-Cr registering up to 20°, although dB/dz values were only 3.1 and 2.4 T m^{-1} respectively [31]. Heating at 7 T was less than 1 °C, even for cross-linked rods (which form a current loop). More recently magnetically activated self-extending rods have been introduced. These contain a rare earth permanent magnet which may be activated using a remote control unit, thereby removing the need for repeat surgery. In phantom experiments no activation (elongation, contraction, or rotation) was observed in a 1.5 T scanner [32]. An example of a fixation device is considered in Chapter 11.

Stents, coils, and filters

A review of mrisafety.com for intravascular coils, stents and filters revealed 250 which were MR Safe, and 544 as MR Conditional. Most coronary artery or peripheral vascular stents are made from 316L stainless steel or Nitinol, both exhibiting minimal magnetic interactions. Platinum, gold, cobalt alloy, tantalum, and MP35N are occasionally present. The practice of waiting 6–8 weeks post-implantation to allow fibrosis to anchor the stent is not supported by clinical

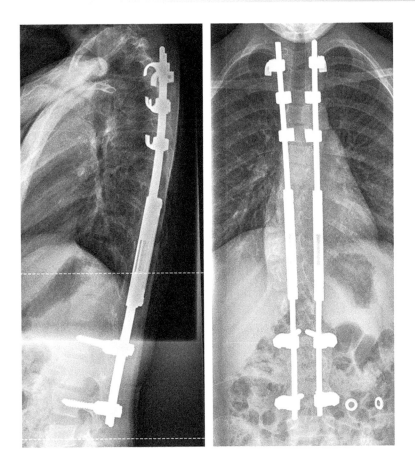

Figure 9.19   X-ray of patient with spinal rods. Source [30]. Reproduced with permission of Elsevier.

evidence [33]. Heating of 1–2° ex-vivo has been reported. Blood cooling will reduce localized tissue heating. The possibility that the dosage rate of drug-eluting stents may be altered has generally been discounted. Most aortic stents have been designated as MR Safe, but a small minority may be ferromagnetic.

Inferior vena cava (IVC) filters are generally MR Safe or Conditional. Patients with non-ferromagnetic IVC filters may be scanned any time after implantation. For the weakly ferromagnetic (stainless steel) filters, a six week period is recommended before scanning.

Older embolization coils were commonly manufactured from stainless steel. Newer ones use platinum, Nitinol, and other metal alloys. Minimal heating has been reported.

Heart valves and annuloplasty rings

Mechanical prosthetic heart valves may contain titanium alloy, MP35N, pyrolytic carbon, Elgiloy, Co-Cr alloy, Nitinol, 316 L and 316 LVM SS. Some annuloplasty rings are non-metallic. The low levels of magnetic interactions and RF heating are likely to be insignificant compared with the in-vivo forces of up to several newtons and the cooling effect of rapidly flowing blood. The influence of Lenz forces has been dismissed [12–14].

Guidewires, catheters, and leads

One important class of devices includes those which may be involved with interventional procedures: catheters, guidewires, and also electrical leads. Phantom experiments show that these are
particularly susceptible to RF heating. For those that are external to the body, the wavelength in
air must be taken into account; significant heating occurs (at 1.5 T) for air lengths of less than
60 cm or for 2.4–3 m. Insertion depths of between 13 and 40 cm (longer for fatty tissues, bone,
and lung) also display enhanced heating. Heating can be minimized by keeping the wire parallel
to B_0 and close to the z-axis. For wires that are off-center heating of up to 1.4 °C per 1 W kg^{-1}
can occur. More significant heating can occur if the patient's tissues are off-center, for example,
a temperature rise of 50 °C per W kg^{-1} at 10 cm off-axis [34].

Medicinal patches

Transdermal medicinal patches often use aluminium foil as backing. With its high electrical
conductivity the foil may heat up significantly within the RF field, possibly causing skin burns or
altering the dosage rate of the medicine. In the case of the pain-relieving opiate Fentanyl a serious overdose could occur. Patches with metal foil backing should be removed prior to
scanning.

Other devices

A number of devices may contain magnets and are unsafe. These include ocular implants, and
tissue expanders. Some penile implants have exhibited significant magnetic deflections.

Tattoos, piercings, cosmetics, and clothing

Tattoo ink may contain iron oxide or other conductive materials which may experience RF heating. Caution is advised when scanning, and some centers apply a cold compress to the relevant
area as a precaution.

Body piercing jewellery is commonly made from 316 L stainless steel. It is recommended that
all piercings are removed prior to entering the MR environment. If this is not possible the items
can be tested using a small hand-held magnet. Secure taping or bandaging may be required to
prevent dislodgment. Signs of excess RF heating should be monitored.

Some cosmetics contain small amounts of ferromagnetic material and can cause image artefacts [35]. Eye make-up should be removed prior to scanning. RF burns may occur from clothing
that contains metallic microfibers [36]. Silver and copper may be incorporated into the garments
for their antibacterial and odor-resisting properties. Both metals are highly conductive with thermal properties that enhance inductive heating. In this example the apparel had an electrical
resistance measured as 10Ω! In one case reported a non-metallic but heat resistant and highly
absorbent material has contributed to the occurrence of a burn [37].

ARTEFACTS

The presence any metal within or close to the imaging field-of-view will cause artefacts which
may impair the diagnostic quality of the images.

Cause of artefacts

Artefacts are caused by the disruption of the magnetic fields, usually the static or RF fields (Figure 9.20). The presence of the metal distorts B_0 changing the local resonant frequency; this can result in signal loss ("drop out") or accumulation ("pile up") and is worse for ferromagnetic objects. The B_1 RF transmit field induces electric current in the metal which will generate a field that opposes B_1 leading to signal loss. Artefacts will be worse for implants with a higher magnetic susceptibility (Figure 9.21a) and if scanned at higher B_0 (Figure 9.21b). Gradient echo sequences exhibit worse artefacts than spin echo (Figure 9.22).

Ferromagnetic objects

The artefacts from ferromagnetic materials typically involve significant geometric distortions accompanied by signal drop-out and signal pile-up sometimes exhibiting interference-like patterns (Figure 9.23) [38]. An unanticipated ferromagnetic metal artefact flags the potential for serious injury if it occurs, e.g., within the eye or brain. In such instances remove the patient slowly and calmly from the magnet. Further investigations with, for example CT, may be indicated, and a positive benefit vs risk analysis must be carried out by the radiologist before proceeding with the MR scans.

Testing for artefacts: ASTM-F2119-07

The ASTM *Standard Test Method for Evaluation of MR Image Artifacts from Passive Implants* [39] involves scanning the device along with a non-magnetic reference object (e.g. a nylon rod) in a bath of weak paramagnetic solution of copper sulphate ($CuSO_4$), manganese chloride ($MnCl_2$), or nickel chloride ($NiCl_2$). Both spin echo and gradient echo sequences are used. The device is scanned in up to three orthogonal orientations, each repeated with a swapping of the phase and frequency encode directions. The artefact is characterized by the largest measured dimension of the artefact region. The images in Figures 9.21 are typical (although are without the reference object).

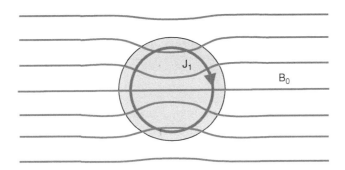

Figure 9.20   The magnetic susceptibility of the object distorts the B_0 field lines changing the local Larmor frequency and causing geometric distortions in the image. The RF B_1 transmit field induces current density J_1 in the metal; this generates a time-varying magnetic field that opposes B_1.

220

(a)

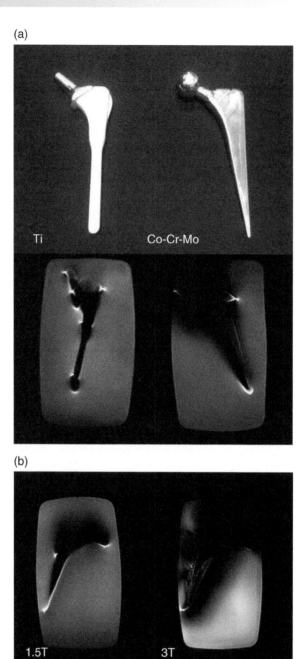

(b)

Figure 9.21   (a) Titanium and Co-Cr-Mo hip implants and corresponding gradient echo images from the ASTM-F2119 artefacts test; (b) the influence of field strength on image artefacts. Courtesy of Charing Cross Hospital, London.

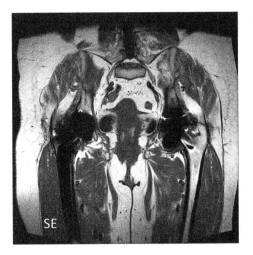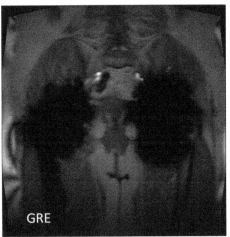

Figure 9.22   MR artefacts from bilateral MR conditional Co-Cr-Mo hip implants from a 1.5 T scanner with spin echo (left) and gradient echo (right). Courtesy of Charing Cross Hospital, London.

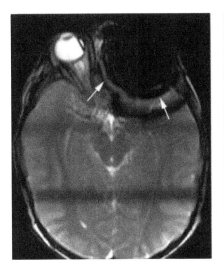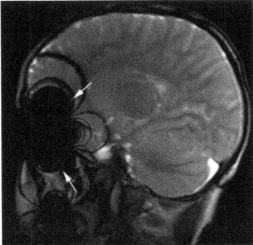

Figure 9.23   Artefact from a ferromagnetic object in the eye. Source [38]. Used with permission of Elsevier.

CONCLUSIONS

This chapter has reviewed the essential interactions of the scanner's magnetic fields with passive implants. For *unsaturated* materials, including diamagnetic, paramagnetic, and weakly ferromagnetic metals, the magnetic displacement force is proportional to:

- the magnetic susceptibility of the object χ
- the value of static magnetic field B_0
- the value of spatial gradient of $B_0 - dB/dz$
- the size, shape, and orientation of the device.

The field-gradient product is the key scanner parameter in determining MR safety.

For *saturated* ferromagnetic objects the magnetic force depends primarily upon the spatial gradient dB/dz, size, and orientation. The key scanner parameter for determining safety is the fringe field spatial gradient dB/dz. You should be familiar with the field and spatial gradient data and plots for the scanners you work with. This information must be supplied by the equipment manufacturer (see Chapter 11). Magnetic torque is small for diamagnetic and paramagnetic materials, but is proportional to the square of the magnetic field B_0^2. The torque is maximal within the bore of the scanner.

Devices made from diamagnetic and paramagnetic materials exhibit minimal magnetic force and torque, including:

- copper
- silver
- gold
- plastics
- platinum
- titanium
- Nitinol
- Elgiloy (Phynox)
- cobalt-chromium-molybdenum.

Martensitic stainless steels are ferromagnetic and always unsafe in the MR environment; austenitic "non-ferromagnetic" stainless steels are weakly ferromagnetic and may exhibit forces approaching or exceeding their weight under gravity.

Metals with lower conductivity: titanium, Nitinol, Elgiloy/Phynox, and 316 stainless steels, exhibit less induction resulting in less Lenz effect resistance to movement, and less RF heating. Figure 9.24 summarizes the properties of implant metals: those with high susceptibility (to the

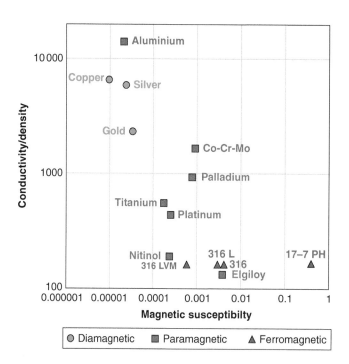

Figure 9.24 Key MRI safety-related properties for metals used in implants. A combination of low susceptibility and conductivity is best.

right) present most risk for translation and torque; those with high conductivity and low suscep-tibility (towards the top left corner) are more likely to experience RF heating.

   The potential for RF heating of tissue around an implant is a real hazard, particularly for objects with dimensions of a half wavelength in tissue. Rules-of-thumb commonly cited for reso-nant lengths do not necessarily apply in tissue. Similarly plots of the B_1 RF field outside the transmit coil volume are *not* an accurate indication of the RF magnetic and electric fields in tissue which can extend well beyond the coil dimensions. Simplistic assumptions about RF behavior are often erroneous!

   The MR Conditions are derived from the various ASTM standard tests. Patient safety is best ensured by scanning within the conditions. Chapter 11 will consider the MR Conditions for specific implants.

Revision questions

1. Which of the following may present a hazard in the scanning of patients with passive implants?
    A. Vibration
    B. RF heating
    C. Magnetic displacement force
    D. Magnetic torque
    E. All of the above.
2. The magnetic translational force for a strongly saturated ferromagnetic object depends upon:
    A. The magnetic field B_0
    B. The static fringe field spatial gradient dB/dz
    C. The object's magnetic susceptibly χ
    D. The shape of the object
    E. All of the above.
3. Which of the following is true? The magnetic torque
    A. Depends upon the static field spatial gradient dB/dz
    B. Depends upon the square of B_0
    C. Is zero at the magnet iso-center
    D. Depends upon the field-gradient product B·dB/dz
    E. Is negligible near the scanner's bore entrance.
4. Which of the following is ferromagnetic?
    A. Nickel
    B. Nitinol (nickel-titanium alloy)
    C. Aluminium
    D. Gold
    E. Niobium-titanium.
5. Which of the following will show the greatest resistance to movement in a field gradient due to the Lenz effect?
    A. Elgiloy
    B. Stainless steel
    C. Cobalt-chromium-molybdenum alloy
    D. Copper
    E. Iron.
6. A patient with a ferromagnetic aneurysm clip is inadvertently introduced into the MR envi-ronment. The most dangerous effect is:
    A. Displacement of the clip due to Lenz's law whilst the couch is moving into the scanner
    B. Magnetic force of attraction in the fringe field gradient

C. Magnetic torque within the bore of the scanner
D. Vibration resulting from the imaging gradients activity
E. RF heating.

7. A ferromagnetic implant that saturates at 1.5 T is introduced into a 3 T scanner by accident. Compared to a 1.5 T scanner with a similar magnitude of static field spatial gradient the attractive force will be approximately:
A. Half
B. The same
C. Double
D. Quadruple
E. None of the above.

8. A non-ferromagnetic metal is introduced into a 3 T scanner by accident. Compared to a 1.5 T scanner with similar magnitude of static field spatial gradients the attractive force will be approximately:
A. Half
B. The same
C. Double
D. Quadruple
E. None of the above.

9. A patient with a non-ferromagnetic implant is introduced into a 3 T scanner. Compared to a 1.5 T scanner with a lower magnitude of static field spatial gradients the magnetic torque will be approximately:
A. The same
B. Slightly higher
C. Double
D. Quadruple
E. None of the above.

10. Which identical device made from the following will have the highest SAR?
A. Titanium
B. Platinum
C. Palladium
D. Silver
E. Nitinol.

11. A passive implant has undergone the ASTM deflection test with a deflection angle less than 45° for a maximum spatial gradient of 7.2 T m^{-1} on a 1.5 T magnet. This means that
A. The implant will deflect to an angle greater than 45° for a 3 T scanner
B. The magnetic force is less than the force due to gravity
C. Scanning the device is safe at 3 T
D. You can safely scan the device on a 1.0 T vertical bore open scanner
E. All of the above.

12. Which of the following is most likely to experience RF heating in MRI:
A. A prosthetic heart valve
B. A coronary stent
C. A cobalt–chromium hip implant
D. A titanium hip implant
E. An external limb fixation frame.

References

1. www.periodictable.com Element Collection Inc. (accessed 17 August 2019).
2. Keyser, P.T. and Jefferts, S.R. (1989). Magnetic susceptibility of some materials used for apparatus construction (at 295 K). *Review of Scientific Instruments* 60:2711–2714.

3. Schenck, J.F. (1996). The role of magnetic susceptibility in magnetic resonance imaging: MRI magnetic compatibility of the first and second kinds. *Medical Physics* 23:815–850.
4. Ho, J.C. and Shellock, F.G. (1999). Magnetic properties of Ni-Co-Cr-base Elgiloy. *Journal of Materials Science: Materials in Medicine* 10:555–60.
5. Powell, J., Papadaki, A., Hand, J., et al. (2012). Numerical simulation of SAR_{10g} induced around Co-Cr-Mo hip prostheses in situ exposed to RF fields associated with 1.5T and 3T MRI body coils. *Magnetic Resonance in Medicine* 68:960–968.
6. Suprihanto, A. (2017). Magnetic properties of austenitic stainless steel 316L and 316LVM after high temperature gas nitriding treatment. *ROTASI* 19:72–75.
7. Soekrisno, R., Suyitno, Dharmastiti, R. et al. (2015). Evaluation of hardness, wear, corrosion resistance and magnetic properties of Austenitic Stainless Steel 316LVM by means short high temperature gas nitriding. *Journal of Chemical and Pharmaceutical Research* 7:28–34.
8. Australian Stainless Steel Development Association. *Magnetic effects of stainless steels*. Brisbane: ASSDA. https://www.assda.asn.au/images/PDFs/FAQs/FAQ3.pdf (Accessed 15 July 2019).
9. Kaye, G.W.C. and Laby, T.H. (1995) *Tables of Physical and Chemical Constants and Some Mathematical Functions 16th edn*. Harlow, UK: Longman.
10. ASTM F2052-15 (2015): *Standard Test Method for Measurement of Magnetically Induced Displacement Force on Medical Devices in the Magnetic Resonance Environment*. West Conshohocken, PA: ASTM International.
11. Klucznik, R., Carrier, D., Pyka, R. et al. (1993). Placement of ferromagnetic aneurysm clip in a magnetic field with fatal outcome. *Radiology* 187:855–856.
12. Condon, B. and Hadley, D.M. (2000). Potential MR hazard to patients with metallic heart valves: the Lenz Effect. *Journal of Magnetic Resonance Imaging* 12:171–176.
13. Graf, H., Lauer, U.A, Schick, F. (2006). Eddy-current induction in extended metallic parts as a source of considerable torsional moment. *Journal of Magnetic Resonance Imaging* 23:585–590.
14. Golestanirad, L., Dlala, E., Wright, G. et al. (2012). Comprehensive analysis of Lenz Effect on the artificial heart valves during magnetic resonance imaging. *Progress In Electromagnetics Research* 128:1–17.
15. Hartwell, R.C. and Shellock, F.G. (1997). MRI of cervical fixation devices: sensation of heating caused by vibration of metallic components. *Journal of Magnetic Resonance Imaging* 7:771–772.
16. Graf, H., Steidle, G. and Schick, F. (2007). Heating of metallic implants and instruments by gradient switching in a 1.5T whole-body unit. *Journal of Magnetic Resonance Imaging* 26:1328–1333.
17. Nagy, Z., Oliver-Taylor, A., Kuehne, A. et al. (2017) Tx/Rx head coil induces less RF transmit-related heating than body coil in conductive metallic objects outside the active area of the head coil. *Frontiers in Neuroscience* 26 January 2017. https://www.frontiersin.org/articles/10.3389/fnins.2017.00015/full
18. ASTM F2213-17 (2017). *Standard Test Method for Measurement of Magnetically Induced Torque on Medical Devices in the Magnetic Resonance Environment*. West Conshohocken, PA: ASTM International.
19. ASTM F2182-11a (2011). *Standard Test Method for Measurement of Radio Frequency Induced Heating On or Near Passive Implants During Magnetic Resonance Imaging*. West Conshohocken, PA: ASTM International.
20. Food and Drug Administration (2014). *Establishing Safety and Compatibility of Passive Implants in the Magnetic Resonance (MR) Environment: Guidance for Industry and Food and Drug Administration Staff*. Silver Spring, MD:FDA.
21. Mcfadden, J.T. (2012). Magnetic resonance imaging and aneurysm clips. *Journal of Neurosurgery* 117:1–11.
22. Shellock, F.G., Tkach, J.A., Ruggieri, P.M. (2003). Aneurysm clips: evaluation of magnetic field interactions and translational attraction by use of "long-bore" and "short-bore" 3.0-T MR imaging systems. *American Journal of Neuroradiology* 24: 463–471.
23. Kangarlu, A. and Shellock, F.G. (2000). Aneurysm clips: evaluation of magnetic field interactions with an 8.0 T MR system. *Journal of Magnetic Resonance Imaging* 12:107–111.
24. Mosher, A.A., Sawyer, J.A., and Kelly, D.M. (2018). MRI safety with orthopaedic implants. *Orthopedic Clinics of North America* 49:455–463.
25. Muranaka, H. Horiguchi, T., Ueda, Y. et al (2010). Evaluation of RF heating on hip joint implant in phantom during MRI examinations. *Nippon Hoshasen Gijutsu Gakkai Zasshi* 66:725–733.
26. Zou, Y-F., Chu, B., Wang, C-B. et al. (2015). Evaluation of MR issues for the latest standard brands of orthopedic metal implants: Plates and screws. *European Journal of Radiology* 84:450–457.

27. McComb, C., Allan, D., and Condon, B. (2009). Evaluation of the translational and rotational forces acting on a highly ferromagnetic orthopedic spinal implant in magnetic resonance imaging. *Journal of Magnetic Resonance Imaging* 29:449–453.

28. Luechinger, R., Boesiger, P., and Disegi, J.A. (2007). Safety evaluation of large external fixation clamps and frames in a magnetic resonance environment. *Journal of Biomedical Materials Research B: Applied Biomaterials* 82:17–22.

29. Liu, Y., Chen, J., Shellock, F.G. et al. (2013). Computational and experimental studies of an orthopedic implant: MRI related heating at 1.5-T/64-MHz and 3-T/128-MHz. *Journal of Magnetic Resonance Imaging* 37:491–497.

30. Davis, W., Allouni, A.K., Mankad, K. et al. (2013). Modern spinal instrumentation. Part 1: normal spine implants. *Clinical Radiology* 68:64–74.

31. Tsukimura, I., Murakami, H., and Sasaki, M. (2017). Assessment of magnetic field interactions and radiofrequency-radiation-induced heating of metallic spinal implants in 7T field. *Journal of Orthopaedic Research* 35:1831–1837.

32. Budd, H.R., Stokes, O.M., Meakin, J, et al. (2016). Safety and compatibility of magnetic-controlled growing rods and magnetic resonance imaging. *European Spine Journal* 25:578–582.

33. Levine, G.N., Gomes, A.S., Arai, A.E., et al. (2007). American Heart Association Statement: Safety of magnetic resonance imaging in patients with cardiovascular devices. *Circulation* 116:2878–2891.

34. Yeung, C.J., Karmarkar, P., and McVeigh, E.R. (2007). Minimizing RF heating of conducting wires in MRI. *Magnetic Resonance in Medicine* 58:1028–1034.

35. Escher, K. and Shellock, F.G. (2013). Evaluation of MRI artifacts at 3 tesla for commonly used cosmetics. *Magnetic Resonance Imaging* 31:778–782.

36. Pietryga, J.A., Fonder, M.A., Rogg, J.M. et al. (2013). Invisible metallic microfiber in clothing presents unrecognized MRI risk for cutaneous burn. *American Journal of Neuroradiology* 34:E47–50.

37. Watari, T. and Tokuda, Y. (2018). MRI thermal burn injury: an unrecognized consequence of wearing novel, high-tech undergarments. *QJM: An International Journal of Medicine* 111:495–496.

38. Platt, A.S., Wajda, B.G., Ingram, A.D. et al. (2017). Metallic intraocular foreign body as detected by magnetic resonance imaging without complications: A case report. *American Journal of Ophthalmology Case Reports* 7:76–79.

39. ASTM F2119-07(2013.) *Standard Test Method for Evaluation of MR Image Artifacts from Passive Implants*. West Conshohocken, PA: ASTM International.

Further reading and resources

Delfino, J.G. and Woods, T.O. (2016). New developments in standards for MRI safety testing of medical devices. *Current Radiology Reports* 4:28. DOI 10.1007/s40134-016-0155-y.

Schaefers, G. and Melzer, A. (2006) Testing methods for MR safety and compatibility of medical devices, *Minimally Invasive Therapy & Allied Technologies* 15:71–75.

Shellock, F.G. (2019) *Reference Manual for Magnetic Resonance Safety, Implants, and Devices: 2019 Edition* (and subsequent years). Los Angeles, CA: Biomedical Research Publishing Group.

Smithells, C.J., Gale, W.F., and Totemeier, T.C. (2003). *Smithells Metals Reference Book*. Jordan Hill, LA: Elsevier Science & Technology. Chapter 20: Magnetic materials and their properties, pp 1254–1277.

www.MagResource.com The Villages FL: MagResource. (accessed 17 August 2019).

www.MRIsafety.com. Shellock R &D Services Inc. (accessed 17 August 2019).

10

Active implants

INTRODUCTION

An active device is one that uses "electrical energy or any source of power other than that directly generated by the human body or gravity" [1]. Not so very long ago the scanning of patients with active implanted medical devices (AIMDs) would have been inconceivable. Devices such as cardiac pacemakers (PM) and cochlear implants (CI) were absolute contraindications for MRI. The 0.5 mT designation of Zone IV or the "MR environment" is based upon the avoidance of the external magnetic field's interference with pacemaker function. Patients with *MR conditional* AIMDs can now be scanned safely, but no active devices qualify as MR safe and some remain MR unsafe. The patient's wellbeing and life may depend upon the devices functioning properly. A significant proportion of the population may have an AIMD and the modern paradigm is to make MRI accessible, so it is important to understand the hazards and how, if scanning, to minimize the risk of complications.

RISKS FROM ACTIVE IMPLANTS

The risks inherent in the MR scanning of active devices include all the risks pertinent to passive devices reviewed in Chapter 9 and summarized in Table 9.1 plus additional risks including:

- Device malfunction
- Therapeutic inhibition
- Excess stimulation
- Damage to the device
- Excessive heating of lead or electrode tips
- Loss of data or communication
- Changing of detection sensitivity
- Voltage induction
- Battery depletion.

Table 10.1 and Figure 10.1 summarize the *additional* risks and possible interactions for AIMDs in the MR environment.

Essentials of MRI Safety, First Edition. Donald W. McRobbie.
© 2020 John Wiley & Sons Ltd. Published 2020 by John Wiley & Sons Ltd.

Table 10.1   Categorization of interactions of active devices with magnetic fields. These are additional to the interactions outlined in Table 9.1.

Effect on the Device	Interaction		
	Static magnetic forces	Low frequency induction	High frequency induction
Device malfunction (including reset)	Static field B_0	Gradient dB/dt RF interference	RF dB/dt
Therapeutic inhibition	Static field B_0	Gradient dB/dt RF interference	RF dB/dt
Magnetization	Static field B_0		
Mechanical force on current carrying leads	Lorentz force		
Excess stimulation	-	Gradient dB/dt RF interference	RF dB/dt
Damage to device components	Static field B_0	Gradient dB/dt RF rectification	RF dB/dt
Battery depletion		Gradient dB/dt	
Localized heating of device or leads	-	Gradient dB/dt, duty cycle	RF frequency, amplitude, duty cycle, SAR Lead length, geometry, and position

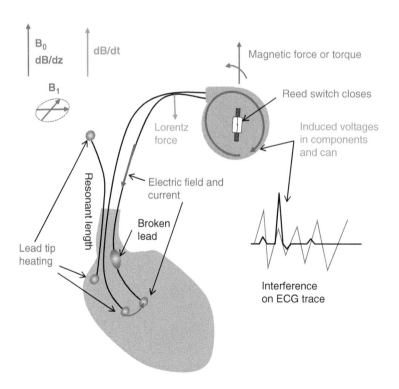

Figure 10.1   AIMD interactions in the MR scanner.

MRI accidents involving active devices

An estimated 13 deaths attributed to the MR scanning of pacemakers has been reported, six occurring in Germany from 1992–2001 on 0.5–1.5 T scanners [2]. Two serious adverse events have been reported for patients with implanted deep brain stimulator (DBS) electrodes [3,4], and from an intracranial pressure transducer [5]. In 2017 the FDA issued a warning about implanted infusion pumps following multiple injuries and deaths [6].

Static magnetic forces

All the static field-related interactions considered in Chapter 9 apply to active devices. Mechanical displacement of both cardiac pacemakers and cochlear implants has occurred [7,8]. The magnetic forces on 5/31 models of pacemakers and 11/13 implanted cardioverter defibrillators (ICDs) exceeded the gravitational force by up to five times, although pacemakers made after 1995 exhibit minimal magnetic forces [9].

Effect on reed switches

The major source of risk from B_0 is for devices which utilize a reed switch (Figure 10.2a) as the "reeds" are made from a soft ferromagnetic nickel–iron alloy which can become magnetized. The separation of the contacts when open is 0.05–0.1 mm. When an external magnet is brought close the two reed contacts become magnetized with opposite polarities, attracting each other, thereby creating an electrical contact. When the magnet is removed the contacts spring back mechanically.

Reed switches are affected by B_0: above 0.7 mT the contacts have been found to close, staying closed to around 50 mT. Above 200 mT 50% of switches tested opened as the force from B_0 exceeded that of the contacts' magnetization [9]. They also demonstrated a directionality with

(a)   (b)

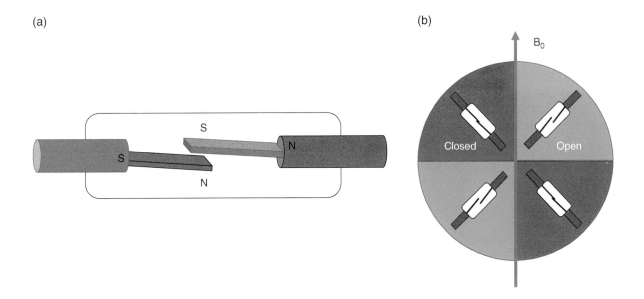

Figure 10.2   Reed switches: (a) reed contacts; (b) directional behavior in B_0.

respect to B_0, making their behavior unpredictable in the MR environment (Figure 10.2b). For 162 different pacemaker models implanted prior to 1998 reed switch activation occurred in the range 0.7–6 mT [2].

Forces on leads

The magnetic force on the leads and electrodes are minimal as these are made from non-ferromagnetic materials such as MP35N (a steel–nickel alloy) or platinum, but the Lorentz force will act upon leads as they carry electrical current within the static field. Example 10.1 shows that, in the worst-case situation of a defibrillating shock delivered within B_0, the force on the lead is significantly less than mechanical forces within the beating heart. Lead dislodgement is therefore unlikely. The electrode used for defibrillation is of helical geometry, so Lorentz forces on opposite half-turns should cancel each other.

Example 10.1   Lorentz force on an ICD lead

A 10 cm section of an MP35N alloy lead lies 90° to the B_0 direction. If the peak current during defibrillation is 2 A, what is the force on the lead in a 3 T scanner?
   The force is (Equation 2.19)

$$F = I d B_0 \sin\theta$$
$$= 2 \times 0.1 \times 3 \times 1 = 0.6 \ N$$

If the lead diameter is 1 mm, the volume of the segment is $\pi \times 0.0005^2 \times 0.1 = 7.85 \times 10^{-8} \ m^3$. The MP35N alloy has a density of 8430 kg m^{-3}; its mass = $8430 \times 7.85 \times 10^{-8} = 6.6 \times 10^{-4}$ kg or 0.66 g. The force due to gravity is 0.0065 N. The Lorentz force on the lead is nearly a hundred times greater than the gravitational force but ten times less than forces within the beating heart.

Induction from gradients' dB/dt

The use of long leads in AIMDs (e.g. pacemaker leads of 35, 42, 52, 58, 65, 85 cm) presents a significant opportunity for Faraday induction of voltages and electrical current from dB/dt. These can cause:

- Inhibition of therapy from induced voltages being misinterpreted as genuine cardiac activity or masking genuine activity
- Overstimulation causing dangerous levels of physiological stress, at worst, ventricular fibrillation, leading to cardiac arrest
- Interference with the mode of operation; e.g. initiating a power reset
- Damage to electronic components
- Heating.

Examples 10.2 and 10.3 examine the magnitude of induction. This is unlikely to result in significant heating, but it can produce spurious voltages significantly greater than the electro-cardiogram (ECG signal).

Example 10.2   Pacemaker lead induced voltage from the gradients

An excess lead length is coiled into 2 turns, radius 3 cm in the pectoral region making an angle of 15° to the z-axis. What voltage is induced voltage by dB/dt = 50 T s^{-1}?
   The area of the loop = $\pi \times 0.03^2 = 0.0028 \ m^2$ but the effective area = $\sin 15 \times 0.0028 = 0.00073$
   The induced voltage is $V = 0.00073 \times 50 \times 2 = 0.073 \ V$
   or 73 mV. This is significantly greater than the ECG signal of ≤ 10 mV.

Induction from the RF dB/dt

RF-induced fields and currents are significantly different to those from the imaging gradients because:

- B_1 is a strongly time-varying magnetic field with temporal variations in the MHz region
- B_1 rotates around the z-axis, orthogonal to B_0 and the gradients throughout the transmit coil volume
- The "wave-like" behavior and antenna effect of conductors whose length is close to an integer number of half-wavelengths in tissue.

Example 10.3   RF induction in a lead

What voltage will be induced in a 2-turn coil of radius 3 cm if B_1=10 µT in a 3 T scanner?
The peak value of B_1 is

$$B_1(t) = B_1 e^{i2\pi f_0 t}$$

$$\left|\frac{dB}{dt}\right|_{max} = |2\pi f_0 B_1|$$

$$= 2 \times \pi \times 128 \times 10^6 \times 10^{-5} = 8042 \ T\,s^{-1}$$

The turns of the lead are nearly normal to the B_1 axis, so the induced voltage is V = 0.0028 × 8042 × 2 = 45.5 V

This is 600 times the gradient-induced voltage in Example 10.2.

Examples 10.2 and 10.3 illustrate that the RF voltages induced in leads are orders of magnitude greater than from the gradients. The antenna effect (see Chapters 2 and 5) can greatly increase local SAR and heating at the electrode tips.

Measurement of lead tip heating

Phantom and in-vitro measurements

ASTM standard F2182-11a [10] for the evaluation of heating arising from an implant uses a gel with thermal properties similar to tissue. Pacemaker and ICD leads have shown temperature increases of 3–63 °C after 75 seconds of scanning [11] at 1.5 T in an isolated porcine heart, causing substantial necrosis around the lead tip. In-vivo temperature increases of 1.5–5.7 °C for PMs and up to 6.9 °C for ICDs were measured in a canine model [12], significantly less than in a phantom (≤35 °C).

Abandoned and broken leads

Abandoned leads may pose a greater heating hazard than those connected to the pulse generator. Figure 10.3 shows temperature increase measurements for leads of various lengths either connected to the PM, capped with an insulator, or left bare within the phantom gel. Except for the

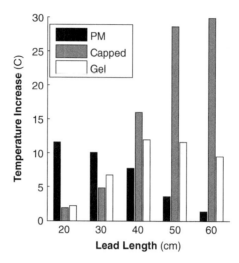

232

Figure 10.3   Capped, uncapped, and terminated PM leads and tip heating. Source [13]. Reproduced with permission of Wiley.

shortest (and not clinically relevant) leads, the PM-terminated leads exhibited less heating. The capped leads exhibited the greatest temperature rise [13]. Abandoned leads act as an open circuit, with a resonance for $\lambda/4$ [14].

Lead configuration

It is difficult to predict the extent of heating given the complexity of physical and geometric configurations possible. Figure 10.4 illustrates the measurement of local SAR and temperature from different arrangements of leads and pacemakers in a phantom for 1 W kg^{-1} whole-body SAR at 64 MHz [15]. In summary:

- A resonant length (25 cm) heats more than non-resonant (10 cm)
- Right and left implantations with geometric symmetry do not necessarily cause the same heating
- A coiled lead is not necessarily worse than a straight lead
- Connection to the pulse generator is not necessarily worse than non-connection
- Bipolar leads may heat up more than unipolar
- Insulated leads are better than bare leads.

Maximum lead tip temperature rises were 30 °C with local SAR (in 1 g of gel) up to 12 000 W kg^{-1} although, for more typical configurations, were around 1000 W kg^{-1}. These complex, often conflicting results demonstrate that making simple assumptions about the effect of RF exposure on leads is unwise.

Broken or intermittent leads present a different level of hazard. The maximum heating occurs when the induced electric field is parallel to the wire direction, with a peak E at the tip. If there is a break, then a strong E-field will develop between the ends (Figure 10.1).

In-vivo temperature measurements

With such large temperature rises shown in phantom experiments and predicted by modeling, it seems inconceivable that PM leads could be exposed to MRI without incurring thermal injury to the heart. Early studies showed temperature rises of up to 6.9 °C for a whole-body SAR of

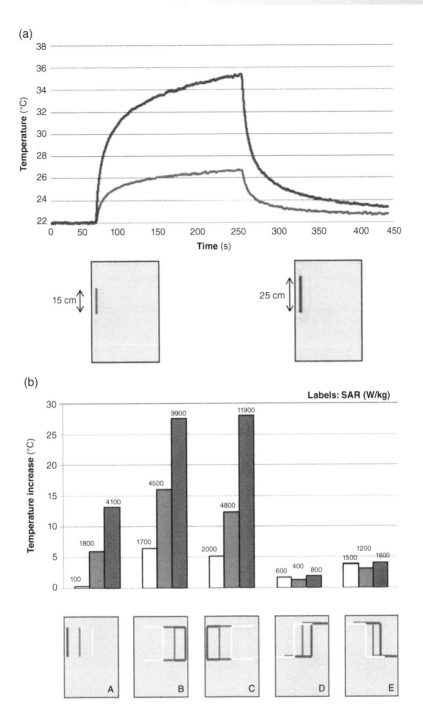

Figure 10.4   Pacemaker lead tip heating (charts) and peak local SAR (labels) from various configurations:

    a. Resonant v non-resonant length
    b. Lead position
    c. Shape and area
    d. With or without pulse generator, uni- v. bipolar leads
    e. Insulation.

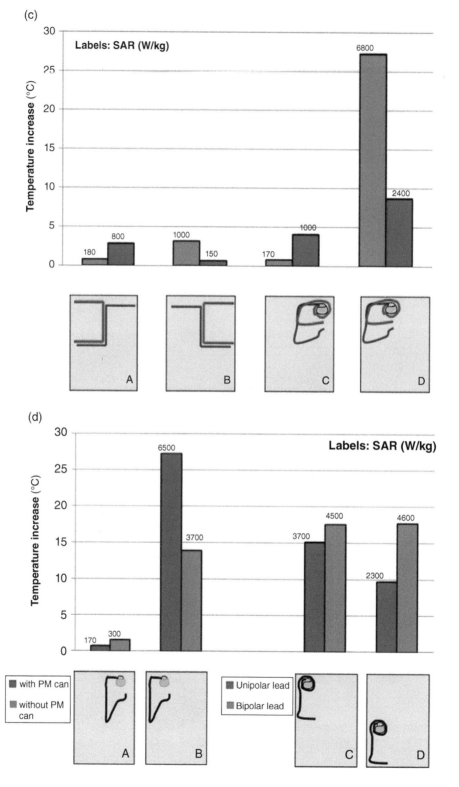

Figure 10.4   (Continued)

(e)

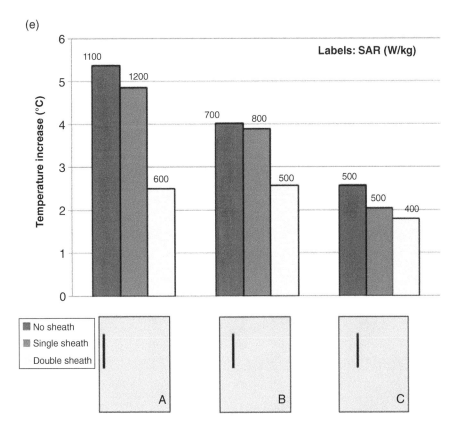

Figure 10.4   (Continued)

0.6 Wkg^{-1} [16]. On this basis, a SAR of 2 W kg^{-1} (limit of Normal Mode) would produce a 23 °C temperature rise, but the paper concluded that MR was safe for patients with pacemakers!

Nevertheless, MRI has been performed on thousands of patients both with MR conditional and other modern pacemakers and ICDs without evidence of significant thermal damage as inferred from the observation of minimal or clinically insignificant changes in pacing parameters. (See next section). A possible reason for this is that the scar tissue around the lead tip is electrically insulating with a conductivity less than 0.001 S m^{-1} compared with around 0.7 S m^{-1} for heart muscle [17] (see Example 10.4). It appears that the injury inflicted upon the heart muscle by the implantation of the lead, once fibrosis forms (after six weeks), acts as protection from further thermal injury arising from tip heating in MRI.

Example 10.4   SAR and scar tissue

Phantom experiments indicate local SAR values of 1000 W kg^{-1} in 1 gram of tissue in the ASTM phantom with electrical conductivity is 0.47 S m^{-1} for a single lead pacemaker. What is the peak SAR in scar tissue surrounding an electrode tip?

From Equation 2.27 SAR $= 0.5\dfrac{\sigma}{\rho}E^2$

Assuming equal densities, the SAR in 1 g of scar tissue is

$$SAR = \frac{0.001}{0.47} \times 1000 = 2.1W\,kg^{-1}$$

PACEMAKERS AND ICDS

Pacemakers (PM) and implanted cardioverter defibrillators (ICD) are designed to treat cardiac arrhythmias. Pacemakers use low energy electrical impulses to treat bradycardia (i.e. slow) arrhythmias and conduction blocks. ICDs treat tachycardia (fast) arrhythmias, ventricular tachycardia and fibrillation, using high energy electrical shocks. All devices consist of a pulse generator (PG) or "can" which includes a lithium battery, and leads. In addition to pacing leads an ICD has shock delivery electrodes (Figure 10.5). The PG is usually implanted in the pectoral region under the collarbone, whilst the leads are routed through the subclavian vein, superior vena cava and embedded into the right atrium (RA) or right ventricle (RV) (Figure 10.6).

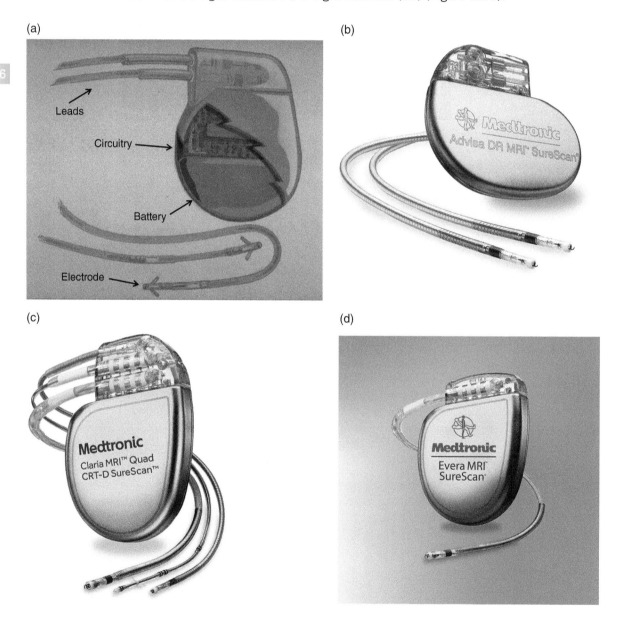

Figure 10.5   Cardiac devices: (a) Pacemaker components; (b) dual lead pacemaker; (c) cardiac resychronizaton therapy (CRT); (d) implantable cardioverter defibrillator (ICD). Reproduced with permission of Medtronic, Inc.

(a)   (b)

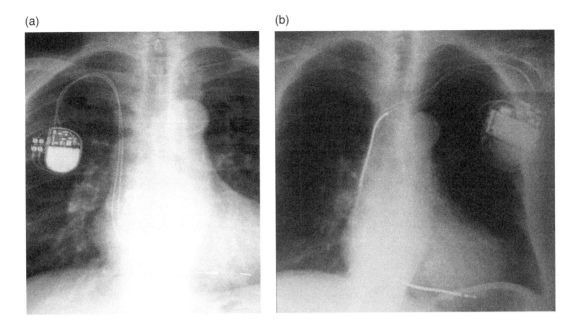

Figure 10.6   Lead placement: (a) dual chamber pacemaker; (b) ICD. Reproduced with permission of Medtronic, Inc.

Pacemakers may be:

- Single chamber, with a lead embedded in either the right atrium or ventricle
- Dual chamber, with leads in the right atrium and right ventricle
- Bi-ventricular, with leads in each ventricle and a third in a vein in the left ventricular wall, for cardiac resynchronization therapy (CRT).

They have four pacing modes:

- Asynchronous (i.e. fixed pacing)
- Single chamber synchronous (or demand mode)
- Dual chamber sequential
- Rate responsive.

Their function can be characterized by the North American and British Generic (NBG) pacemaker mode table [18] using a three to five letter code (Table 10.2). For example, a pacemaker in VOO mode provides ventricular asynchronous pacing: the ventricle is paced at a fixed rate, independent of the heart rate without the PM detecting ("sensing") intrinsic heart activity. The AOO mode is similar but with atrial pacing. OOO is a complete disabling of the device function. A key feature is the operation of the reed switch. When the switch is closed the pacemaker reverts to asynchronous mode. This feature, known as "magnet mode", is useful to temporarily suspend pacing in the presence of significant external interference. It is triggered using a small hand-held magnet external to the chest.
    ICDs have a similar coding scheme, but often a short form is used [19]:

- ICD-S: provides shocking only;
- ICD-B: bradycardia with pacing;
- ICD-T: tachy- and bradycardia, and shocking.

Table 10.2   NBG coding for pacemakers (1st three letters only).

I	II	III
Chambers paced	**Chambers sensed**	**Response to sensing**
O = None	O = None	O = None
A = Atrium	A = Atrium	T = Triggered
V = Ventricle	V = Ventricle	I = Inhibited
D = Dual (A & V)	D = Dual (A & V)	D = Dual (T & I)

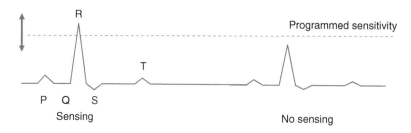

Figure 10.7   Sensing and under-sensing of the ECG waveform.

ICDs have shorter battery life, due to their requirement to deliver high energy stimuli.

A key feature of the pacemaker/ICD is the detection of the ECG signal, known as "sensing" (Figure 10.7). Under-sensing occurs when the PM does not detect intrinsic cardiac activity and carries on pacing, resulting in competitive rhythms that could cause ventricular fibrillation. Over-sensing is where the PM erroneously interprets other activity as R-waves, possibly from the detection of signals originating from muscle (EMG) or from external interference from the MR pulse sequence. Over-sensing in demand mode may inhibit pacing (Figure 10.8) [20].

The successful delivery of a pacing stimulus resulting in the depolarization and subsequent contraction of the atria or ventricles is referred to as "capture". There is a strength–duration curve for pacing (Figure 10.9) where the required stimulus, or capture threshold, is a function of the pulse duration. Shorter pulses require a higher voltage to achieve capture. Capture thresholds change over time, particularly in the six weeks post implantation, known as "lead maturation" (Figure 10.10). This is related to the fibrosis processes that form scarring around the embedded lead tip, changing its electrical impedance.

MR conditional pacemakers and ICDs

In 2007 Medtronic introduced *EnRythm*, the first MR conditional pacemaker [21]. To function safely in the MR environment, several design changes were made:

- Ferromagnetic parts were replaced
- The reed switch was replaced with a more predictable Hall effect sensor
- Additional electromagnetic interference (EMI) prevention circuitry was added to reduce induced voltages from the gradients and RF
- The leads were designed to minimize RF-induced heating
- MRI-specific programmable pacing modes were introduced.

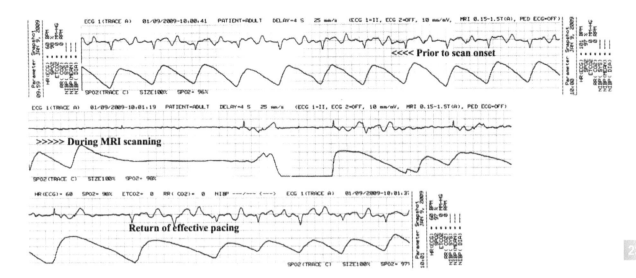

Figure 10.8 Over-sensing in demand mode during MRI due to the reed switch being open resulting in inhibition of pacing. Source [20]. Reproduced with permission of Oxford University Press.

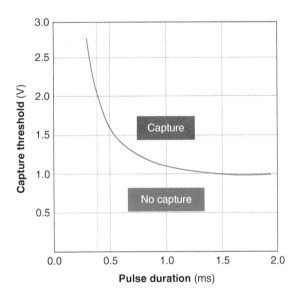

Figure 10.9 Strength-duration curve for pacing.

The MRI programmable modes offer either asynchronous pacing (AOO, VOO, DOO) or inhibit (OOO) modes and may suspend ECG data recording.

Scanning procedure

The scanning of patients with MR conditional pacemakers and ICDs can be performed safely provided appropriate procedures are in place. Firstly, the device and its leads need to be identified. The leads and pulse generator must be from the same manufacturer in order to be MR

(a)

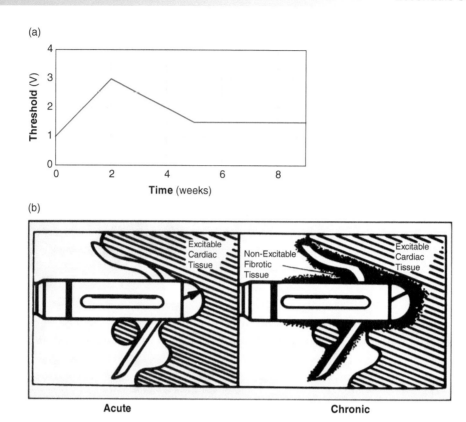

Acute   Chronic

Figure 10.10   Lead maturation: (a) change in capture (pacing) threshold over time post implantation; (b) formation of fibrosis around lead tip. Reproduced with permission of Medtronic, Inc.

conditional. There may be a number of configurations of an MR conditional generator with existing non-conditional leads that have subsequently been shown to work safely in the scanner. Check the status of the specific combination of PM and leads with the implant manufacturer. The identity of the can and the leads may be confirmed by chest X-ray if required.

Prior to its introduction into the MR environment the PM or ICD must be interrogated by a cardiac physiologist to establish the patient's cardiac characteristics and select the appropriate pacing mode. ECG sensing is disabled to avoid interference from the gradient and RF pulses. For non-PM dependent patients pacing may be disabled (OOO), whilst for PM-dependent patients the device is set to an asynchronous mode (AOO, VOO, or DOO).

During the scan the patient should be monitored using ECG, blood pressure measurement, or pulse oximetry. After the scan is completed and the patient has been removed from the MR environment the PM is interrogated again and reprogrammed by the cardiac physiologist. At all times there should be preparedness for patient rescue, with an external defibrillator available. It is helpful to work from checklists, observing written procedures that clearly identify the staff required to be present and their duties. The MR technologist/radiographer should only perform the scanning; cardiac staff are responsible for the device preparation, programming, physiological monitoring, and emergency resuscitation if required.

Complying with the conditions

It is essential to comply with the MR conditions, including static field B_0, static field spatial gradient dB/dz, and RF limits: SAR or B_{1+}RMS. Some devices have an overall scan time limit. There may be restrictions on the anatomical location of the scan, a scan exclusion zone, and on patient presentation, usually restricted to supine. Table 10.3. summarizes the MR conditions of devices on the market at the time of writing. It is essential to check for the latest published conditions for each device. Not all devices have regulatory approval in all countries. Manufacturer web addresses are given in Further reading and resources at the end of the chapter.

Contraindications

Contraindications for MRI include:

- Incompatible leads and pulse generator: the leads and PG must be MR conditional in combination, and from the same manufacturer
- PM implanted for less than six weeks
- PM implanted in sites other than the left or right pectoral region
- Previously implanted (active or abandoned) medical devices, leads, lead extenders or adaptors (Figure 10.11)
- Broken or intermittent leads
- Imaging or spectroscopy for nuclei other than hydrogen
- Patients with pacing capture thresholds greater than 2.0 V at a 0.4 ms pulse width
- Battery at end of life (EOL)
- Patient position other than supine
- Patients with fever.

If any of the above apply, the patient cannot be scanned. Even with compliance with all the conditions, there are still inherent risks: for example, competitive rhythms when in asynchronous mode, or bradycardia when in demand mode. It is essential that appropriately trained cardiology staff are present to deal with adverse events.

"Legacy" pacemakers

Recently, the scanning of so-called "legacy" pacemakers (we would call them "MR unsafe" or "non-conditional") has become more prevalent [22–24], attracting Medicare reimbursement in certain circumstances in the USA.

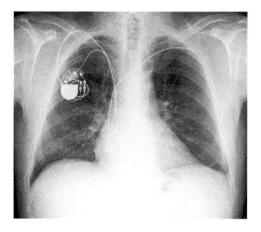

Figure 10.11   Patient pacemaker and abandoned lead. Source: Getty Images.

Table 10.3 MR conditional pacemakers and ICDs. Always check the most recent specific conditions for each device that apply in your country. Manufacturer details are given in Further reading and resources.

Manufacturer	Abbot (St Jude)	Biotronik	Boston Scientific	Medtronic	Sorin
Designation	MRI-Ready	ProMRI	ImageReady	MRI/SureScan	
Pacemakers	Accent, Assurity, Endurity CRT: Quadra Allure	Ecuro[1], Edora 8, Eluna 8, Epyra 6/8, Estella[1], Enticos 4, Enitra 8, Entovis[1], Etrinsa 6/8, Evia[1], Evity 6/8	Accolade[2], Altrua, Advantio, Essentio[2] Formio, Ingenio, Proponent[2], Vitalio CRT: Valitude[2], Visionist[2]	Advisa, Astra, Attesta, Azure, Enrhythm[3], Micra, Ensura, Revo[3], Sphera CRT: Claria, Amplia, Compia, Percepta, Serena, Solara	KORA 100, KORA 250
ICDs	Ellipse, Fortify Assura, Quadra Aussura/MP	Acticor 7, Idova 7, Iforia 5/7, Ilesto 5/7, Inlexa 3, Ilivia 7/Neo 7, Intica 5/7/Neo, Inventra 7, Iperia 5/7, Itrevia 5/7, Ilesto5/7, Lumax 740/640, Rivacor 3/5/7	Autogen, Charisma, Dynagen, Inogen, Origen, Perciva, Resonate, Vigilent	Evera, Primo, Visia	
Leads	Tendril, Durata, Optisure, Quartet, IsoFlex Optim	Safio, Solia, Setrox, Siello, Sentus, Corox, Linox, Plexa, Protego	Fineline II, Ingevity, Reliance, Acuity	CapsureFix, Novus, Sprint Quattro, Secure MRI	Beflex, VEGA, XFINE
B_0 (T)	1.5	1.5 and 3 (device and lead dependent)	1.5 3 certain models[2]	1.5 or 3	1.5
B_0 spatial gradient (T m⁻¹)	≤30	not specified	≤50	≤20 Micra ≤25	not specified
$B_{1+\text{RMS}}$ (µT)	Not specified	Not specified	Not specified	≤2.8 (3 T, inferior to C7)[4]	≤3.2 chest if BMI>23[5]
WB SAR (W kg⁻¹)	Model dependant	≤2	≤2 ≤4 Ingevity leads	≤2 Micra ≤4	≤2 ≤1.0 in chest if BMI>23[5]
Head SAR (W kg⁻¹)	≤3.2	≤3.2	≤3.2	≤3.2	≤3.2
Slew rate (T m⁻¹ s⁻¹)	≤200	≤200	≤200	≤200	≤200
Gradient amplitude (mT m⁻¹)	Not specified	Not specified	Not specified	Not specified	≤50
Thorax exclusion	no	no for most at 1.5 T yes for some at 3 T	no	Revo	KORA 100
Cummulative scan time limit	Model dependant	< 30 mins	no	no	≤40 min out of chest ≤20 min chest[5]

[1] For Evia, Entovis, Estella and Ecuro models up to incl. serial number 66237094 a maximum slew rate of 125 T m⁻¹ s⁻¹ per axis applies. [2] Accolade, Essentio, Proponent, Valitude, Visionist 1.5 T or 3 T with appropriate leads. ICDs 1.5 T only. [3] Revo, Enrhythm 1.5 T only. [4] Micra $B_{1+\text{RMS}}$ not specified. [5] KORA 250 only.

"Modern" pacemakers, said to be those manufactured after 2000 [12,20], contain less ferromagnetic components and are designed to better withstand electromagnetic interference (EMI). The ubiquity of mobile telephony and WiFi has made this essential. Consequently, such devices *may* be able to maintain limited function during scanning. Modern pacemakers do not use the reed switch for programming as this is done using RF telemetry and "magnet mode" can be overridden. The PM may incorporate alternative switching devices: Hall effect sensors or giant magneto-sensitive resistors with more predictable behavior in the magnetic field [25]. PM batteries may last 5–15 years (average 6–7) so current implanted devices are likely to be "modern". However, the leads may not be, or there may be abandoned leads from a previous device.

The MagnaSafe Registry trial performed non-thoracic 1.5 T MRI according to a strict protocol on 1000 pacemaker-dependent and non-dependent patients, and 500 non-ICD-dependent patients, with devices implanted after 2001. There were no deaths, lead failures, loss of capture during MRI, or ventricular arrhythmias. There was one ICD pulse generator failure, six instances of atrial arrhythmia, and six PM electrical resets. All adverse events were treated successfully with no harm to the patients. Decreases in P- and R-wave amplitudes occurred in less than 1% of cases. An increase in pacing voltage of >0.5 V was seen in 0.7% of PMs and 0.5% of ICDs. 3.3% of PM and 4.2% of ICD leads experienced an impedance change of 50 Ω or more [23].

Other studies have shown similar outcomes for 1.5 T scanning, including the thoracic region leading to a consensus that, provided the appropriate protocols and safety measures are in place, these patients can now be scanned, with any changes in device function being manageable [26]. Consensus statements on the MR scanning of conventional pacemakers have been made by US Heart Rhythm Society [24] and British Society of Cardiovascular Imaging in conjunction with the Royal College of Radiologists [27]. The pre-scan work-up is similar to that for MR conditional pacemakers: for PM-dependent patients reprogramming into asynchronous mode, for non-PM-dependent patients programming inhibited modes, and disabling tachycardia therapies in ICD patients [28]. Contraindications are similar as for MR conditional PMs, but they include B_0 greater than 1.5 T and PM/ICDs manufactured prior to 2000. Scanning of patients with pacemakers and ICDs is never totally without risk. The decision to scan requires risk-benefit analysis, inappropriateness of alternative imaging modalities, patient consent, staff preparedness for patient rescue, and exceptional collaboration between cardiac and imaging departments.

NEUROSTIMULATORS

Neurostimulation or neuromodulation systems commonly encountered include deep brain stimulation (DBS), spinal cord stimulation (SCS), vagus nerve stimulation (VNS), sacral nerve stimulation (SNS), and gastric electric stimulation (GES) [29–33] (Table 10.4 and Figure 10.12). Neurostimulators typically comprise three implanted components: the electrodes, extension leads, and the implanted pulse generator (IPG); with an external programming unit linked by RF telemetry or Bluetooth. The IPG cases are commonly made from titanium or titanium alloy. IPG battery life ranges from 3–10 years. Systems with rechargeable batteries can last up to fifteen years.

The risks from MRI arise mainly from induced voltage and current from the gradients and RF. These include parasitic neurostimulation and thermal injury from heat induction. Heating of neural tissue can produce reversible damage in the range 42–44 °C with irreversible damage above 45 °C. Many neurostimulators are MR unsafe. The online device database ("the list") on the website www.mrisafety.com has details of MR unsafe and conditional neurostimulation systems.

Table 10.4   Neuro-stimulation systems. References are to recent review papers.

Stimulator	For treatment of	Implantation	Stimulus duration and frequency
DBS Deep brain stimulation [29]	Parkinson's disease, essential tremor, dystonia.	*Electrodes*: thalamus, sub-thalamic nucleus or globus pallidus; *IPG*: pectoral.	2–100 Hz, typically > 90 Hz
SCS Spinal cord stimulation [30]	Chronic pain	*Electrodes*: usually thoracic spine.	400 μs pulses; 8–200 Hz; typically 40–60. High frequency stimulation: 10 kHz.
VNS Vagus nerve stimulation [31]	Epilepsy, depression	*Electrodes*; left cervical vagus; *IPG*: pectoral under collarbone.	500 μs pulses; 20–30 Hz
SNS Sacral nerve stimulation [32]	Incontinence	*Electrodes*: sacral nerve via S3 or S4 foramen; *IPG*: subcutaneously above the buttocks.	400 μs pulses; 5–50 Hz, typically ~ 15 Hz.
GES/GNS Gastric electrical/neural stimulation [33]	Gastric paresis: chronic nausea and vomiting	*Electrodes*: stomach muscle; *IPG*: abdomen.	400 μs pulses, delivered in pairs.

Deep brain stimulator (DBS)

MRI is required for accurate positioning of the electrodes using a stereotactic frame and also to verify the correct location of the electrodes post-implantation. In the two known instances of injury to DBS patients from MRI both occurred in a 1 T scanner. In one instance the IPG was disconnected with external leads [3], whilst the for the other the IPG was implanted abdominally and the body transmit coil used for a lumbar spine scan [4]. In both cases MRI was not performed in accordance with the implant manufacturer's safety guidance.

Following these incidents the implant manufacturer (Medtronic) imposed an RF limit of 0.1 W kg^{-1} head SAR (previously 0.4 W kg^{-1}) for the transmit receive (T/R) head coil only. As this limit is quite restrictive on the scan parameters it has been challenged by some authors [34]. In-vitro studies show electrode temperature increases of 1 °C per 0.045 W kg^{-1} whole-body SAR or 1.2 W kg^{-1} local SAR [35]. A more conservative increase to 0.2 W kg^{-1} for both body and head transmission on a 1.5 T scanner has been proposed for one particular device[1] [36]. EM simulations suggest 0.7–3.5 °C electrode tip heating from an average head SAR of 0.1 W kg^{-1} in accordance with the MR conditions [37].

The placement of the lead with respect to the plane of maximum B$_1$ interaction is critical. Electrode length currently is 40 cm; excess length is coiled subcutaneously around the skull burr hole, connected to an extension (usually 51 cm long but 66 and 91 cm leads are also available) and fed down to the IPG. Excess extension lead is usually coiled around or underneath the IPG can. An alternative configuration has no coiling at the burr hole site with the extension cable excess coiled at the IPG (Figure 10.13). With body coil transmit this latter configuration may produce more electrode tip heating (>25 °C) than the former (~6 °C) [38].

---

[1] Specifically the Medtronic *ActivaPC* DBS with 3389 electrodes.

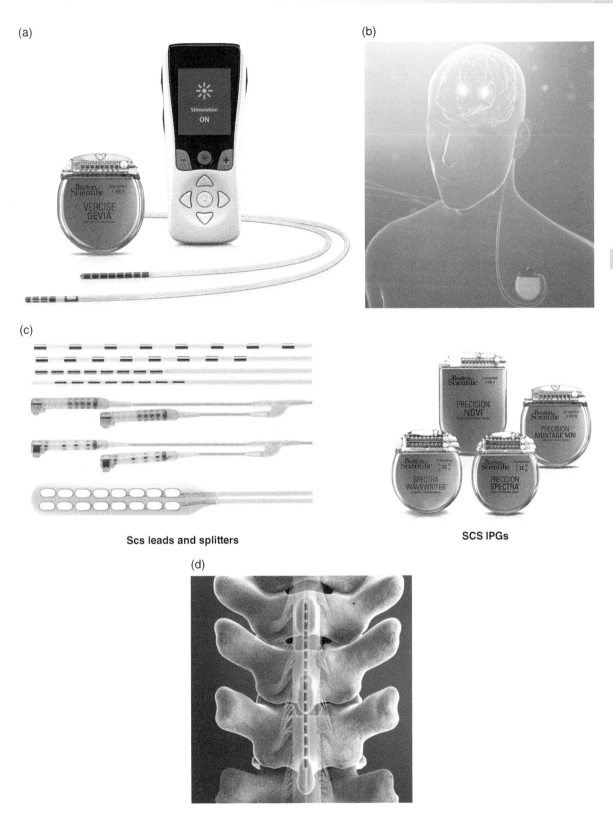

Scs leads and splitters

SCS IPGs

Figure 10.12   Neurostimulators: (a) Deep brain stimulator system; (b) DBS and lead/electrode placement; (c) spinal cord stimulator pulse generators, leads and splitters; (d) spinal cord electrode placement spinal cord. Reproduced with kind permission from Boston Scientific, Inc.

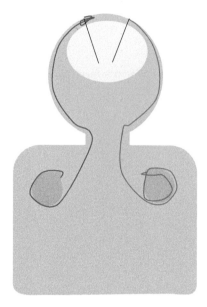

Figure 10.13   Lead/electrode configurations for DBS stimulators.

Example 10.5   DBS electrode

A DBS electrode has 25 cm of unused length. What is the difference in induced current if this is coiled into 1, 2, or 3 loops?
For 1 loop the radius will be

$$r_1 = \frac{25}{2\pi} = 4\,cm$$

The induced current will be proportional to the number of turns multiplied by the area:

$$i_1 \propto \pi \times 0.04^2 = 0.005$$

For two loops the radius is 2 cm and the current is:

$$i_2 \propto 2 \times \pi \times 0.02^2 = 0.0025$$

For three loops the radius is 1.3 cm and the current is:

$$i_2 \propto 3 \times \pi \times 0.013^2 = 0.0017$$

This is three times less than for a single loop. It is better to have more, smaller loops than fewer larger ones.

B_{1+}RMS

The introduction of B_{1+}RMS as an RF metric reduces the approximation, uncertainty, and potential error (e.g. by entering the wrong patient weight) inherent in SAR estimations (see Chapters 1 and 5). B_{1+}RMS is independent of patient size, is calibrated according to flip angle, and relates more directly to the induced fields and currents.

MR conditions

For each device follow the manufacturer's instructions. These may include:

- The anatomical location of the IPG(s) and lead/electrode configurations
- Pre-scan interrogation of the DBS system
- Absence of broken electrodes
- Output of each IPG disabled
- Post-scan interrogation/reprogramming of the DBS system.

Prior to MRI, patients should be instructed to report any unusual sensations experienced during the scan. Patients should be monitored throughout the scan visually and/or verbally.

Specific conditions

Since 2015 FDA approval has been granted for full body (i.e. using the body transmit coil) MRI for certain devices. Some DBS systems have differing MR conditions depending upon connection status of the electrodes and leads to the pulse generator. Conditions for particular models are shown in Table 10.5. Remember that not all devices have been approved as MR conditional in every country. Check the information appropriate to your location. Some DBS systems are MR unsafe. Consulting www.MRIsafety.com is a good start, but for each system you need to obtain the up-to-date conditions specified by the implant manufacturer.

MYTHBUSTER:

Different regulatory approval or MR conditions may apply in different countries. MR safety is not the same worldwide.

Other neurostimulators

Many neurostimulators are MR conditional. Some may be scanned at 3 T. Some are unsafe in the MR environment.

Vagus nerve stimulators (VNS)

Measurement of VNS electrode heating for head coil transmission has been shown as minimal (0.2 °C), but body coil exposure (whole-body SAR = 1.4 Wkg^{-1}) resulted in temperature increases in a phantom of 11.5–14.5 °C at a VNS electrode tip with the IPG attached [39]. Some MR conditional VNS systems have been safely scanned at 1.5 and 3 T using a head T/R coil [40].

The conditions may include scan exclusion zones and SAR or B_{1+}RMS limits. Pre-MRI preparation includes device interrogation, disabling output and magnet mode, and confirmation of the IPG location (e.g. between vertebrae C7–T8). Interrogation and reprogramming of the device are required post-MRI. Do not let the patient's small magnet used to control the device enter the MR environment. Some VNS systems only permit head coil transmission. Table 10.6 summarizes the conditions for some devices.

Table 10.5 MR Conditions for various deep brain stimulation systems. Always check the most recent specific conditions for each device that apply in your country. Manufacturer details are given in Further reading and resources.

Manufacturer	Abbot (St Jude)	Boston Scientific	Medtronic	
DBS system	*6660 Infinity 5* *6662 Infinity 7*	*Vercise Gevia 16 ImageReady*	*37602 Activa SC* *7428 Kinetra,* *7426 Soletra*	*37 612 Activa RC* *37 603 Activa SC* *37 601 Activa PC*
Leads	*6170, 6171, 6172, 6173* Extensions: *6371, 6372*	*2201* *2202* Extensions: *NM-3138-55*		
B_0 (T)	1.5 T closed bore[1] H imaging or spectroscopy only			
B_0 Spatial gradient (T m^{-1})	30	40	19	
Transmit coil	Head, body or extremity quadrature	Head or body quadrature	Head transmit only quadrature	Body transmit quadrature
B_{1+}RMS (µT) leads only	≤ 2.6 head coil ≤ 2.2 body coil iso-center inferior to C1: ≤ 1.3	≤ 2.0		≤ 2.0
B_{1+}RMS (µT) Full system	≤ 1.7 head coil ≤ 1.0 body coil	≤ 1.8 iso-center above T5[1]; ≤ 2.0 iso-center below T5.		≤ 2.0
SAR if B_{1+}RMS not available (W kg^{-1})	≤ 0.1	≤ 0.1	≤ 0.1	≤ 0.1
Gradient slew rate (T m^{-1} s^{-1})	200 per axis	200 per axis	200 per axis	200 per axis
Cumulative scan time (min)	30	30	No limit	30

[1] B_{1+}RMS ≤ 1.2 iso-center above T12 if *DB-2202* leads present (full system).

Spinal Cord Stimulators (SCS)

Occasional heating of the IPG, increased intensity of stimulation, lead impedance increase, and loss of telemetry have been reported from body MRI of patients with SCS systems [41]. Follow the MR conditions observing any coil or location exclusion, SAR or B_{1+}RMS limits, device preparation and reprogramming. Table 10.7 shows MR conditions for some devices. Some are MR unsafe, e.g., *Freedom 4A* (Stimwave Inc, Pompano Beach, FL USA) or *Itrel 3 Model 7425* (Medtronic, Minneapolis, MN USA).

Sacral nerve stimulators (SNS)

These may be MR conditional for head coil transmit only. Check the manufacturer's documentation for the specific conditions that apply to each model. Some are MR unsafe. (e.g. Medtronic *InterStim Twin* and some serial numbers of *InterStim 3023*). See Table 10.8.

Gastric electro-stimulators (GES)

These are MR unsafe. Possible hazards include dislodgement leading to internal injury, heating of the IPG, and overly strong stimulation [42].

Table 10.6   MR conditions for vagus nerve stimulation systems. Always check the most recent specific conditions for each device that apply in your country. Manufacturer details (LivaNova) are given in Further reading and resources.

VNS system	Aspire HC 105 Aspire SR 106 SenTiva Model 1000	Pulse Model 102, Pulse Duo Model 102R, DemiPulse Model 103, DemiPulse Duo Model 104
B_0 (T)	1.5 or 3 T closed bore, horizontal, cylindrical field	
B_0 Spatial gradient (T m^{-1})	30	
Exclusion Zone	Head or extremity T/R coil: C7–T8 Body coil: C7–L3	Head or extremity T/R coil: C7–T8
Transmit coil	Head, body, extremity	Head, extremity
B_{1+}RMS (μT)	Not specified	
SAR (W kg^{-1}) if B_{1+}RMS not available	Head 3.2 Body 2.0	Head 3.2
Gradient slew rate (T m^{-1} s^{-1})	200 per axis	
Cumulative scan time (min)	Head/extremity T/R coil: no restrictions. Body coil: 15 min in 30 min period.	No restrictions

COCHLEAR IMPLANTS

A cochlear implant (CI) is a device which stimulates the auditory nerve to replace the function of damaged hair cells [43]. They are often implanted in young children from 6–12 months. The CI consists of implanted and external components (Figure 10.14):

- Internal: the electrode array, RF receiver, and magnet to hold the external part in place
- External: microphone, speech processor, battery, and coil.

Power is supplied to the internal components by induction via the external coil.

MR conditional cochlear implants

Cochlear implants used to be an absolute contraindication for MRI unless the magnet was surgically removed prior to scanning. More recently implant manufacturers have produced devices labeled as MR conditional (Table 10.9). There is considerable variation in the extent, completeness and possible accuracy of this information, and some manufacturers have been known to publish contradictory information in the past.

The main complications in MRI arise from the magnetic force and torque on the internal magnet from B_0. To address this, manufacturers advise bandaging around the head to keep the magnet in place, often supplying a kit to achieve this. For fields above 1.5 T surgical removal of the internal magnet is generally required. For head scans ferromagnetic artefacts can be severe, potentially degrading the diagnostic value of the examination.

The external components are generally MR unsafe and must not be brought into the MR environment.

Table 10.7　MR conditions for spinal cord stimulators. Always check the most recent specific conditions for each device that apply in your country. Manufacturer details are given in Further reading and resources.

Manufacturer	Abbot (ST. Jude)	Boston Scientific	Medtronic	Nuvectra	StimWave
Designation		ImageReady	Surescan		
SCS SYSTEM	3660 Proclaim 5 Elite, 3662 Proclaim 7 Elite, 3772 Prodigy MRI, 3664 Proclaim DRG	Precision Spectra, Precision Montage	97 702, 97 712-97 716, 37 701-37 704, 37 711-37 714, 7479B, 7427N, 7424S[2]	Algovita	Freedom 8A, Freedom 4, Freedom 4A
B_0 (T)	1.5	1.5	1.5	1.5	1.5[3] or 3
B_0 Spatial gradient ($T\,m^{-1}$)	≤ 30	≤ 40	≤ 19	≤ 20	Freedom 8A ≤ 10, Freedom 4 ≤ 30
Transmit coil	3660/3662: Any. 3664/3772: Head or extremity T/R only	Spectra: Head transmit only quadrature. Montage: Any.	Head or body quadrature (depends on device)	Head only	Head or body quadrature
B_{1+RMS} (µT)		≤ 2.0 Montage[1]			
SAR ($W\,kg^{-1}$) if B_{1+RMS} not available	3660/3662 ≤ 0.8 wb (Octrode); ≤ 0.1 wb (Penta); Head/extremity T/R: normal mode. 3664/3772: normal mode	Spectra: ≤ 3.2 head. Montage: 3.2 head ≤ 2 wb Montage ≤ 0.2 wb Montage (depends on leads/IPG)	≤ 3.2 head ≤ 2 wb	≤ 3.2 head	Freedom 8A: 1.5 T: ≤ 2 wb 3 T head ≤ 2 3 T torso ≤ 0.3 Freedom 4: ≤ 2.9 wb Freedom 4A[3]: ≤ 1.0 wb
Gradient slew rate ($T\,m^{-1}\,s^{-1}$)	≤ 200 per axis	≤ 200 per axis	≤ 200 per axis	≤ 200 per axis	≤ 200 per axis
Gradient dB/dt ($T\,s^{-1}$)	Not specified	Not specified	Not specified	≤ 42	Not specified
Cumulative scan time (min)	≤ 30 min	No limit	≤ 30 min	≤ 30 min	No limit

[1] dependent upon lead configuration.
[2] Itrel 3 Model 7425 susceptible to reset and not recommended for MRI.
[3] Freedom 4A 1.5T only, SAR dependent upon stimulator implantation.

Table 10.8 MRI conditions for sacral nerve stimulators. Always check the most recent specific conditions for each device that apply in your country. Manufacturer details are given in Further reading and resources.

Manufacturer	Axonics	Medtronic
SNS system	*Neurostimulator (1101) Tined Lead (1201/2201)*	*InterStim 3023* (eligble serial nos. only), *InterStim II 3058*
B_0 (T)	1.5 or 3 T	1.5
B_0 Spatial gradient (T m^{-1})	≤ 25	≤ 19
Transmit coil	Head, body or extremity Quadrature (circular polarization)	Head only Quadrature (circular polarization)
B_{1+}RMS (μT)	1.5 T: ≤ 3.0 3 T: ≤ 1.0	Not specified
SAR (W kg^{-1}) if B_{1+}RMS not available	1.5 T: ≤ 0.85 wb 3 T: ≤ 0.6 wb Head T/R: ≤ 3.2	Head ≤ 3.2
Gradient slew rate (T m^{-1} s^{-1})	≤ 200 per axis	≤ 200 per axis
Cumulative scan time (min)	Body: 30 min Head T/R: No limit	No restrictions

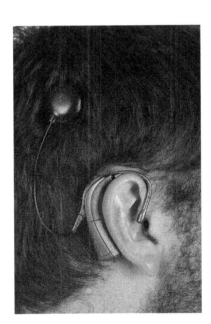

Figure 10.14 Cochlear implant external placement. Source: Elizabeth Hoffmann/ Getty Images.

Adverse events

Despite the use of bandages there are numerous reports of magnet dislodgement, polarity reversal (by flipping), and unbearable patient pain. Table 10.10 shows an adverse incidence rate of around 30% from scanning patients with CIs [44–47]. Case reports of CI dislodgement also abound [48–54]. So don't say you haven't been warned!

Table 10.9 MR conditional cochlear implants. Always check the most recent specific conditions for each device that apply in your country. Manufacturer details are given in Further reading and resources.

Manufacturer	Cochlear	Advanced Bionics	Med-EL
Cochlear Implant (internal component only)	*Nucleus C1500 series, C1422, C124REH/ RE/R series*	*HiRes 90K/90K Advantage/Ultra/ Ultra 3D*	*Concerto, Sonata, Mi1200 Synchrony[1], Mi1200 Synchrony PIN[1], Synchrony ST[1], Synchrony ABI series, Pulsar[2], C40 series[2]*
B_0 (T)	1.5[3] 3.0 (remove magnet)	1.5 3.0 (remove magnet)	0.2, 1.0, 1.5 3[1]
B_0 Spatial gradient (T m^{-1})	≤ 20	≤ 20	Not specified
B_{1+}RMS (µT)	Not specified	Not specified	Not specified
Head SAR (W kg^{-1})	≤ 1	≤ 3.2 ≤ 2.6 3 T	≤ 3.2 ≤ 1–2 landmark specific 3 T
WB SAR (W kg^{-1})	≤ 1, 1.5 T ≤ 0.5, 3 T	≤ 2 wb ≤ 3.2 head	≤ 2 ≤ 1–2 landmark specific 3 T
Gradient slew rate (T m^{-1} s^{-1})	Not specified	≤ 200	Not specified
Gradient dB/dt (T s^{-1})	Not specified	≤ 30.0 RMS ≤ 34.4 RMS *Ultra 3D* ≤ 150 peak	Not specified
Other		Remove external components	
Artefact with magnet 1.5 T	11.8–11.9 cm	4.1–6.5 cm	Not specified
Artefact without magnet 3 T	3.4–5.7 cm	1.4–3.2 cm	Not specified
Bandage required?	Yes	Yes	Yes[2]

[1] *Mi1200 Synchrony, Mi1200 Synchrony PIN, Synchrony ST* have the rotating magnet and do not require magnet removal at 3 T.
[2] *Pulsar* and *C40* series require 0.4mm bone underneath the implant to withstand magnetic forces and must not be scanned within 6 months of implantation.
[3] Since January 2020 Cochlear recommends magnet removal at 1.5 T.

Table 10.10 Adverse events involving cochlear implants and MRI. Number of events/patients in study.

B_0 (T)	Device Movement	Magnet Polarity reversal	Incomplete scan	Other	Incident rate (%)	Reference
1.5	1/14		2/14		21.4	[44]
1.5, 3	1/18	1/18	5/18		27.8	[45]
1.5	3/19	1/19	2/19		31.6	[46]
1.5	1/13	3/13		1/13[1]	30.8	[47]

[1] reduced magnet strength

Most importantly, the patient must be properly counseled prior to scanning, and a thorough risk-benefit analysis undertaken. Surgical remedies to magnet displacement can result in complications such as infection. The definition of MR conditional that the "device poses no additional risk to the patient when introduced to the MR environment under specified conditions" is hard to reconcile with cochlear implants. Some CI devices are labeled as MR unsafe (e.g. *C122M* models of the Nucleus 22 series without a removable magnet). A promising innovation is the use of a rotating magnet which will simply align with the B_0 field (see note 1 in Table 10.9).

Example 10.6   Cochlear implant magnet

The maximum torque on a small CI type magnet (diameter 12 mm, thickness 2.4mm) in a 1.5 T system is 0.2 N-m. What is the force required on a bandage to prevent movement?

$$Torque = Force \times length$$

$$F_\tau = \frac{0.2}{0.006} = 33.3\,N$$

If the magnet has a density 8000 kg m^{-3} the force due to gravity is

$$F_g = 9.8 \times \pi \times 0.006^2 \times 0.0024 \times 8000 = 0.021\,N$$

The maximum torque from a 1.5 T MR magnet is 1570 times the force from gravity. The pressure required to keep the magnet in place is

$$p = \frac{F_t}{area} = \frac{33.3}{\pi \times 0.006^2} = 295\,000\,N\,m^{-2}$$

The total force to be exerted on a 10 cm width bandage around a head of circumference 60 cm is

$$F = 295\,000 \times 0.6 \times 0.1 = 17\,700\,N$$

This is equivalent to almost two tonnes of weight. It seems unlikely that the bandage is going to be very effective! This example is originally from [55].

ENDOSCOPIC CAMERAS

Endoscopic cameras or video capsule endoscopy (VCE) systems ("pillcams") are ingestible devices that transmit endoscopic images of the gastro-intestinal (GI) tract. They are small, easily swallowed, and should be excreted normally. In rare instances they may get trapped by GI stenosis. Despite a few instances of no harm resulting from inadvertent MR scanning of patients with these devices [56], they are MR unsafe and may result in bowel injury or perforation if introduced into the MR environment. If a patient scheduled for an MRI cannot positively confirm that they have passed the device, they should contact their physician for evaluation and possible abdominal X-ray to confirm its absence prior to MRI [57].

IMPLANTABLE INFUSION PUMPS

Implantable infusion pumps or implantable drug delivery systems (IDDS) are used for the intravascular or intrathecal (into CSF) delivery of drugs: often morphine, ziconotide or fentanyl for pain relief, or baclofen to treat muscle spasticity. The use of an IDDS allows for lower dosage, controlled delivery, and patient mobility. The pump is usually implanted subcutaneously in the abdomen and the drug delivered via a catheter. Issues that may arise for these systems in MRI include:

- Heating
- Possible increased rate of drug delivery
- Delivery of the entire contents in one dose- with potentially fatal outcome

- Torque on the device
- Demagnetization of the pump magnet
- Cessation of drug delivery whilst in the MR magnet
- Delay in the restart of pumping after removal from the MR magnet.

A number of pumps are MR unsafe. Table 10.11 shows the MRI information for some MR conditional devices. There are some vital additional non-MR conditions such as emptying the device of its medicine prior to MRI, ensuring the correct orientation of the device with respect to B_0, or setting the flow rate to zero.

Before scanning, a physician must confirm that the patient can withstand cessation of the drug delivery whilst the MRI examination takes place. Afterwards they must check the patient for signs of overdosing. Staff must be prepared in the event that resuscitation or the use of drug reversal agents are required.

254 Adverse events

Between 2013–2019 there were six fatal incidents in the USA involving implantable infusion devices and MRI reported to the FDA on their MAUDE (Manufacturer and User Facility Device Experience) database. Four of these occurred as the result of drug overdose following failure to empty the device prior to MRI. One involved a full discharge from an unknown device. The sixth involved a significant device stall after MRI but the cause of death was undetermined. In view of the number reports of MR-related patient injury or death the FDA issued a statement about safety concerns regarding implantable infusion pumps in the MR environment [6].

Table 10.11   MR conditional implantable infusion systems. Always check the most recent specific conditions for each device that apply in your country. Manufacturer details are given in Further reading and resources.

Manufacturer	Codman	FlowOnix	Medtronic
Implantable infusion system	*3000[1]*	*ProMetra, ProMetra II*	*SynchroMed, SynchroMed II, SynchroMed EL, IsoMed[3]*
B_0 (T)	1.5, 3	1.5	1.5[3], 3
B_0 Spatial gradient (T m^{-1})	≤ 40	≤ 4.1 Europe conditions ≤ 19 US conditions	≤ 19
Transmit coil	any	any	any
B_{1+}RMS (μT)	not specified	not specified	not specified
SAR (W kg^{-1})	≤ 2.0 wb	≤ 2.0 wb for 10 min.	≤ 2.0 wb
Temperature increase (°C)	<6.5 after 15 min[2]	No limit	<1 after 20min, 1 W kg^{-1} 1.5 T <1.7 after 20min, 3 Wkg^{-1} 3 T for *SynchroMed EL*
Gradient slew rate (T m^{-1} s^{-1})	≤ 150 per axis	Not specified	≤ 200 per axis
Gradient dB/dt (T s^{-1})	Not specified	Not specified	≤ 20 *SynchroMed EL*
Other conditions		Empty pump	Device orientation restrictions

[1] Discontinued from April 2018
[2] Can increase flow by 50%
[3] *isoMed* 1.5 T only

MYTHBUSTER:

The most common cause of MR accident deaths in recent years is not from pacemaker malfunction or projectiles, but from drug overdosing by implantable infusion pumps, usually as a result of failure to follow the instructions for using the device in the MR environment.

KEEPING WITHIN THE CONDITIONS

Keeping within the MR conditions ensures the safe scanning of patients with active implants. It is essential to use the most current information provided by the implant manufacturer that is applicable in your country.

Static field and static field spatial gradient

Only scan patients with active devices at the static fields specified in the conditions. Do not assume that a device which is conditional at 1.5 T will be so at other, even lower, field strengths. RF induced electric field and heating may not follow a simple pattern of behavior: they may be worse at lower frequencies (lower B_0). Conditions often specify horizontal closed-bore systems only; other open or vertical field systems may interact differently with the AIMD. Active devices are more likely to contain ferromagnetic components than passive ones so always follow the dB/dz spatial gradient conditions.

Gradient slew rate and dB/dt

Most AIMDs have a slew rate (SR) condition (in $T\ m^{-1}s^{-1}$). Check whether these are per axis (the usual case) or a combined value, the so-called "effective" SR. If the condition stated is less than or equal to your scanner slew rate specification, then compliance is ensured for all sequences. Sometimes the condition is given in terms of a maximum dB/dt ($T\ s^{-1}$). This can be problematic as most scanners (except Philips) do not report this value. If the scanner has "implant mode" software it may be possible to limit dB/dt to pre-set values. If this is not available, then the selection of low acoustic noise gradients, low SAR RF pulses, longer TE or inter-echo spacing, smaller receive bandwidth (greater water-fat pixel shift), and larger fields-of-view should reduce the gradient dB/dt.

SAR and B_{1+}RMS

Restricting SAR and B_{1+}RMS to within the implant's conditions is crucial to safe scanning. For details about steps to control SAR and B_{1+}RMS see Chapter 5. In order of effectiveness the following actions should be followed:

- Use low SAR RF pulses or hyperechoes if available
- Reduce the flip angle
- Reduce the number of echoes and slices
- Increase TR.

For a given pulse sequence these changes will reduce SAR more effectively than B_{1+}RMS which is proportional to the square root of SAR. For example, halving B_{1+}RMS will reduce SAR by a factor of four for the same pulse sequence.

Be aware that different scanners use different methods to estimate SAR and there is considerable uncertainty in the scanner-reported values [58]. These are based upon simple models of the patient, e.g. as a set of cylinders of differing lengths and diameters to represent the head, body, and extremities. It is therefore good practice to allow an additional safety margin for the SAR. The SAR reported on the console also depends upon user-entered data: weight, height, and sex – so always enter these values accurately.

B_{1+}RMS is arguably a better parameter as a scan condition, as it relates more directly to induced electric fields and currents in active devices and leads. It is also independent of patient size, unlike SAR, offering more reliable control of the RF exposure. For some devices it will be easier to control B_{1+}RMS than SAR because the uncertainties around SAR often result in more stringent conditions. Example exercises in controlling SAR and B_{1+}RMS are given in Chapter 11.

Always observe any transmit coil restrictions in the conditions. Be aware that the MR safety labeling does not currently include parallel transmission, only quadrature or circular polarization. Parallel transmission can result in significant increases in the RF power induced in an implant [59]. Also observe any patient presentation conditions (e.g. supine) and scan exclusion zones. SAR conditions are sometimes dependent on the patient position.

MYTHBUSTER:

Using parallel transmission (RF shim) is contrary to the MR conditions and can result in increased SAR.

The fixed parameter option

The fixed parameter option or "FPO:basic" is a set of MR exposure parameters that have been agreed by implant manufacturers and MRI manufacturers to ensure the safety of active implants during MRI scanning. It is derived from the standard ISO/TS 10974:2018 *Assessment of the safety of magnetic resonance imaging for patients with active implants* [1]. A device labeled as FPO:B is guaranteed to function safely subject to certain pre-defined field limits on the scanner. These limits are specified in IEC60601-2-33 [60] and are detailed in Table 10.12. They apply only for 1.5 T cylindrical closed-bore whole-body scanners operating at around 64 MHz using quadrature excitation from the body coil.

Table 10.12   Field limits for the Fixed Parameter Option: basic [1, 60]

Field	Peak value	RMS value
Static field B_0 (T)	1.5	1.5
Gradient dB/dt (T s^{-1})	≤ 100	≤ 56
RF field B_{1+} (μT)	≤ 30	≤ 3.2

Active implant scanning policy

The scanning of patients with active implants will usually involve other medical disciplines: cardiology, neurology, pain management, etc. It is essential that your hospital has robust written policies and procedures for dealing with these patients. This will need to address the actions and responsibilities of each staff group from referral and booking to the discharging of the patient from the MR department. The responsibility of radiographers and MR technologists is to conduct the MRI examination safely observing all the MR conditions. However, other professionals have a major role in ensuring patient safety by interrogating, programming and reprogramming the device, checking the patient's medical condition, and responding to unanticipated device changes or patient emergencies. The use of device-specific checklists is a good way to ensure that all procedures are observed, and all safety measures taken.

257

CONCLUSIONS

The scanning of patients with active implants presents the greatest challenge in clinical MRI, often requiring an unprecedented degree of cooperation and coordination between different clinical departments. Inappropriate scanning of patients with AIMDs can result in serious injury or death. The interactions of the device with the scanner's magnetic fields include all those that are pertinent for passive devices (magnetic force and torque, vibration, heating) but also include more complex and unpredictable effects: device inhibition or overstimulation, device damage, loss of data, loss of telemetric communication, electrical reset, battery depletion, electric shock, drug overdosing or under-dosing, and localized thermal injury to vital neurological structures. These adverse events can be avoided by strict observance of the MR conditions, including those related to patient and device preparation and management.

Finally, an observation regarding the off-label scanning of devices currently labeled as unsafe, or exposure to fields in excess of the conditions. Leading experts in MRI safety have observed that small anecdotal studies (e.g. of cochlear implants, DBS systems, or pacemakers) where no harm is reported or recognized is not the same as proving safety [55,61]. Quoting from the FDA's approach to device evaluation [62]:

> "… failing to identify an adverse event is not equivalent to demonstrating safety—especially when only a limited number of patients are studied."

Appropriate levels of safety can only be established by sound basic science and large-scale clinical trials in the context of an effective regulatory framework. Justified off-label scanning of AIMDs requires significant clinical, radiological, radiographic, engineering, MR physics, and EM modeling resources. Most centers do not possess this. Rather keep to the conditions, follow strict protocols, and don't make assumptions about AIMD safety in MRI or act beyond your technical knowledge or scope of practice.

Revision questions

1. Which of the following is true regarding active implants?
   A. All active devices use electrical energy
   B. All active devices can be safely scanned in MRI
   C. All active devices contain an implanted battery
   D. Active devices are less ferromagnetic than passive devices
   E. An active device cannot be introduced into the MR environment.

2. Risks inherent in the MR scanning of active devices include:
   A. Therapeutic inhibition
   B. Excess stimulation
   C. Damage to the device
   D. Excessive heating of lead or electrode tips
   E. All of the above.

3. Active implants can be safety scanned in MRI as long as:
   A. They are outside the transmit coil volume
   B. High slew rate gradients are not used
   C. You use a transmit-receive head coil
   D. You use parallel transmit
   E. You follow the appropriate conditions.

4. In which of the following is not a contraindication for MRI with an MR conditional pacemaker?
   A. There are abandoned leads
   B. The capture threshold is less than 2 volts for a 0.4 ms pulse width
   C. Scanning in a 1 T vertical field scanner
   D. Pulse generator and leads are both MR conditional but from different manufacturers
   E. The pacemaker was implanted four weeks earlier.

5. A neurostimulator has a B_{1+}RMS condition of 2 µT. Your next pulse sequence exceeds this. To comply with the condition, you could:
   A. Increase TR
   B. Use low SAR RF pulses
   C. Increase the slice thickness
   D. Reduce flip angle
   E. Change the field of view.

6. In a horizontal bore MRI system, a deep brain stimulator extension lead is coiled under the scalp. Which lead configuration is likely to experience the least induced power from the RF?
   A. One large loop concentric with B_0, lying in an axial plane
   B. Smaller loops but with more turns concentric with B_0, lying in an axial plane
   C. One large loop orthogonal to B_0, lying in a sagittal plane
   D. Smaller loops but with more turns lying in a coronal plane
   E. They are all the same because the head SAR does not change.

7. You attended an MR safety course where a presentation showing that conventional cardiac pacemakers have been safety scanned in MRI. How does this change *your* practice?
   A. We can now scan conventional pacemakers because they are all safe
   B. No change; they are still contraindicated in MRI
   C. As long as we know the make and model, we can scan at 1.5 T
   D. We can scan them if we use the Fixed Parameter Option
   E. Scanning may be undertaken "off-label" in specialist institutions only after a positive benefit v risk analysis under a strict protocol, appropriate clinical authorization and supervision, with patient consent.

8. Since 2012 what is the major cause of death from MRI-related adverse events?
   A. Injuries from projectiles
   B. RF burns from neurostimulator electrodes
   C. Drug overdose from implantable infusion pumps
   D. Pacemaker malfunctions
   E. Organ perforation from video capsule endoscopic devices.
9. Which of the following adverse events may occur when scanning patients with cochlear implants in MRI?
   A. Internal magnet polarity reversal
   B. Magnet dislodgement
   C. Demagnetization of the internal magnet
   D. All of the above
   E. None as long as the device is MR conditional and you follow the conditions.
10. The Fixed Parameter Option:
   A. Means that all implants can be safety scanned in MRI
   B. Controls the scanner SAR to acceptable levels
   C. Applies at all scanner B_0 values
   D. Limits the RF and gradient dB/dt values to predefined values
   E. Is a special implant-friendly pulse sequence.

References

1. International Standards Organization (2018). ISO/TS 10974. *Assessment of the Safety of Magnetic Resonance Imaging for Patients with an Active Implantable Medical Device*. Geneva: ISO.
2. Irnich, W., Irnich, W., and Bartsch, C. (2005). Do we need pacemakers resistant to magnetic resonance imaging? *Europace* 7:353–365.
3. Spiegel, J., Fuss, G.F., Backens, M. et al. (2003). Transient dystonia following magnetic resonance imaging in a patient with deep brain stimulation electrodes for the treatment of Parkinson disease. Case report. *Journal of Neurosurgery* 99:772–774.
4. Henderson, J., Tkach, J., Phillips, M., et al. (2005). Permanent neurological deficit related to magnetic resonance imaging in a patient with implanted deep brain stimulation electrodes for Parkinson's Disease: Case report. *Neurosurgery* 57:E1063.
5. Tanaka, R., Yumoto, T., Shiba, N. et al. (2012). Overheated and melted intracranial pressure transducer as cause of thermal brain injury during magnetic resonance imaging: case report. *Journal of Neurosurgery* 117:1100–1109.
6. Food and Drug Administration (2017). *Safety Concerns with Implantable Infusion Pumps in the Magnetic Resonance (MR) Environment: FDA Safety Communication*. Silver Spring, MD: FDA. https://www.fda.gov/medical-devices/safety-communications/safety-concerns-implantable-infusion-pumps-magnetic-resonance-mr-environment-fda-safety (accessed 4 July 2019).
7. Nazarian, S., Hansford, R., Roguin, A. et al. (2011). A prospective evaluation of a protocol for magnetic resonance imaging of patients with implanted cardiac devices. *Annals of Internal Medicine* 155:415–410.
8. Luechinger, R., Duru, F., Scheidegger, M. et al. (2001). Force and torque effects of a 1.5-tesla MRI scanner on cardiac pacemakers and ICDs. *Pacing and Clinical Electrophysiology* 24:199–205.
9. Luechinger, R., Duru, F., Zeijlemaker, V. et al. (2002). Pacemaker reed switch behaviour in 0.5, 1.5, and 3.0 Tesla magnetic resonance imaging units: are reed switches always closed in strong magnetic fields? *Pacing and Clinical Electrophysiology* 25:1419–1423.
10. ASTM F2182-11a (2011). *Standard Test Method for Measurement of Radio Frequency Induced Heating On or Near Passive Implants During Magnetic Resonance Imaging*. West Conshohocken, PA: ASTM International.
11. Achenbach, S., Moshage, W., Diem, B. et al. (1997). Effects of magnetic resonance imaging on cardiac pacemakers and electrodes. *American Heart Journal* 134:467–473.

12. Roguin, A., Zviman, M.M., Glenn, R. et al. (2004). Modern pacemaker and implantable cardioverter/defibrillator systems can be magnetic resonance imaging safe: In vitro and in vivo assessment of safety and function at 1.5 T. *Circulation* 110:475–482.

13. Langman, A., Goldberg, I., Finn, P. et al. (2011). Pacemaker lead tip heating in abandoned and pacemaker-attached leads at 1.5 tesla MRI. *Journal of Magnetic Resonance Imaging* 33:426–431.

14. Irnich, W. (2010). Risks to pacemaker patients undergoing magnetic resonance imaging examinations. *Europace* 12:918–920.

15. Mattei, E., Triventi, M., Calcagnini, G. et al. (2008). Complexity of MRI induced heating on metallic leads: Experimental measurements of 374 configurations. *BioMedical Engineering OnLine* 7:11. doi:10.1186/1475-925X-7-11

16. Sommer, T., Vahlhaus, C., Lauck, G. et al. (2000). MR imaging and cardiac pacemakers: in-vitro evaluation and in-vivo studies in 51 patients at 0.5 T. *Radiology* 215:869–879.

17. Langman, D., Goldberg, I., Judy J. et al. (2012). The dependence of radiofrequency induced pacemaker lead tip heating on the electrical conductivity of the medium at the lead tip. *Magnetic Resonance in Medicine* 68:606–661.

18. Bernstein, A., Daubert, J-C., Fletcher, R, et al. (2002). The revised NASPE/BPEG generic code for antibradycardia, adaptive-rate, and multisite pacing. *Journal of Pacing and Clinical Electrophysiology* 25:260–264.

19. Bernstein, A., Camm, A., Fisher, J. et al. (1993). North American Society of Pacing and Electrophysiology policy statement. The NASPE/BPEG defibrillator code. *Pacing and Clinical Electrophysiology* 16:1776–1780.

20. Gimbel, J. (2009). Unexpected asystole during 3T magnetic resonance imaging of a pacemaker-dependent patient with a "modern" pacemaker. *Europace* 11:1241–1242.

21. Sutton, R., Kanal, E., Wilkoff, B.L. et al. (2008). Safety of magnetic resonance imaging of patients with a new Medtronic EnRhythm MRI SureScan pacing system: clinical study design. *Trials* 9:68. doi: 10.1186/1745-6215-9-68.

22. Do, D. and Boyle, N. (2016). *MRI in Patients with Implanted Devices: Current Controversies*. Washington: American College of Cardiology. https://www.acc.org/latest-in-cardiology/articles/2016/08/01/07/15/mri-in-patients-with-implanted-devices (accessed 29 June 2019).

23. Russo, R., Costa, H., Silva, P. et al (2017). Assessing the risks associated with MRI in patients with a pacemaker or defibrillator. *New England Journal of Medicine* 376:755–764.

24. Indik, J.H., Gimbel, J.R., and Abe, H. (2017). 2017 HRS expert consensus statement on magnetic resonance imaging and radiation exposure in patients with cardiovascular implantable electronic devices. *Heart Rhythm* 14 e97–e153.

25. Jacob, S., Panaich, S., Maheshwari, R. et al. (2011). Clinical applications of magnets on cardiac rhythm management devices. *Europace* 13:1222–1230.

26. Nazarian, S. and Halperin, H. (2013). Performing MRI in patients with conventional (non-MR conditional) cardiac devices. In: *MRI bioeffects, safety, and patient management* (Ed. F.D. Shellock and J.V. Crues III) pp. 388–401. Los Angeles, CA: Biomedical Research Publishing Group.

27. British Society of Cardiovascular Imaging (2019). *MRI for patients with pacemakers and implantable cardioverter-defibrillators*. London: BSCI. https://bsci.org.uk/standards-and-guidelines/mri-and-pacemakers-icd/ (accessed 29 June 2019).

28. Nazarian, S., Hansford, R., Roguin, A. et al. (2011). A prospective evaluation of a protocol for magnetic resonance imaging of patients with implanted cardiac devices. *Annals of Internal Medicine* 155:415–410.

29. Pycroft, L., Stein, J., and Aziz, T. (2018). Deep brain stimulation: An overview of history, methods, and future developments. *Brain and Neuroscience Advances* 2:1–6.

30. Verrills, P., Sinclair, C. and Barnard, A. (2016). A review of spinal cord stimulation systems for chronic pain. *Journal of Pain Research* 9:481–492.

31. Johnson, R.L and Wilson, C.G. (2018). A review of vagus nerve stimulation as a therapeutic intervention. *Journal of Inflammation Research* 11:203–213.

32. Oerlemans, D.J. and Van Kerrebroeck, P.E. (2008). Sacral nerve stimulation for neuromodulation of the lower urinary tract. *Neurourology and Urodynamics* 27:28–33.

33. Lal, N., Livemore, S., Dunne, D. et al. (2015). Gastric electrical stimulation with the Enterra System: A systematic review. *Gastroenterology Research and Practice* Volume 2015, Article ID 762972.

34. Larson, P., Richardson, R., Starr, M. et al. (2008). Magnetic resonance imaging of implanted deep brain stimulators: Experience in a large series. *Stereotactic and Functional Neurosurgery* 86:92–100.

35. Finelli, D., Rezai, A., Ruggieri, P. et al. (2002). MR imaging-related heating of deep brain stimulation electrodes: in vitro study. *American Journal of Neuroradiology* 23:1795–1802.

36. Kahan, J., Papadaki, A., White, M. et al. (2015). The safety of using body-transmit MRI in patients with implanted deep brain stimulation devices. *PLOS ONE* DOI:10.1371/journal.pone.0129077.

37. Cabot, E., Lloyd, T., Christ, A. et al. (2013). Evaluation of the RF heating of a generic deep brain stimulator exposed in 1.5T magnetic resonance scanners. *Bioelectromagnetics* 34:104–113.

38. Rezai, A.R, Finelli, D., Nyenhuis, J.A. et al. (2002). Neurostimulation systems for deep brain stimulation: in vitro evaluation of magnetic resonance imaging-related heating at 1.5 tesla. *Journal of Magnetic Resonance Imaging* 15:241–250.

39. Shellock, F.G., Begnaud, J., and Inman, D.M. (2006). Vagus nerve stimulation therapy system: In vitro evaluation of magnetic resonance imaging-heating and function at 1.5 and 3 tesla. *Neuromodulation* 9:204–213.

40. de Jonge, J.C., Melis, G.I., Gebbink, T.A. et al. (2014). Safety of a dedicated brain MRI protocol in patients with a vagus nerve stimulator. *Epilepsia* 55:e112–e115.

41. De Andres, J., Valía, J.C., Cerda-Olmedo, G. et al. (2007). Magnetic resonance imaging in patients with spinal neurostimulation systems. *Anesthesiology* 106:779–786.

42. Manker, S.G. and Shellock, F.G. (2013). MRI safety issues and neuromodulation systems. In: *MRI bioeffects, safety, and patient management* (Ed. F.D. Shellock FD and J.V. Crues JV III) pp 424–460. Los Angeles, CA: Biomedical Research Publishing Group.

43. Lenarz, T. (2018). Cochlear implant – state of the art. *GMS Current Topics in Otorhinolaryngology, Head and Neck Surgery* Vol. 16.

44. Tam, Y. C., Graves, M. J., Black, R.T. et al. (2010). Magnetic resonance imaging in patients with cochlear implants and auditory brain stem implants. *Cochlear Implants International* 11 sup.2:48–51.

45. Kim, B., Park, J., and Kim, J. (2015). Adverse events and discomfort during magnetic resonance imaging in cochlear implant recipients. *JAMA Otolaryngology Head & Neck Surgery* 141: 45–53.

46. Carlson, M.L, Neff, B.A., Link, M.J. et al. (2015). Magnetic resonance imaging with cochlear implant magnet in place: Safety and imaging quality. *Otology & Neurotology* 36:965–971.

47. Young, N.M., Rojas, C., Deng, J. et al. (2016). Magnetic resonance imaging of cochlear implant recipients. *Otology & Neurotology* 37:665–671.

48. Yun, J.M., Colburn, M.W., and Antonelli, P.J. (2005). Cochlear implant magnet displacement with minor head trauma. *Otolaryngology Head & Neck Surgery* 133:275–277.

49. Deneuve, S., Loundon, N., and Leboulanger, N. (2008). Cochlear implant magnet displacement during magnetic resonance imaging. *Otology & Neurotology* 29:789–790.

50. Jeon, J.H., Bae, M.R., Chang, J.W. et al. (2012). Reversing the polarity of a cochlear implant magnet after magnetic resonance imaging. *Auris Nasus Larynx* 39:415–417.

51. Cuda, D., Murri, A. and Suggo, G. (2013). Focused tight dressing does not prevent cochlear implant magnet migration under 1.5T MRI. *Acta Otorhinolaryngologia Italica* 33:122–136.

52. Keereweer, S., Van der Schroeff, M.P., and Pullens, B. (2014). Case report: Traumatic displacement of a cochlear implant magnet. *Annals of Otology, Rhinology & Laryngology* 123:229–231.

53. Hassepass, F., Stabenau, V., Maier, W. et al. (2014). Revision surgery due to magnet dislocation in cochlear implant patients: an emerging complication. *Otology & Neurotology* 35:29–34.

54. Leong, W. and Yuen, H. (2018). Dislocation of cochlear implant magnet during 1.5 tesla magnetic resonance imaging despite head bandaging, and its repositioning using an endoscopic approach. *Journal of Laryngology and Otology* 132:943–945.

55. Erhardt, J., Fuhrer, E., Gruschke, O. et al. (2018). Should patients with brain implants undergo MRI? *Journal of Neural Engineering* 15.4:041002.

56. Bandorski, D., Kurniawan, N., Baltes, P. et al. (2016). Contraindications for video capsule endoscopy. *World Journal of Gastroenterology* 22:9898–9908.

57. Food and Drug Administration (2012). *De novo classification request for PillCam Colon 2 capsule endoscopy system*. Silver Spring, MD:FDA. http://www.accessdata.fda.gov/cdrh_docs/reviews/k123666.pdf. (accessed 4 July 2019).

58. Baker, K.B, Tkach, J.A., Phillips, M. et al. (2006). Variability in RF-induced heating of a deep brain stimulation implant across MR systems. *Journal of Magnetic Resonance Imaging* 24:1236–1242.

59. Córcoles, J., Zastrow, E., and Kuster, N. (2017). On the estimation of the worst-case implant-induced RF-heating in multi-channel MRI. *Physics in Medicine and Biology* 62:4711–4727.
60. International Electrotechnical Commission (2105). *Medical Electrical Equipment – Part 2–33: Particular Requirements for the Safety of Magnetic Resonance Equipment for Medical Diagnosis*. IEC 60601-2-33 3.3 edn. Geneva:IEC.
61. Kanal, E. (2015). Magnetic resonance imaging in cochlear implant recipients: pros and cons *JAMA Otolaryngology Head & Neck Surgery* 141:52–53.
62. Faris, O.P. and Shein, M. (2006). Food and Drug Administration perspective: magnetic resonance imaging of pacemaker and implantable cardioverter-defibrillator patients. *Circulation* 114:1232–1233.

Further reading and resources

Erhardt, J., Fuhrer, E., Gruschke, O. et al. (2018). Should patients with brain implants undergo MRI? *Journal of Neural Engineering* 15.4:041002.

Fitzpatrick, D. (2015). *Implantable electronic medical devices*. Amsterdam: Academic Press, Elsevier.

Manker, S.G. and Shellock, F.G. (2013). MRI safety issues and neuromodulation systems. In: *MRI bioeffects, safety, and patient management* (Ed. F.D. Shellock and J.V. Crues III) pp. 424–460. Los Angeles, CA: Biomedical Research Publishing Group.

Shinbane, J.S. and Summers, J. (2013). MRI and cardiac devices: MR conditional pacemakers and implantable cardioverter defibrillators In: *MRI bioeffects, safety, and patient management* (Ed. F.D. Shellock and J.V. Crues III) pp. 402–423. Los Angeles, CA: Biomedical Research Publishing Group.

Thornton, J.S. (2017). Technical challenges and safety of magnetic resonance imaging with in situ neuromodulation from spine to brain. *European Journal of Paediatric Neurology* 21:232–241.

www.magresource.com

www.mrisafety.com

Manufacturers' technical manuals and MRI information

(all accessed 1 August 2019)

Abbot (formerly St. Jude), Chicago IL, USA: https://manuals.sjm.com/

Advanced Bionics, Sonova CA, USA: https://advancedbionics.com/us/en/home/professionals/hires-ultra-3d-mri-safety.html

Axonics, Irvine CA, USA: http://www.axonicsmodulation.com/mri/

Biotronik, Berlin, Germany: https://manuals.biotronik.com

Boston Scientific, Marlborough MA, USA: http://bostonscientific.com/manuals

Cochlear, Sydney, Australia: https://www.cochlear.com/us/en/home/ongoing-care-and-support/device-support/mri-and-medical-considerations

Codman (a Johnson and Johnson company) New Brunswick NJ, USA: https://www.jnjmedicaldevices.com/en-US/codman-pumps

FlowOnix, Mount Olive Township NJ, USA: https://flowonix.com/healthcare-provider/mri-information

LivaNova, London, UK: https://www.livanova.com/en-US/Home/Products-Therapies/Resources.aspx

MedEl, Innsbruck, Austria: https://s3.medel.com/documents/AW/AW37154_10_Manual-Medical-Procedures-EN-English-SGP.pdf

Medtronic, Minneapolis MN, USA: http://manuals.medtronic.com/content/dam/emanuals/crdm/CONTRIB_151926.pdf

NuVectra, Plano TX, USA: https://nuvectramedical.com/us/patient/mri/

Sorin pacemakers, Microport CRM, Paris, France: http://crm.microport.com/product

Stimwave, Pompano Beach FL, USA: http://stimwave.com/mobile/mri/

11

Would you scan this? Understanding the conditions

INTRODUCTION

This chapter explains how to interpret and implement the MR safety information, the "Conditions", provided by implant manufacturers, and will review, through examples, the practical aspects of scanning passive and active implanted medical devices. Information on specific types, makes, and models of implant are available from other well-established sources of specialist information such as MRIsafety.com [1], MagResource.com [2], or "the List" [3]. Additionally, general advice on classes of device may be available from national guidance documents [4-8].

For the aspiring MRSO or MRMD this chapter should be read in conjunction with Chapters 9 and 10. Those wishing to act as an MRSE should also be conversant with the material in Chapter 2 and Appendix 1.

MRI CONDITIONS

The development of the MRI safety conditions and labeling of medical devices through standard ASTM-F2503 (universally accepted as standard IEC-625700) [9] has placed the task of safely scanning patients with implants on a more scientific and consistent footing.

MR device safety definitions

The three designated MR safety definitions for devices are:

- **MR Safe** means that the device poses no risk to the patient in the MR environment. Image quality may be affected
- **MR Conditional** means that the device poses no additional risk to the patient when introduced to the MR environment under specified conditions
- **MR Unsafe** means that the device may not be introduced into the MR environment as it poses significant risk to the patient and/or staff.

Essentials of MRI Safety, First Edition. Donald W. McRobbie.
© 2020 John Wiley & Sons Ltd. Published 2020 by John Wiley & Sons Ltd.

The approved symbols were shown in Figure 1.29. The terms refer exclusively to safety, but where there is metal image quality may be affected (Chapter 9, page 218).

"Sub-conditions"

Practitioners who use the MRIsafety.com web resource or Shellock's "List" [3] will encounter categories of "sub-conditions" grouped together according to the manufacturer information available, common sets of generic conditions, or the specific nature of the hazard (Table 11.1). This table is for illustrative purposes only; the examples given are neither fully inclusive nor exclusive. For each actual device check with the manufacturer's information and/or MRIsafety. com or equivalent devices database.

Device labeling

Typical labeling of a passive device is:

Non-clinical testing has demonstrated that the DEVICE NAME *is MR Conditional. It can be scanned safely under the following conditions:*

1. *A static magnetic field of less than or equal to 3.0 T;*
2. *Spatial gradient field of less than or equal to 7.2 T/m (720 G/cm);*
3. *Maximum whole-body averaged Specific Absorption Rate (SAR) of 2 W/kg for 15 minutes of scanning. In non-clinical testing the* DEVICE NAME *produced a temperature rise of less than or equal to 0.5 °C at a maximum MR system-reported whole-body SAR of 2 W/kg on a 3 T MR* SYSTEM NAME/MODEL *scanner.*

Table 11.1 Shellock 'subconditions'. Examples are not exclusive. For each device check the current manufacturer's MR safety information

Condition	Meaning	Examples
MR safe	Device has undergone testing to demonstrate its safety at the stated B_0 – by default 1.5 T; or is made from non-metallic materials: ceramic, glass, plastics.	Some stents, clips, staples, small devices made from titanium or titanium alloy.
Conditional 1	Weakly ferromagnetic only; generally acceptable for scanning due to weak interactions.	Prosthetic heart valves
Conditional 2	Weakly ferromagnetic and firmly incorporated into tissue within six weeks of implantation; generally acceptable for scanning.	Coils, filters, stents, clips
Conditional 3	Transdermal patch with metal foil which may heat up.	Medicinal patches, e.g. for insulin.
Conditional 4	Device with ferromagnetic parts but which has not been evaluated for MR safety.	Halo vest or cervical fixation devices.
Conditional 5	Follow manufacturer's specific conditions only.	Infusion pumps, MR conditional pacemakers, other active devices.
Conditional 6	Tested to ASTM Standards; follow conditions.	Orthopedic implants, coils, filters, stents, aneurysm clips
Conditional 7	Device not intended to be in the bore of the magnet.	Drip stands, wheelchairs, infusion pumps, anesthetic equipment.
Conditional 8	ASTM F2503 labelled for 1.5 T and 3 T closed bore scanners only.	Orthopedic implants, coils, filters, stents, aneurysm clips
MR Unsafe 1	Ferromagnetic with a high risk of movement or dislodgement. Do not introduce to the MR environment.	MR unsafe wheelchairs, trolleys, gas tanks.
MR Unsafe 2	Main risk due to induced currents and/or excessive heating.	MR unsafe external fixation devices, cardiac pacemakers, implantable cardioverter defibrillators.

The current ASTM requirement is to use SI units: T m^{-1}, usually written as "T/m". Older implant information may use G cm^{-1}, written as "G/cm." To convert between units, 1 T m^{-1} = 100 G cm^{-1}.

The device manufacturer's website should contain the most up-to-date information. Note that the published conditions can sometimes change. In many cases the patient will carry an implant card, stating the make, model, and implantation date, and sometimes information regarding the conditions.

UNDERSTANDING FRINGE FIELD SPATIAL GRADIENT MAPS

When it comes to interpreting the conditions for a particular implant, the spatial gradient condition appears to be the most problematical. Confusion may occur with the *imaging gradients* G_x, G_y, G_z which are only present during scanning. The spatial gradient referred in the conditions is a consequence of the static field B_0 and is present at all times for a superconducting or permanent MRI magnet. Denoted dB/dz, it is several hundred times stronger than the imaging gradients and is responsible for the translational force. One of the most important aspects of practical MR safety is to interpret the spatial gradient information provided by your MR manufacturer. This can be found in the *Compatibility Data* statement that the MR manufacturer is required to provide on the extent and spatial distribution of magnetic fields [10], specifically:

- The position where the spatial gradient of the main magnetic field B_0 is a maximum, the values of B_0 and the spatial gradient of B_0 (dB/dz) at that location – where the translational force on a saturated ferromagnetic object is a maximum.
- The position where the product of the magnitude of the B_0 and its spatial gradient (B·dB/dz) at that location- where the translational force on any other object is a maximum.

The location of these two maxima may or may not be the same. Because of rotational symmetry, the locations of the maxima lie on a circle close to the bore entrance (Figure 11.1). MR manufacturers usually choose to provide more information than this, but each does so in their own way.

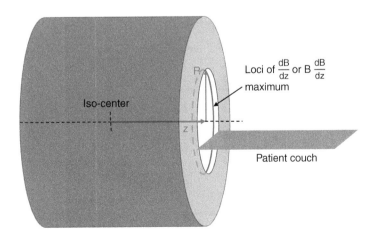

Figure 11.1 Examples of typical locations of maximum spatial gradient dB/dz and maximum field-gradient product B·dB/dz at an axial distance z and radial distance R from the iso-center.

Spatial gradient maps on General Electric scanners

General Electric (Milwaukee, WI, USA) provides spatial gradient information in both tabular and concentric cylindrical form.

Tabular form

The radial and axial positions of the peak values of B_0, dB/dz and their product and the values themselves are given in tabular form. Table 11.2 shows data for the 3 T TLC magnet. Note that for GE systems you need to know the type number of the magnet.

For example, for a paramagnetic object the maximum attractive force occurs at the location of the maximum product value of 38.7 T^2 m^{-1}, occurring 73 cm along the z-axis from the iso-center at a radial distance (towards the inner surface of the bore) of 36 cm. Due to the rotational symmetry the maximum force occurs a locus of points lying on a circle of radius 36 cm concentric with the z-axis, 73 cm from the iso-center – at both ends (Figure 11.1). At this location B_0 is 3.6 T and dB/dz is 10.7 T m^{-1}.

For a saturated ferromagnetic object, the maximum force will be at the point of maximum gradient dB/dz (12.4 T m^{-1}) on a circle of radius 51 cm from the bore axis, 92 cm along z from the iso-center. Note that you need to know the diameter and length of the bore in order to properly visualize these locations.

Concentric cylindrical form

The concentric cylinder representation provides the maximum B_0, dB/dz, and product (B·dB/dz) values within notional cylindrical volumes concentric with the scanner bore, plus their positions along the z-axis from the iso-center. Table 11.3 shows data published for the 3 T "TLC" magnet. A separate table (not shown) provides the data for cylinder diameters of 50, 55, 60 and 70 cm.

Table 11.2 Tabular form of GE compatibility data for the 3 T TLC magnet.

Parameter	Radial location R (m)	Location along z (m)	B_0 (T)	dB/dz (T m^{-1})	Max B·dB/dz (T^2 m^{-1})
Peak B	0.35	0.64	3.9	7.2	28.2
Peak gradient	0.51	0.92	1.8	12.4	22.6
Peak product	0.36	0.73	3.6	10.7	38.7

Table 11.3 Example data for General Electric 3 T TLC magnet.

	Cylinder diameter									
	z-axis		20 cm		30 cm		40 cm		60 cm	
	Peak	R, z (m)	Peak	R, z (m)	Peak	R, z (m)	Peak	R, z (m)	Peak	R, z (m)
B_0 (T)	3.0	0.000 0.250	3.0	0.100 0.358	3.0	0.150 0.460	3.0	0.200 0.530	3.3	0.300 0.610
dB/dz (T m^{-1})	5.1	0.000 0.880	5.3	0.100 0.880	5.6	0.150 0.880	6.2	0.200 0.845	8.3	0.300 0.825
B·dB/dz (T^2 m^{-1})	10.6	0.000 0.790	11.3	0.100 0.785	12.3	0.150 0.765	14.0	0.200 0.785	22.4	0.300 0.740

From Table 11.3 above the maximum spatial gradient within a 40 cm diameter is 6.2 T m^{-1} occurring 84.5 cm from the iso-center. Figure 11.2a shows such a diagram for the 3 T TLC magnet. Currently this is not provided; you have to draw it yourself!

Example 11.1   Prosthetic heat valve.

A mitral pericardial prosthesis (heart valve) is stated to have the following MR conditions:

- Static magnetic field of less than or equal to 3.0 T
- Spatial gradient field of less than or equal to 720 G/cm.

Can we scan this patient within the conditions on the GE TLC magnet whose data is given in Tables 11.2 & 11.3?
   Firstly, we need to convert from Gauss per cm (G/cm) to Tesla per meter (T/m).
   1 T = 10 000 G and 1 m = 100 cm. To convert from G cm^{-1} to T m^{-1} divide by 100:

$$720\frac{G}{cm} = 720 \times \frac{100}{10\ 000} = 7.2\ T\ m^{-1}$$

267

Secondly, does our magnet have values of spatial gradient which exceed this? Yes, from Table 11.2 the maximum spatial gradient is 12.4 T m^{-1} (shaded cell). This occurs 92 cm along z from the iso-center at a radial distance of 51 cm which is out of the bore. Clearly this exceeds the condition of 7.2 T m^{-1}.
   Thirdly, is the implant likely to pass through a gradient greater than 7.2 T m^{-1}? Looking at the shaded cell in Table 11.3 the maximum dB/dz within a 40 cm diameter is 6.2 T m^{-1}. This occurs 20 cm from the z-axis radially. The heart valve is unlikely to lie in this position. To confirm this graphically look at Figure 11.2b which has the patient outline superimposed upon the concentric contours. The maximum gradient in the heart region is less than 5.6 T m^{-1}.

Conclusion: *introducing the patient into the scanner will not result in the implant being exposed to a spatial gradient greater than 7.2 T m^{-1}. We are compliant with the MR conditions.*

Example 11.2   Prosthetic hip joint

Can we safely (within the conditions) introduce a patient for a routine brain examination with the following hip implant into the GE TLC magnet whose data is given in Tables 11.2 & 11.3?
   MR Conditions:

- Static magnetic field of 1.5 or 3 T
- Spatial gradient field of 9.3 T/m (value extrapolated) or less
- Spatial gradient field product of 39 T^2/m (value extrapolated) or less.

Looking at Table 11.2, the peak gradient is 12.4 T m^{-1}, so we need to consider the concentric circles shown in Figure 11.2. dB/dz is 8.3 T m^{-1} up to 30 cm radially from the iso-center, so the hip implant will lie in a region not exceeding the spatial gradient condition.
   We now need to consider the spatial gradient field product condition. From Table 11.2, the peak product is 37.8 T^2 m^{-1}. This is less than the stated condition.

Conclusion: *we can scan within the MR conditions.*

Spatial gradient maps on Philips scanners

Philips Medical Systems (Best, the Netherlands) provide the spatial gradient information in two ways. On older systems dB/dz is indicated on a set of concentric cylinders coaxial to the bore. More recently contour maps are provided.

(a)

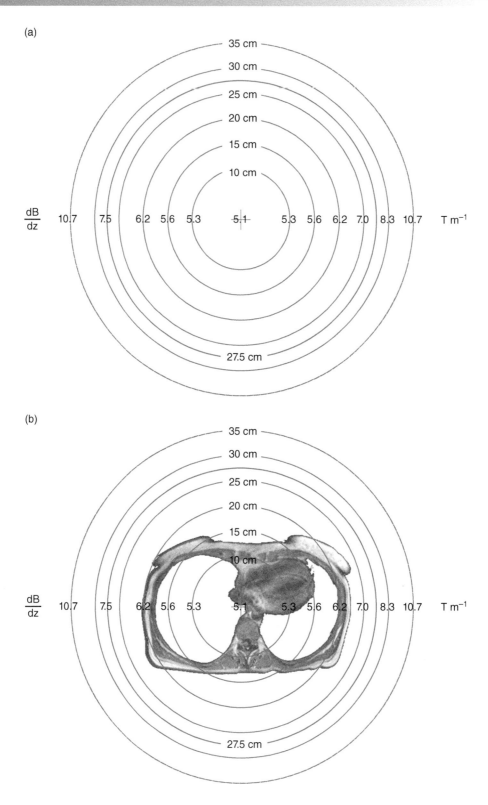

Figure 11.2   Concentric cylindrical representation of the spatial gradient dB/dz for the General Electric 3T TLC magnet derived from Table 11.3; (b) the same showing the position of a patient as reference in Example 11.1.

Concentric cylindrical representation

In this representation the maximum value of dB/dz occurring with cylindrical volumes centred on the bore axis z with radii 20, 30, 40, and 50 cm are shown (Figure 11.3a). The maximum dB/dz within each cylinder is shown in tabular form. For example, on an Achieva 1.5 T scanner these are 2.5 T m^{-1} along the z-axis, rising to 3.6 Tm^{-1} on the 50 cm radius cylinder. Also shown is the position of the patient couch top relative to these cylinders. In this representation it is not possible to know exactly where along the z-axis the maximum value occurs. Also provided are the maximum values of the magnitude of B, dB/dz, and product B·dB/dz with the locations indicated on a side view diagram of the scanner (Figure 11.3b).

Example 11.3   Aortic stent

An aortic stent is stated to have the following MR conditions:

- Static magnetic field of less than or equal to 3.0 T
- Spatial gradient field of less than or equal to 525 G/cm.

Can we scan the patient within the conditions on the Achieva 1.5 T and 3 T scanners?
From Figure 11.3a the maximum dB/dz is only 3.6 T m^{-1} (360 G cm^{-1}) for the 1.5 T scanner. Therefore, we are within the conditions for this scanner. However, the 3 T scanner has dB/dz of up to 5.1 T m^{-1} at a radial distance of 10 cm. Somewhere between a radial distance of 10 cm and 15 cm from the z-axis the condition of 5.25 T m^{-1} will be exceeded. Figure 11.3c shows an outline of the patient superimposed on the 3 T concentric plot. The orange area indicates the region of uncertainty as to compliance with the condition.

Conclusion: *scanning at 1.5 T presents no issues; at 3 T is it possible that the dB/dz condition may be slightly exceeded.*

dB/dz field maps

Philips also provide field contour maps (Figure 11.4) in either a side elevation or top down view. In both cases the plane shown passes through the iso-center. In the example shown, an Ingenia 3 T scanner, a patient entering the scanner will fully pass through dB/dz contours of up to 3 T m^{-1}. The position of maximum spatial gradient is indicated by the letter "A" with a value of 17 T m^{-1}.

Example 11.4   Prosthetic hip joint

Can we safely (within the conditions) introduce a patient with the following hip implant into the scanner shown in Figure 11.4 for a routine brain examination?
MR conditions:

- Static magnetic field of 1.5 or 3 T
- Spatial gradient field of 9.3 T/m (value extrapolated) or less
- Spatial gradient field product of 39 T^2/m (value extrapolated) or less.

From Figure 11.4a we see that 9.3 T m^{-1} is exceeded close to the bore entrance but that the implant will lie in a region where the spatial gradient is less than 10 T m^{-1}.

Conclusion: *we can scan within the conditions.*
As a point of interest, the use of the extrapolated value indicates that the device has not actually been tested within a 9.3 T m^{-1} spatial gradient, but at lower value, and the ASTM F2502 allowance for extrapolating to higher field invoked. See Chapter 9.

(a)

Achieva	1.5 T		3 T	
	T/m	gauss/cm	T/m	gauss/cm
Patient axis	2.5	250	4.9	490
20 cm diameter cylinder	2.6	250	5.1	510
30 cm diameter cylinder	2.8	280	5.5	550
40 cm diameter cylinder	3.1	310	6.0	600
50 cm diameter cylinder	3.6	360	7.0	700

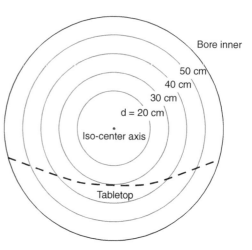

(b)

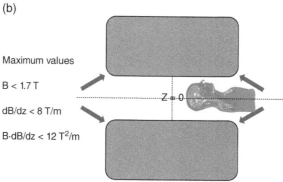

Maximum values

$B < 1.7$ T

$dB/dz < 8$ T/m

$B \cdot dB/dz < 12$ T^2/m

(c)

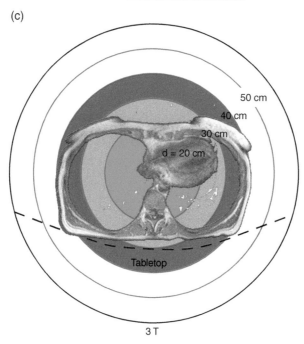

Figure 11.3 (a) Maximum spatial gradients occurring within concentric cylinders; (b) location of maximum dB/dz and B·dB/dz for Philips scanners; (c) 3T scanner plot with patient position superimposed.

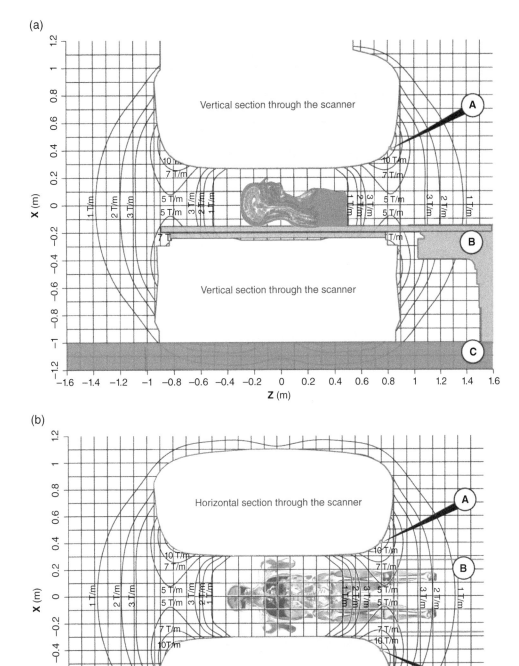

Figure 11.4 (a) Side view of dB/dz spatial gradient contour map as depicted for Philips scanners showing patient position; (b) top down view. Contour maps reproduced courtesy of Royal Philips.

Spatial gradient maps on Siemens scanners

Siemens Healthineers (Erlangen, Germany) provide data on the B_0 fringe field, its spatial gradient dB/dz, and the product B·dB/dz in the form of contour maps. For each field parameter both side and top down views are provided.

dB/dz map

Figure 11.5a shows the side view for the Magnetom Skyra 3 T scanner. The map shows one quadrant of the cross-section shown as a blue plane in the scanner avatar. The contour map corresponds to the darker blue section, one quarter of the field. The iso-center is located at coordinates (0,0) 20 cm above the top of the patient couch. The maximum dB/dz occurs at the point marked "⊗" and is 11 T m^{-1}. Because of the rotational symmetry, the maximum translational force on a saturated ferromagnetic object will occur on a circle around the bore opening. Each line represents a contour of dB/dz, so as the patient travels along the couch mechanism they will pass though regions of 0.3, 0.5, 1, and 3 T m^{-1}, with part of their body possibly passing through 5 T m^{-1}.

Figure 11.5b shows the top view with the patient position indicated. The iso-center (0,0) is at the top left-hand corner. The dark blue plane in the scanner avatar indicates the quadrant shown in the map. We can see more clearly that part of the patient is likely to pass through 5 T m^{-1}. The maps have rotational symmetry, the contours rotating about the z-axis to form three dimensional volumes.

B_0 map

Siemens also provide B_0 contour maps (Figure 11.6). On the 3 T Skyra the maximum B_0 occurs at the point marked "⊗" and is 3.4 T. The field at the bore entrance is about 2 T. A top down view is also provided. The iso-center and patient positions are as before.

B_0·dB/dz product map

Additionally, Siemens provide B·dB/dz product maps (Figure 11.7) also with the side and top down quadrant views. The maximum product occurs at the point "⊗" and is 26.5 T m^{-2} on a locus of points forming a circle around the inside of the bore. At these points the translational force on any object, other than one comprised of saturated ferromagnetic material, will be a maximum. With a field of 2 T at the bore entrance the 10 T^2 m^{-1} contour shape is similar to the 5 T m^{-1} dB/dz contour. Again, picture the contours as three-dimensional shapes by rotation about the bore axis z.

Example 11.5   MR Conditional aortic stent

A CP stent used for aortic stenting in paediatric patients is stated to have the following MR conditions:

- Static magnetic field of less than or equal to 3 T
- Spatial gradient field of less than or equal to 3.9 T/m
- Spatial gradient field product of 39 T^2/m (value extrapolated) or less.

Which of the scanners featured above in this chapter would ensure scanning within the conditions?
   The GE 3 T scanner detailed in Tables 11.2 & 11.3 and Figure 11.2 has a spatial gradient along the iso-center on 5.1 T m^{-1}. This exceeds the condition.
   The Philips 3 T scanner in Figure 11.3 has a similar value of 4.9 T m^{-1}, also exceeding the condition. However, the Philips 1.5 T scanner's gradient contours show a maximum of 3.6 T m^{-1}. The scanner in Figure 11.4 shows contours for 3 and 5 T m^{-1}. You need to interpolate these to estimate where the 4 T m^{-1} contour may lie. It seems likely that for a small child the 3.9 T m^{-1} condition may be exceeded.
   Looking at the Siemens scanner in Figure 11.5 there are contours for 3 and 5 T m^{-1}. You need to interpolate these to estimate where the 4 T m^{-1} contour may lie. It seems likely that this may impinge upon the stent's position at some point.

Conclusion: *Only the 1.5 T scanner can be said to definitively comply with the MR conditions.*
   Does this mean we cannot scan at all on the 3 T scanners? We will review this later.

(a)

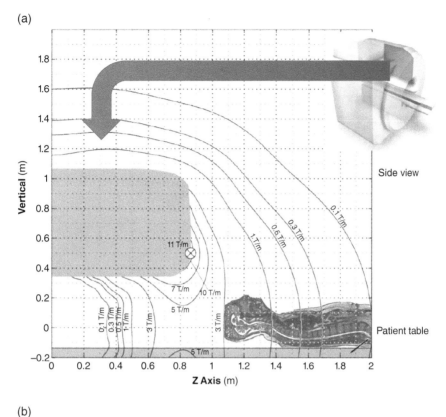

(b)

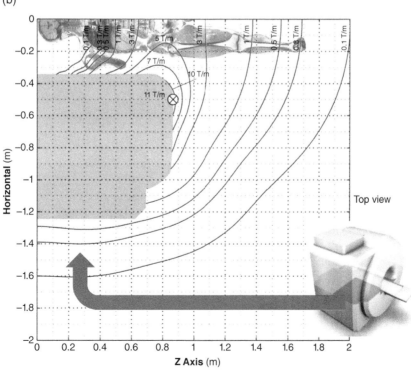

Figure 11.5 (a) Side view of dB/dz spatial gradient contour map as depicted for Siemens scanners showing patient position; (b) top down view. Contour maps reproduced with permission of Siemens.

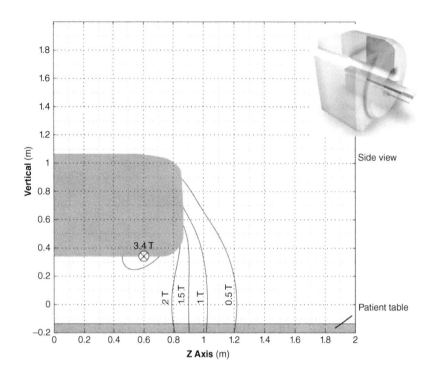

Figure 11.6 B₀ contour map for a Siemens Skyra 3T scanner: side view only. Reproduced with permission of Siemens.

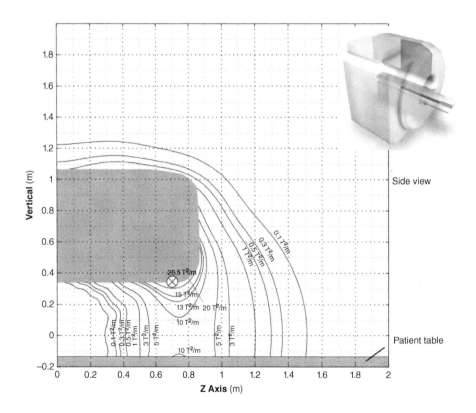

Figure 11.7 B·dB/dz product contour map for a Siemens Skyra 3T scanner: side view only. Reproduced with permission of Siemens.

Field strength and bore diameter

Does a higher B_0 always result in greater spatial gradients? We saw in Figure 11.3 an instance where the spatial gradients are approximately double for 3 T compared with the same model at 1.5 T. This is not necessarily always the case. The Siemens 1.5 T Aera and 3 T Skyra both have a maximum dB/dz of 11 T m^{-1}, although the contours of the 3 T scanner extend further in space.

MYTHBUSTER:

Do not assume that all scanners of the same field strength have the same spatial gradients. Do not assume *anything*; check the Manufacturer's Compatibility Data for your scanner, noting the magnet model number where relevant.

UNDERSTANDING RF CONDITIONS

The RF conditions also sometimes cause confusion. These are stated either in terms of a maximum SAR, usually the whole-body SAR, or B_{1+}RMS. Be aware of certain devices which may have a condition related to the choice of transmit coil, e.g. a transmit/receive head coil for a deep brain stimulator (DBS).

SAR

Often the SAR condition will coincide with the Normal Mode, i.e. a whole-body SAR of 2 W kg^{-1}. The SAR limit usually applies for 15 minutes of scanning, generally taken to mean "per sequence." The 15-minute scan duration relates to the FDA criteria for significant risk [11] which specifies SAR measurement over 15 minutes. Some active implants have a cumulative scan time limit relating to the whole examination (see Tables 10.3–10.8). MR scanners calculate SAR continuously over six minutes. The RF conditions also report the heating measured in non-clinical testing according to ASTM F-2182 [12]. Heating in tissue where there is good blood perfusion is likely to be less than in a phantom. The SAR reported may either be measured by calorimetry in the ASTM phantom or "as reported from the MR scanner console". Be aware that there are variations in how different scanners estimate SAR.

Controlling SAR

For a given patient, SAR depends upon scanner and sequence parameters:

$$\text{SAR} \propto B_0{}^2 \alpha^2 \frac{N_{echoes} N_{slices}}{t_p\, TR} \tag{11.1}$$

For Fast or Turbo Spin Echo (FSE/TSE), the most efficient way to reduce SAR is generally to change parameters in the following order:

1. Use a lower SAR RF pulse (this increases pulse length t_p significantly).
2. Reduce flip angle α (for a refocusing pulse this gives about 10% SAR reduction per 10°).
3. Reduce number of slices and/or echoes (SAR scales linearly with the product of N_{slices} and N_{echoes}).
4. Increase TR (only suitable for sequences giving T_2-weighted contrast).

For 3 T scanners with "Hyper-echoes", this option proves a very good way of reducing SAR in TSE sequences. For gradient echo sequences it may be more efficient to change the flip angle first but be aware of the effect of this on image contrast. Chapter 5 contains a more complete discussion.

Example 11.6   MR conditional aortic stent

A CP (Cheatham Platinum) stent used for aortic stenting in pediatric patients is stated to have the following RF condition:

- Maximum average whole-body specific absorption rate (SAR) of 1.1 W/kg for less than or equal to 20 minutes of scanning as read from the scanner console.

You are scanning at 3 T and the patient weight is 25 kg, height 120 cm. Your protocol includes a T_2-weighted sequence with

- Turbo/fast spin echo, TE = 120 ms
- Turbo factor/no. echoes = 16
- TR = 4000 ms
- Inter-echo spacing: 10 ms (RF pulse type: normal)
- Flip angle 170°
- 20 slices.

At pre-scan the scanner indicates the First Level Mode with an estimated SAR of 1.84 W kg^{-1}, exceeding the condition.

What parameter changes are required to reduce the SAR to within the MR conditions?

Use the SAR calculator (https://drdonaldmcrobbie.com/sar-and-b1rms-calculator/) [13] starting with the parameters above (including changed patient details and B$_0$) without adversely affecting the anatomical coverage or changing the contrast.

The easiest way to comply with the condition is to reduce the flip angle. This requires a reduction to 125°.

However, the most efficient way to reduce SAR is to change to low SAR RF pulse and reduce the flip angle to 160°.

The following works, but it is not the only way to achieve the required SAR: RF pulse → low SAR, flip angle → 160°. Mathematically these changes can be calculated from Equation 11.1

$$SAR_{new} = 1.84 \times \frac{1}{1.5} \times \left(\frac{160}{170}\right)^2 = 1.09 \, W \, kg^{-1}$$

B$_{1+}$RMS

Active implants may also carry a limit in terms of B$_{1+}$RMS. This is more easily relatable to induced voltages in the device components. B$_{1+}$RMS does not depend upon patient geometry or magnetic field B$_0$. However, the induced voltages will depend upon the MR frequency; 1 μT B$_{1+}$RMS at 128 MHz will induce double the voltage than at 64 MHz (assuming no resonant or antenna effect).

For a given patient, B$_0$ and specified RF pulse shape B$_{1+}$RMS scales with the square root of SAR

$$B_{1+RMS} \propto \alpha \sqrt{\frac{N_{echoes}N_{slices}}{t_p \, TR}} \tag{11.2}$$

For spin echo sequences changing the RF pulse type may be more effective than changing flip angle (as was the case for SAR). For low flip angle gradient echo sequences, changing flip angle becomes more important.

Example 11.7   MR conditional pacemaker

The pacemaker has the following MR conditions:

- For 1.5 T: whole-body averaged specific absorption rate (SAR) must be less than or equal to 2 W kg^{-1}.
- For 3 T: B_{1+}RMS must be less than or equal to 2.8 μT.

The patient has weight 90 kg (198 lb) and height 1.76 m (5′9″). The default sequence parameters are:

- T_2-weighted Turbo/fast spin echo
- Turbo factor/no. echoes 16
- TR 4000
- Inter-echo spacing 10 ms (fast RF pulse)
- 24 slices.

The estimated SAR is 3.04 W kg^{-1} in the First Level Controlled Mode.

Use the SAR calculator (https://drdonaldmcrobbie.com/sar-and-b1rms-calculator/) starting with the parameters shown above to make changes suitable for scanning the implant at 1.5 T and 3 T.

For 1.5 T scanning: The easiest way to comply with the condition is to reduce the flip angle. This requires a reduction to 145°. From Equation 11.1:

$$SAR_{new} = 3.04 \times \left(\frac{145}{180}\right)^2 = 1.98 \ W \ kg^{-1}$$

Alternatively (but not exclusively): RF pulse → normal, TR → 4360 ms results in 1.39 W kg^{-1} (TR can be increased for T_2-weighted sequences without degrading the image contrast).

$$SAR_{new} = 3.04 \times \frac{0.5}{1} \times \frac{4000}{4360} = 1.39 \ W \ kg^{-1}$$

For 3T scanning: The pre-scan reported B_{1+}RMS is 5.2 μT. A flip angle of 90° would provide the required B_{1+}RMS but is impractical, so try the following (not exclusively):

RF pulse type → normal, flip angle → 150°, echoes → 15, TR → 4300 ms. This gives a SAR of 2.8 μT, compliant with the MR Conditions. Note that we are still scanning in the First Level Mode.

From Equation 11.2

$$B_{1+RMS} = 5.2 \times \frac{150}{180} \times \sqrt{\frac{0.5}{1} \times \frac{15}{16} \times \frac{4000}{4300}} = 2.8 \ μT$$

This is not affected by patient size or weight, so the parameters can be stored in a scanning protocol and used whenever this implant is present.

Transmit coil

Active implants may restrict scanning to the use of a local transmit or transmit–receive coil. For example, deep brain stimulators often have this condition. If you do not have the coil specified, you cannot scan.

Example 11.8   Deep brain stimulator – using SAR

The MR conditions for scanning a patient with a deep brain stimulator (DBS) are:

- 1.5 T closed bore only
- 0.1 W kg^{-1} whole body SAR
- Gradient slew rate limited to 200 T/m/s.

Modify the following T$_2$-weighted sequence to comply with the B$_{1+}$RMS condition:

- Turbo/fast spin echo, TE =120 ms
- Turbo factor/no. echoes 16
- TR 4000
- Inter-echo spacing 10 ms (fast RF pulse)
- 24 slices.

Use the SAR calculator (https://drdonaldmcrobbie.com/sar-and-b1rms-calculator/) [13] starting with the parameters shown above to make changes suitable for scanning the implant at 1.5 T or calculate from Equation 11.2. Assume the patient weighs 80 kg with height 1.76 m. The initial pre-scan SAR is 2.7 W kg^{-1}.
Suitable (but not exclusive) changes would be:
RF pulse type → low SAR, flip angle → 120°, echoes → 4. This gives a SAR of 0.1 W kg^{-1}, compliant with the MR Conditions. Note the increased scan time to achieve this SAR.

$$SAR_{new} = 2.7 \times \frac{0.5}{1.5} \times \left(\frac{120}{180}\right)^2 \times \frac{4}{16} = 0.1\,W\,kg^{-1}.$$

Example 11.9   Deep brain stimulator – using B$_{1+}$RMS

The DBS device in Example 11.8 has a B$_{1+}$RMS condition ≤ 2.0 µT. Modify the sequence above to comply. Compare these parameters with those you derived using the SAR only condition?

Suitable (but not exclusive) changes would be:
RF pulse type → low SAR, flip angle → 150°, echoes → 12, TR → 4500 ms. This gives a B$_{1+}$RMS of 2.0 µT, compliant with the condition.

$$B_{1+RMS} = 5.2 \times \frac{150}{180} \times \sqrt{\frac{0.5}{1.5} \times \frac{12}{16} \times \frac{4000}{4500}} = 2\mu T$$

It is much easier to comply with the B$_{1+}$RMS condition. It will also be valid for different patients.

GRADIENT SLEW RATE CONDITION

Example 11.8 raises a new conditional requirement relating to the (imaging) gradient switching. The principal effect of gradient dB/dt is induction of voltages and currents in the device and leads, potentially resulting in loss of therapy by inhibition or by over stimulation with potentially serious health consequences.

The gradient condition may be expressed as a slew rate (SR) in T m^{-1} s^{-1} or as dB/dt, for example, 20 T s^{-1}. Interpreting these can be problematical as the scanner may not report these values. The maximum slew rate per gradient axis is a key scanner specification. For example, a scanner with a specified SR of 150 T m^{-1} s^{-1} would at a first glance appear to comply with the conditions. However, with oblique slices using two or more gradient axes the combined SR can exceed this. Manufacturers used to call this the "effective slew rate." If each axis has equivalent specifications, the maximum gradient amplitude with all three axes at their maximum value is $\sqrt{3}$ (=1.73) times the single axis maximum. A slew rate specified as 150 T m^{-1} s^{-1} per axis could actually reach 260 T m^{-1} s^{-1} in an extreme situation. One way to ensure lower gradient slew rates is to select a low acoustic noise waveform, if available. Other means to reduce scanner noise explored in Chapter 6 will also help. Additionally, some scanner software designed to assist with implant scanning (e.g. *Implant Suite*, *ScanWise*) may report or restrict gradient dB/dt.

MORE EXAMPLES

In this section we consider some classes of device in general. For specific safety information and the MR conditions you should consult the device manufacturer's data sheets or suitable databases of MR safety of devices.

Example 11.10   External fixation system

The MR conditions for a tibial external fixation frame are stated as:

- Static magnetic field of 1.5 Tesla only
- Maximum spatial gradient magnetic field of 90 mT/cm or less
- Maximum MR system reported whole body averaged SAR of 2 W/kg
- The fixation system must remain outside the scanner bore
- Under the scan conditions defined above, the maximum expected temperature rise is less than 6 °C.

Looking at the scanners considered in this chapter are there likely to be any restrictions on anatomical regions we can scan?
  Convert to $T\,m^{-1}$. 90 mT/cm = 0.09/0.01 = 9 T/m.
  Then consult the spatial gradient maps. None of the 1.5 T scanners spatial gradients exceed the condition but there may be restrictions on patient position.

Example 11.11   External fixation system – induced voltage

Estimate the induced electric field, current density and average SAR in tissue between the fixation screws for the above device if scanning with a whole body SAR of 2 W kg^{-1} on a 1.5 T scanner?
  The maximum B_{1+}RMS for a patient can be estimated from the SAR calculator [13]. Assume 80 kg, 1.76 m. For example, using the "fast" RF pulse option B_{1+}RMS is 4.4 μT (peak B_1 is 20.88 μT, duty cycle D is 0.05).
  The geometry of the device presents a large conduction loop for the RF (Figure 11.8). If one section of the device has length l = 30 cm; with fixation pins of length 10 cm, then we can simply calculate the peak induced voltage as:

$$V_{ind} = area \times \frac{dB}{dt}$$

$$= 0.3 \times 0.1 \times 2\pi \times 64 \times 10^6 \times 20.88 \times 10^{-6} = 252\ V$$

The peak electric field within tissue is

$$E_{pk} = 252/0.3 = 840\ V\,m^{-1}.$$

The average local SAR will be given by

$$SAR = \frac{\sigma_{tissue}}{2\rho} D \times E_{pk}^{\,2}$$

For muscle (Table 5.2) this gives an average

$$SAR = \frac{0.688}{2 \times 1090} \times 0.05 \times 840^2 = 11.1\ W\,kg^{-1}.$$

This will be much greater at the ends of the fixing pins. Excessive heating is possible. Full EM modeling is required to properly evaluate the local SAR [14]. Remember that materials that are insulating for DC currents can act as dielectric media at radiofrequencies.

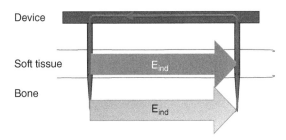

Figure 11.8   Geometry of an external fixation device. B_1 is into the page, inducing large current in the metal and strong electric fields between the pins.

Example 11.12   Magnetically activated spinal extension device

A patient with this device can be scanned in an MR system meeting the following conditions:

- Static magnetic field of 1.5 Tesla (1.5 T)
- Maximum spatial field gradient of 3000 gauss/cm (30 T/m)
- Maximum MR system reported, whole body averaged specific absorption rate (SAR) of 0.5 W/kg at 1.5 T.

Under the scan conditions defined above, the device is expected to produce a maximum temperature rise of no greater than 3.7 °C after 15 minutes of continuous scanning.
   Modify the following T_2-weighted sequence to comply with the SAR condition:

- T2w Turbo/fast spin echo, TE = 120 ms
- Turbo factor/no. echoes = 16
- TR = 4000
- Inter-echo spacing: 10 ms (Fast RF pulse)
- 24 slices.

Use the SAR calculator [13] starting with the parameters shown above to make changes suitable for scanning the implant at 1.5 T. The patient weights 80 kg (176 lb) and has height 1.76 cm. Pre-scan SAR is estimated as 2.7 W kg^{-1}.
   The following is not the only way to achieve the SAR condition.
   RF pulse → low SAR, Flip angle → 150°, No. echoes → 13, TR → 4100 ms results in 0.5 W kg^{-1}

$$SAR_{new} = 2.7 \times \frac{0.5}{1.5} \times \left(\frac{150}{180}\right)^2 \times \frac{13}{16} \times \frac{4000}{4100} = 0.5\,W\,kg^{-1}$$

Occasionally you may come across a set of MR conditions which do not make sense or appear to be contradictory. This may arise if the device was tested for translation on a 1.5 T system with a lower spatial gradient, then subsequently tested on a 3 T system with higher dB/dz. What are we to do in these situations? Have a look at Example 11.13.

Example 11.13   Urinary control system

The MR conditions are stated as:

1.5 T: Spatial gradient of 4.5 T/m or less
          maximum whole-body averaged SAR of 1.5 W/kg for 15 minutes or less as assessed by calorimetry, highest
          temperature change ≤ 0.4 °C
3 T: Spatial gradient of 7.2 T/m or less
          maximum whole-body averaged SAR of 2.9 W/kg for 15 minutes or less as assessed by calorimetry, highest
          temperature change ≤ 2 °C.

Which of the scanners considered in this chapter would be suitable for scanning a patient with this device? Do you notice anything odd about the conditions?

Discussion: *Before you go plunging into the fringe field gradient maps, consider how is it possible for the spatial gradient limit to be higher at 3 T than 1.5 T? From Chapters 2 and 9 we recognize that whilst magnetic forces are complex, depending upon shape, state of saturation, etc., the force must be linear with dB/dz. In short, the device manufacturer has got it wrong; the dB/dz limit at 1.5 T should be as stated for 3 T (if not higher).*
   What has happened with the SAR condition?
   It is possible that, using the ASTM phantom, it was difficult to achieve a higher SAR at 1.5 T than reported in the conditions. Clearly the 1.5 W kg^{-1} is lower than the usual 2 W kg^{-1} recommended for testing, however with RF exposures we should not jump to conclusions too readily. There may be reasons, e.g. wavelength resonance effects, which are not obvious.

Conclusion: *we can scan a patient with this device on any of the scanners considered in this chapter, but we should exercise caution with the SAR, keeping to the stated RF conditions.*

OFF-LABEL SCANNING

Scanning with exposures in excess of the conditions or where they are unknown is considered to be "off-label." Off-label is a description more commonly applied to the use of an approved or licensed medicine in an unapproved way, for example, to treat a condition the drug is not intended for, or with a dosage different to that which is specified on the "label" [15]. Off-label treatments or medications are not illegal; however certain additional constraints apply. For example, in the UK's guidance [16] for off-label medicinal products, a prescriber should:

- *Be satisfied that an alternative, licensed medicine would not meet the patient's needs before prescribing an unlicensed medicine*
- *Be satisfied that such use would better serve the patient's needs than an appropriately licensed alternative before prescribing a medicine off-label*
- *Be satisfied that there is a sufficient evidence base and/or experience of using the medicine to show its safety and efficacy*
- *Take responsibility for prescribing the medicine and for overseeing the patient's care, including monitoring and follow-up*
- *Record the medicine prescribed and, where common practice is not being followed, the reasons for prescribing this medicine; [you may wish to] record that you have discussed the issue with the patient.*

Communication with the patient is essential to ensure informed consent can be given [17].
How should we interpret this for MRI? The following may help. You should:

1. Be satisfied that an alternative diagnostic test would not meet the patient's needs before proceeding with the MRI.
2. Be satisfied that MRI better serves the patient's needs than an alternative examination.
3. Be satisfied that there is a sufficient evidence base and/or experience of using MRI in this situation to show its safety and efficacy.
4. Take responsibility for the examination and for overseeing the patient's care, including monitoring and follow-up; this is the responsibility of the *radiologist*.
5. Record the details of the examination and, where common practice is not being followed, the reasons for proceeding, recording that you have discussed the issue with the patient.

The majority of these are the responsibility of the radiologist. The MR technologist or MRSO and MRSE may be consulted regarding the third point, and the technologist will optimize the scanning protocol (minimizing SAR, B_{1+RMS}, etc.), and record the parameters.

Specific examples of off-label MRI include the scanning of patients with "legacy" pacemakers, or with an external fixation device within the scanner bore, or at a B_0 greater than the conditions, or the administration of gadolinium contrast in excess of the standard dosage.

WHAT TO DO WHEN YOU DO NOT KNOW THE CONDITIONS?

Not knowing the conditions does not mean you cannot scan, but there are a few practical considerations to be made in addition to those above. Complying with the conditions ensures that the patient can be scanned safety, but this does not necessarily mean that the device is *unsafe* for exposures that exceed the conditions. For example, if a passive implant has a spatial gradient condition of 7.2 T m⁻¹, this could be interpreted in two ways:

- The device deflected less than or equal to 45° in a spatial gradient of 7.2 T m⁻¹ in a magnet which offered higher spatial gradient values
- The figure 7.2 T m⁻¹ was the maximum value available on the test scanner; the device *may* deflect less than 45° at higher spatial gradients.

Unfortunately, we are not told the deflection angle. Some devices will have their spatial gradient condition "extrapolated." This means that they were tested to a lower value of spatial gradient and the limiting condition was calculated mathematically from the observed deflection angle.

Know the material

If you know the implant material you can assess the likely risk involved in scanning. This can be balanced by the responsible radiologist or physician against the potential benefit from proceeding with the examination, or the risk inherent in *not* proceeding.

Example 11.14   Exceeding the spatial gradient condition I

The conditions for a prosthetic heart valve are:

- Static magnetic field of 3 T or less
- Maximum spatial gradient of 7.2 T m⁻¹.

The composition of the material (weight percentage) is stated as:

Cobalt 40%;	Chromium 20%;	Nickel 15%;	Molybdenum 7%;	Manganese 2%;
Carbon < 0.1%;	Beryllium < 0.1%;	Iron 5.8%.		

Can we scan this device if the maximum spatial gradient it may experience *in situ* in the scanner is 9 T m⁻¹?

Discussion: *we can identify the material as Elgiloy/Phynox, a paramagnetic alloy with a susceptibility in the range 0.002–0.005. In Figures 9.12–13 we saw a sphere of this material deflecting around 17°. From Equation 9.3 we can estimate the magnetic force as a fraction of its weight:*

$$\frac{F_m}{mg} = \tan\alpha \approx \tan 17° = 0.3$$

In a spatial gradient of 9 Tm⁻¹ the magnetic force to gravity ratio is:

$$\frac{F_m}{mg} \approx 0.3 \times \frac{9}{7.2} = 0.375$$

The estimated magnetic force is 0.375 of the object's weight. In this example we postulate that the device was only tested up to 7.2 T m⁻¹ and that the risk–benefit analysis may favour scanning over not scanning. Technically this is still "off-label" so the considerations in the previous section should be addressed.

Know the physics (or ask an MRSE)

If we are dealing with an implant with a low magnetic susceptibility (this includes most of the implant materials listed in Table 9.3), the maximum twisting force on a weakly ferromagnetic or paramagnetic object of length l is

$$F_{torque,max} = \frac{1}{2l\mu_0} \chi^2 V B_0^2 \qquad (11.3)$$

This will be the case for any object deflecting up to 45° in the deflection test. The maximum translational force will be

$$F_{trans,max} = \frac{\chi}{\mu_0} V B_0 \frac{dB}{dz} \qquad (11.4)$$

The ratio is

$$\frac{F_{torque}}{F_{trans}} = \frac{1}{2l} \chi B_0 \bigg/ \frac{dB}{dz} \qquad (11.5)$$

We can use this to assess the risk of twisting of the device.

Example 11.15   Exceeding the spatial gradient condition II (advanced)

Can we scan the following device if the maximum spatial gradient it may experience is 12 T m⁻¹?
   The conditions are:

- Static magnetic field of 3 T or less
- Maximum spatial gradient of 9 T m⁻¹ (extrapolated)
- No information about the material.

Discussion: *In this case an estimation of the spatial gradient limit has already been carried out by invoking extrapolation in the deflection test. We do not know the material; therefore, we must assume that at 9 T m⁻¹ the magnetic force may equal the force due to gravity. Under this assumption we can estimate that the ratio of magnetic to gravitational force in our scanner may be up to*

$$\frac{F_m}{mg} \le \frac{12}{9} = 1.33$$

The force may be up to 33% more than that due to gravity.
   We should also consider the magnetic torque. If the long axis of the object is parallel to B_0 the torque will be close to zero. Otherwise, we do not know the value of χ - but we can make a worst-case estimate.
   Assume from the deflection test that the magnetic and gravitational forces are equal at 9 T m⁻¹. From Equation 11.4 and using $m = \rho V$

$$\frac{1}{\rho V g} \frac{\chi}{\mu_0} V B_0 \frac{dB}{dz} \le 1$$

χ/ρ is the mass susceptibility and will have a maximum value

$$\chi_\rho \le \frac{9.8 \mu_0}{B_0 \frac{dB}{dz}}$$

In the example the worst case $B_0 \frac{dB}{dz}$ is $3 \times 9 = 27$ T^2 m^{-1} so an upper limit on the mass susceptibility is

$$\chi_\rho \leq \frac{9.8 \times 4\pi \times 10^{-7}}{27} = 4.6 \times 10^{-7}$$

To estimate the torque, we still need the volume susceptibility χ. We do not know the material, but iridium has the highest density of implant materials at 22 560 kg m^{-3}. The worst-case value of χ is

$$\chi \leq 22\,560 \times 4.6 \times 10^{-7} = 0.01$$

From Equation 11.3 we can then estimate the force due to torque if we know the object's length. For example, if the device is 1 cm long

$$F_{torque,max} \leq \frac{0.01}{0.02} \times \frac{3}{9} \times 1.33mg = 0.22mg$$

The twisting force is not more than one fifth of the device's weight.

Know your institutional policies

It is important that your institution has written policies on MR safety, including how to deal with implants. Be aware of these and follow them at all times. Accidents occur when procedures are bypassed or ignored.

Also be aware of and observe the appropriate levels of responsibility and delegation. It helps to have the MR safety roles in place: the MR Medical Director who holds the ultimate and legal responsibility for the patient's wellbeing, the MR Safety Officer, and the MR Safety Expert (see Chapter 14).

Ensure a risk–benefit analysis is carried out. The MRSO, aided by the MRSE, can assess the risks to assist the MRMD or supervising radiologist to carry the analysis and arrive at a considered clinical decision. This will also help with communication with the patient and for obtaining consent. This is off-label scanning. Following clear guidelines is essential for the patient's physical and your professional safety.

Know your scanner

Be sure to have access to your scanner's spatial gradient maps and understand their interpretation. Revisit the examples in the chapter, but for your own scanner. Be adept at controlling SAR and B_{1+}RMS. Be able to make appropriate sequence choices, e.g. substituting low SAR sequences if required. Know the scanner hardware: for example, which coils are transmit–receive. Remember, if your scanner has parallel transmit, that this mode is *not* compatible with the MR conditions.

Know your limitations

Lastly, know your limitations. We cannot know everything about MR safety, so recognize when you just do not know and when to seek help. Kruger and Dunning [18], in a seminal social psychology paper "Unskilled and unaware of it: how difficulties in recognising one's own incompetence lead to inflated self-assessments," identified that the less you know about a subject, the more confident you may feel about it. Basically, you lack the expertise to realize how little you may have! Conversely, people with greater knowledge are more aware of the potential complexities, and consequently may doubt their own expertise. This is a good place to be in MR safety, always questioning, never assuming.

CONCLUSIONS

Scanning within the MR conditions will achieve the maximum level of protection for your patients. The important skills to develop are:

- Understanding the conditions
- Interpreting spatial gradient data
- Controlling SAR and B_{1+}RMS
- Understanding the implications of off-label scanning
- Knowing your physics, your scanner, your institutional policies, and your limitations.

Revision questions

1. A passive implant has a MR condition of maximum spatial gradient of 7.2 T/m. Your scanner's maximum spatial gradient is 11 T/m. What do you do?
   A. Scan anyway because your radiologist gets annoyed if you don't
   B. Do not scan. It is too dangerous
   C. Scan anyway, because you have an MRSO certificate and you know best
   D. Check Facebook to see what others say, and follow their advice
   E. Check your spatial gradient map to see where the implant may lie.
2. In the MR conditions RF heating is measured over:
   A. 10 seconds
   B. 5 minutes
   C. 6 minutes
   D. 10 minutes
   E. 15 minutes.
3. Which of the following is not part of the MR conditions?
   A. Static field
   B. Spatial gradient field
   C. Imaging gradient amplitude
   D. Whole-body SAR
   E. B_{1+}RMS.
4. Which of the following is most relevant for a paramagnetic or unsaturated weakly ferromagnetic object?
   A. Static field B_0
   B. Spatial gradient field dB/dz
   C. Imaging gradient slew rate
   D. Static field-spatial gradient product B·dB/dz
   E. B_{1+}RMS.
5. In a typical closed bore magnet
   A. The maximum spatial gradient occurs at the iso-center
   B. The maximum spatial gradient occurs near the bore entrance
   C. The maximum torque is experienced close to the bore entrance
   D. The maximum translational force occurs at the iso-center
   E. The maximum field-gradient-product occurs near the iso-center.

6. An implant has a condition for the spatial gradient to be less than or equal to 120 mT/cm. This is equal to:
   A. 1.2 T/m
   B. 12 T/m
   C. 12 G/m
   D. 120 G/m
   E. 12 T/m/s.

7. The scanner console informs you that the B_{1+}RMS is 5 μT. The MR condition states 4 μT. Which of the following parameter changes will ensure compliance with the condition?
   A. Reducing the number of slices from 20 to 16
   B. Reducing the number of echoes from 10 to 8
   C. Increasing TE from 80 ms to 100 ms
   D. Reducing the flip angle from 180° to 140°
   E. Increasing TR from 4000 ms to 5000 ms.

8. The scanner console informs you that the whole-body SAR is 2 W kg^{-1}. The MR condition states 1 W kg^{-1}. Which of the following parameter changes does *not* ensure compliances with the condition?
   A. Reducing the number of slices from 20 to 10
   B. Reducing the number of echoes from 10 to 5
   C. Doubling the length of the RF pulses
   D. Reducing the flip angle from 180° to 140°
   E. Increasing TR from 4000 ms to 8000 ms.

References

1. www.MRIsafety.com Shellock R &D Services Inc. (accessed 1 August 2019).
2. www.MagResource.com The Villages FL: MagResource. (accessed 1 August 2019).
3. Shellock F.G. (2019) *Reference Manual for Magnetic Resonance Safety, Implants, and Devices: 2019 Edition (and subsequent years)*. Los Angeles, CA: Biomedical Research Publishing Group.
4. Kanal, E., Barkovich, A.J., Bell, C.M. et al. (2013). ACR Guidance Document on MR Safe Practices: 2013, American College of Radiology Expert panel on MR Safety. *Journal of Magnetic Resonance Imaging* 37:501–530.
5. ACR Committee on MR Safety (2019). ACR Guidance Document on MR Safe Practices: Updates and Critical Information 2019. *Journal of Magnetic Resonance Imaging* https://doi.org/10.1002/jmri.26880
6. Medicines and Healthcare Products Regulatory Agency (2015). *Safety Guidelines for Magnetic Resonance Imaging Equipment in Clinical Use*. London: MHRA https://assets.publishing.service.gov.uk/government/uploads/system/uploads/attachment_data/file/476931/MRI_guidance_2015_–_4-02d1.pdf (accessed 17 July 2019)
7. Royal Australian and New Zealand College of Radiologists (2017). *MR safety guidelines*.: Sydney: RANZCR https://www.ranzcr.com/college/document-library/ranzcr-mri-safety-guidelines (accessed 14 March 2019).
8. Society and College of Radiographers and the British Association of Magnetic Resonance Radiographers (2019). *Safety in Magnetic Resonance Imaging*. London: SCOR and BAMRR.
9. ASTM F2503-13 (2015): *Standard Practice for Marking Medical Devices and Other Items for Safety in the Magnetic Resonance Environment*. West Conshohocken, PA: ASTM International. West Conshohocken, PA: ASTM International.
10. International Electrotechnical Commission (2105). *Medical Electrical Equipment – Part 2–33: Particular Requirements for the Safety of Magnetic Resonance Equipment for Medical Diagnosis*. IEC 60601-2-33 3.3 edn. Geneva: IEC
11. Food and Drug Administration (2014). *Criteria for significant risk investigations of magnetic resonance diagnostic devices*. Rockville, MD: Center for Devices and Radiological Health, FDA.

12. ASTM F2182-11a (2011). *Standard Test Method for Measurement of Radio Frequency Induced Heating On or Near Passive Implants During Magnetic Resonance Imaging.* West Conshohocken, PA: ASTM International.

13. https://drdonaldmcrobbie.com/sar-and-b1rms-calculator/ (accessed 1 August 2019).

14. Liu, Y., Chen, J., Shellock, F.G. et al. (2013). Computational and experimental studies of an orthopedic implant: MRI related heating at 1.5-T/64-MHz and 3-T/128-MHz. *Journal of Magnetic Resonance Imaging* 37:491–497.

15. Food and Drug Administration (2018). Understanding Unapproved Use of Approved Drugs Off Label. https://www.fda.gov/patients/learn-about-expanded-access-and-other-treatment-options/understanding-unapproved-use-approved-drugs-label Silver Spring, MD: FDA. (accessed 5 May 2019).

16. Medicines and Healthcare products Regulatory Agency (2014). https://www.gov.uk/drug-safety-update/off-label-or-unlicensed-use-of-medicines-prescribers-responsibilities. London: MHRA (accessed 5 May 2019).

17. General Medical Council (2008). *General Medical Council Good Practice in Prescribing Medicines.* London: GMC.

18. Kruger, J. and Dunning, D. (1999). Unskilled and unaware of it: how difficulties in recognizing one's own incompetence lead to inflated self-assessments. *Journal of Personality and Social Psychology* 77:1121–1134.

Further reading and resources

MR manufacturer Compatibility Data

Shellock F.G. (2019) *Reference Manual for Magnetic Resonance Safety, Implants, and Devices: 2019 Edition (and subsequent years).* Los Angeles, CA: Biomedical Research Publishing Group.

www.MagResource.com

www.MRIsafety.com.

12

Location, location, location: suite design

INTRODUCTION

MRI safety starts before your scanner is installed. It begins with the design of the MR suite or facility. A compromised design makes the task of ensuring the safety of patients, staff, and visitors more difficult. Guidance for the safe design of MR facilities has been in existence from the late 1980s and early 1990s [1,2] but it took the tragic projectile-related fatality of 2001 to galvanize the North American MR community into producing guidance that other less experienced MR centers could adopt, the 2002 American College of Radiology (ACR) "White paper on MRI safety" [3]. Despite the widespread availability and recognition of this advice, it is beyond comprehension that some MRI facilities being built today do not comply with the design principles it advocates.

ACR ZONING SCHEME

The key point of design is the control of access to the magnet. The ACR Zoning system designates four distinct areas or zones, defined by the activities that take place in each, and by their access from categories of persons:

- **Zone 1**: A freely accessible public area with no restrictions, e.g. a hospital corridor
- **Zone 2**: The interface between public and controlled areas, e.g. a reception area under the supervision of MR staff, but readily accessible to patients and hospital staff. MR safety screening usually occurs here. Interception and safe storage of all removable ferromagnetic or potentially ferromagnetic objects should take place in this area
- **Zone 3**: A restricted area accessible only to fully trained and authorized MR personnel. It is physically demarcated with secure entry. Non-MR staff and patients may only enter under the supervision of MR staff after screening. Safety signage is prominent
- **Zone 4:** The magnet or MR examination room is subject to similar security and access restrictions as Zone III. It is contained within Zone III with no other access. Safety signage is required on entrance. Supervision of the entrance is maintained by MR trained staff.

Essentials of MRI Safety, First Edition. Donald W. McRobbie.
© 2020 John Wiley & Sons Ltd. Published 2020 by John Wiley & Sons Ltd.

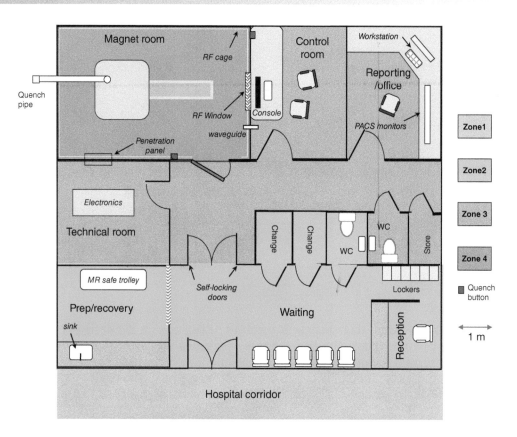

Figure 12.1   ACR Zoning system for a small MR suite.

Figure 12.1 shows an example of the four Zones. The ACR Zoning system has been adopted widely throughout the world [4–7].

Alternative schemes

UK-MHRA

The United Kingdom's Medical Devices Directorate (now MHRA) first published guidance on MR suite layout in 1993 [2], preceding the ACR Zoning scheme by nearly a decade. In the current version [8] the following definitions are given (Figure 12.2):

- **MR Controlled Access Area**: equivalent to the ACR Zone III with similar security and access restrictions
- **MR Environment**: an area encompassing both the Faraday-shielded volume and the 0.5 mT fringe field contour. Whilst similar to Zone IV, it may include regions outside the magnet room
- **MR Projectile Zone**: designated by the 3 mT fringe field contour. Sites that restrict the introduction of ferromagnetic objects into the MR Environment are not required to designate this zone.

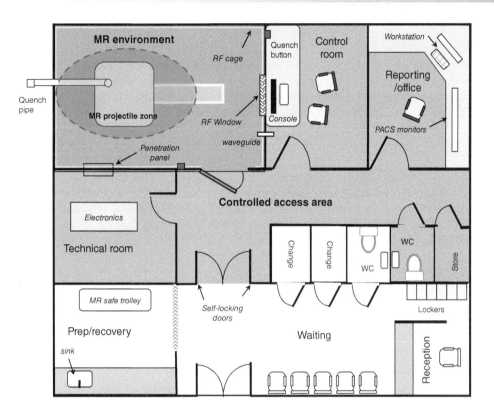

Figure 12.2   Controlled Access Area and MR Environment as for UK guidance [8].

IEC60601-2-33

The International Electrotechnical Commission (IEC) standard [9] is mostly concerned with the operation and safe function of MR equipment. It cites the need for a "Controlled Access Area" based upon field limits and also references the ACR Zones without specifying which approach should be used.

Europe

The European Society of Radiology and the European Federation of Radiographer Societies [7] joint paper on patient safety in medical imaging recommends following ACR guidance. The MRI Working Group in the Netherlands [10], in response to the European Union Physical Agents Directive (currently [11]) produced guidance on safe working with MRI. Whilst not defining the areas, it catergorizes types of room where specific risks exist:

- Controlled access area: scanner room, where the fringe field exceeds 0.5 mT
- Controlled access area: outside the scanner room, where the fringe field exceeds 0.5 mT
- Technical areas outside the controlled access area, where the fringe field is less than 0.5 mT.

These are broadly in line with the MHRA scheme.

FRINGE FIELD

The Zone IV/Controlled Access Area/MR Environment (we will simply call it "Zone IV") is usually defined by the extent of the 0.5 mT contour (previously called "the 5 Gauss line") or a suitable physical barrier, e.g. the walls of the MR room. The word "contour" better describes this region than "line" because it forms a three-dimensional volume, with rotational symmetry about the magnet axis (Figure 12.3).

The purpose of Zone IV is threefold:

* To restrict access of unauthorized persons not trained in MR safety
* To prevent the introduction of MR unsafe items which may become dangerous projectiles
* To prevent the inadvertent exposure of magnet-sensitive devices or equipment. In particular the value of 0.5 mT was selected to ensure that MR-unsafe cardiac pacemakers remain unaffected by the field.

Where the 0.5 mT contour extends beyond the physical barriers of the building, an exclusion zone must be established with suitable barriers and signage.

The extent of the fringe field is one of the principal design considerations. Magnetic shielding may be required if the field extends beyond the magnet room into adjacent areas. Magnetic shielding uses sheets of iron and is both heavy and expensive. It also affects the shim of the magnet. Consideration must be given to floors immediately above or below the scanner. Magnet-sensitive equipment should be suitably excluded (Table 12.1). The influence of nearby ferromagnetic items on the scanner's B_0 uniformity or homogeneity should be considered (Table 12.2).

After installation the fringe field should be confirmed using a suitable magnetometer, as the presence of steel structures in the building can distort the field contours. This may be carried out by the MR manufacturer or by a medical physicist/ MRSE (Figure 12.4).

HELIUM EXHAUST AND QUENCH PIPE

A key aspect of the installation is the provision made for the exhaust of helium gas: the "quench pipe." A "quench" occurs when the magnet's windings lose their superconductivity, resulting in a catastrophic and rapid loss of the field, heating of the windings, and the vaporizing or "boil off" of the helium liquid as gas (see Chapter 1).

Quench

A magnet quench may occur in a controlled manner as a safety feature used, for example, in the event of a serious or life-threatening projectile incident or a major fire in the magnet room. It may also occasionally happen spontaneously as an accident (see https://youtu.be/1R7KsfosV-o, accessed 25 May 19). In a quench the magnetic field collapses over 20–30 seconds. The helium boils off with one liter of liquid typically expanding as 800 liters of gas. The exhaust system has to be capable of handling this volume of high-pressure gas. As the helium encounters the atmosphere it condenses into a fog. It is lighter than air, so will rise – like steam – but very cold. In the event of a leakage into the magnet room, the helium fog will accumulate from the ceiling downwards. If this happens, evacuate the room, keeping low to avoid inhaling the helium gas.

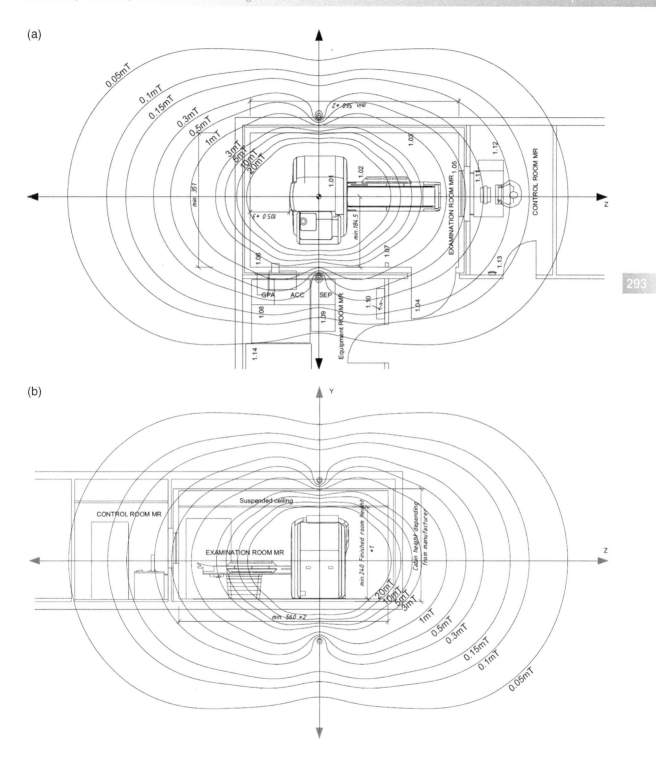

Figure 12.3 Fringe field contours for a 1.5T MRI installation: (a) top view; (b) side view. Reproduced with permission of Siemens Healthineers.

Table 12.1   Typical safe operating distances for the avoidance of interference with various items of equipment.

Fringe field (mT)	Item	Typical Minimum distance (m) 1.5 T		Typical Minimum distance (m) 3 T	
		On axis	Radially	On axis	Radially
10	Oxygen monitors, Laser imager	2.2	1.6	2.6	1.8
3	Magnetic media, LCD displays	2.8	2.0	3.3	2.2
1	Computer hard disks, X-ray tubes	3.4	2.2	4.3	2.4
0.5	Conventional pacemakers	4.0	2.5	4.6	2.6
0.2	CT Scanners	4.9	3.0	5.6	3.2
0.1	Gamma cameras, Image intensifiers, PET scanners	5.6	3.3	6.8	3.9
0.05	Linear accelerators	6.8	3.9	8.2	4.6

Table 12.2   Typical distances for the avoidance of interference with B_0 homogeneity.

Item	Distance (m)	
	Radial	Axial
Wheelchair /trolley	5	6
Car	6	8
Truck	7	10
Train	40	40

Example 12.1   Quench

Looking at the MR room in Figure 12.1 compare the volume of helium gas released in a quench with the volume of the room. Assume that the magnet cryostat contains 1000 L of liquid helium and the the ceiling height is 3.5 m.

The dimensions of the room are 5.5 × 3.5 m. The volume of the room is

$$V_{room} = 5.5 \times 3.5 \times 3.5 = 67.4\,m^3$$

The volume of the gas is

$$V_{gas} = 1000 \times 800 = 800\,000L$$

One liter equals 0.001 m³ so the volume of helium gas is 800 m³, enough to fill 12 MR rooms!

(a)

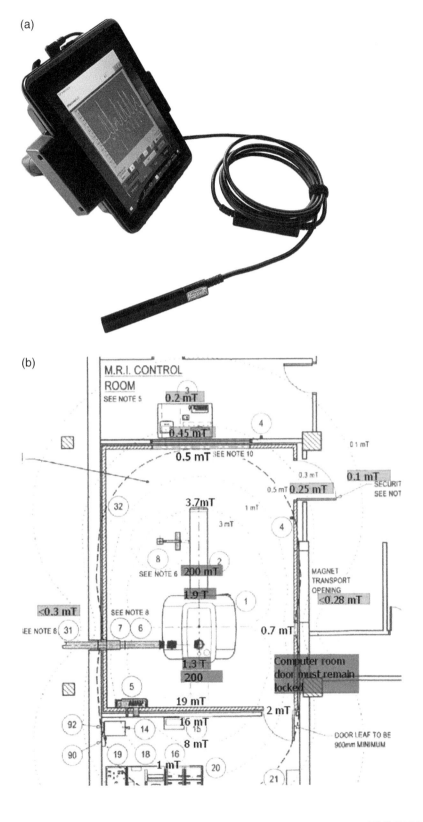

(b)

Figure 12.4   Confirming the fringe field: (a) Handheld 3-axis magnetometer THM1176, image courtesy of Metrolab (technology@metrolab.com); (b) spot check measurements of the fringe field.

Cryogen hazards

Helium is an odorless, non-toxic inert gas. The risks arise mainly from the cold or the displacement of air.

Cold injuries

Cold injuries or frostbite may result from contact with the helium (gaseous or liquid) or cryogen system components such as pipework. Only cryogen-trained personnel should have any contact with cryogenic equipment – usually restricted to MR maintenance engineers. The risks are mitigated by using personal protective equipment (PPE): gloves, facemasks, and overalls.

Asthma induction and asphyxiation

Persons susceptible to asthmatic episodes may suffer an attack if quantities of cold air or helium are inhaled. In an extreme case where leaked helium gas displaces the air in the room, there is a risk of asphyxiation. This is mitigated by the proper maintaining of the helium exhaust system, the deployment of an oxygen level monitor, and rapid air replenishment through appropriate ventilation.

Oxygen condensation

The boiling point of oxygen is -183 °C (90 K); it will liquefy below this temperature. Cold helium coming into contact with air may cause oxygen condensation. This condensate may form on the surfaces of items which otherwise would not be inflammable, rendering them as potential fire hazards.

Quench pipe / helium exhaust system

The helium exhaust system must comply with the MR manufacturer's specifications. Pipework leading to the external atmosphere should follow as short and direct a path as possible, avoiding areas where moisture may be trapped. The outlet should be to an external area, sufficiently remote from occupied areas, windows, and doors (Figure 12.5). The pipe's outlet should be designed to prevent rainwater ingress, or birds nesting! A restricted area surrounding the quench pipe outlet should be designated by signage and, where potentially accessible, by a physical barrier, e.g. fencing.

An annual inspection of the quench pipe and vent is recommended [8]. Responsibility for maintenance of the quench pipe may rest with the MR manufacturer or the hospital/clinic. MR cryostats and associated equipment are pressurized systems and may be subject to national regulations, e.g. [12].

The MR room door should open outwards to enable its use in the event of a pressure build-up following a helium accumulation in the room. Should this not be possible, then a pressure-release mechanism, such as a "cat flap" or pressure-equalizing waveguides should be installed. In the past one MR vendor provided a hammer to shatter the glass of the RF viewing window as a means of pressure equalization in an emergency. This is not a suitable solution.

SECURITY

The security of Zones III and IV is paramount. Both zones require lockable doors with restricted access, e.g. by swipe card or keypad. Only suitably trained personnel should have access for entry. A staffed Zone II is also beneficial, enabling the interception of unauthorized persons or

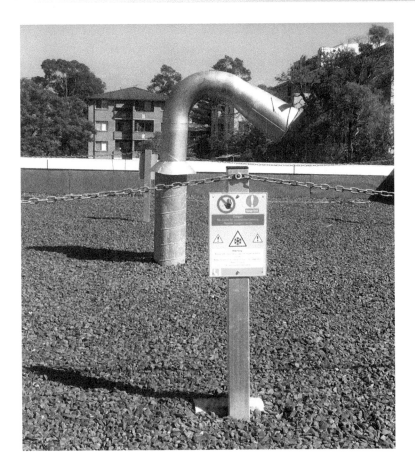

Figure 12.5   Quench pipe outlet. Image from the Australian MR Linac, Liverpool, New South Wales.

unsafe equipment. There should be clear visual surveillance of the Zone IV entrance, the MR room door, at all times by staff in the control room. The magnet room door should open in such a way as permits full view of any persons attempting entrance. A temporary barrier using retract-able tape or a plastic chain is recommended for times when the door remains open.

SAFETY FEATURES

The scanner and MRI suite have a range of safety features.

Quench button

The "quench button" or emergency run down unit (ERDU) initiates a magnet quench, resulting in the loss of the magnetic field. Its use is restricted to seriously injurious or life-threatening projectile incidents or major fire within the room. A quench is a serious occurrence, entailing significant financial expense through scanner downtime, helium refill, and re-ramping/shim-ming. Clear policies on when to quench and on who may authorize a quench are required (Chapter 14).

Quench buttons are usually situated in the control room and in the magnet room. It is important that these are accessible in the event of a serious fire. The electrical control wires of the quench system should be fire-resistant. Appropriate labeling of the quench button is essential.

Emergency stop button

This button has a different function to the quench button. Its purpose is to switch off all electrical supply to the scanner. It does *not* initiate a quench (the magnet will remain cold for days/hours without the cryo-cooler operating). An electrical-off switch may be required by local electrical safety regulations. A manual release "mushroom" button is often used. The emergency stop button can be used in the case of an electric shock or trapping incident. There will usually be an emergency-off button in the control room, magnet room, and technical room.

Couch release

The scanner will also have a manual couch release mechanism which can be used to extract the patient table in the event of an electrical failure or medical emergency. Check your user documentation or ask your MR applications specialist about its location and function.

Intercom

An intercom enables staff in the control room to talk to and listen to the patient, and vice versa. This may operate through the patient headphones or via loudspeakers in the magnet room.

Patient alarm

The scanner has a patient alarm, usually a hand-held squeeze or "panic" button to alert staff to a patient-initiated call.

CC camera, RF window

Visual supervision of the patient is extremely important. The scanner should be suitably positioned to enable clear lines of sight through the scanner bore from the console in the control room. Closed circuit (CC) cameras may be positioned at the far end of the bore to enable visual monitoring of the patient's head.

Acoustic attenuation

Suitable sound proofing of the magnet room is required. An acoustic noise survey should be conducted at installation. Refer to Chapter 6 and relevant national regulations on noise at work.

Magnet room door interlock

Some MR systems employ an electrical interlock on the magnet room door. This may prevent or interrupt scanning when activated. Staff need to be aware of its functionality.

Signage

Signage is a key aspect of MR safety. Appropriate signs are defined in IEC60601-2-33 [9] or national guidance [8]. Figure 12.6a shows examples of signage appropriate for the entrance of

298

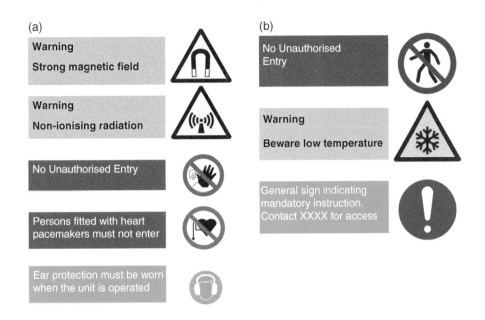

Figure 12.6   Signage: (a) suitable for the magnet room door/ entrance to Zone IV; (b) suitable for the vicinity of the quench pipe output.

the MR room. These include warnings about the strong magnetic field, RF exposure, the use of lasers, the imperative for hearing protection, and prohibited items. Sites may wish to add signage indicating the Zones. These should follow national or international symbol conventions. In the international scheme the following applies:

- Red circle with strike-out: prohibition
- Yellow triangle, edged with black: warning of a hazard
- Blue circle: mandatory instructions.

Figure 12.6b shows signage appropriate for the vicinity of the quench pipe outlet.

Ferromagnetic detection systems

Some sites may deploy ferromagnetic detection systems mounted sentinel-style at door entrances (Figure 12.7a). As these are sensitive to all ferromagnetic materials, they should be positioned away from moving ferromagnetic parts, e.g. in door handles or locks, or from electromagnetically activated door release systems which may interfere with the detector's function. To be effective, the location of the ferromagnetic detection system should be considered at the design stage. Additionally, metal in staff clothing and shoes may need to be restricted. MR safe wheelchairs and trolleys may have steel axles or bearings which may set off the alarm. Alternatively, a stand-alone screening device can be used on ambulant patients (Figure 12.7b). These can be positioned in ferromagnetic "quiet" zones. Prior to scanning, the patient is asked to perform a 360° rotation to ensure the absence of ferromagnetic objects. An overview of the function and use of ferromagnetic detection systems is given in reference [13]. Patient screening is considered later in Chapter 14.

(a)

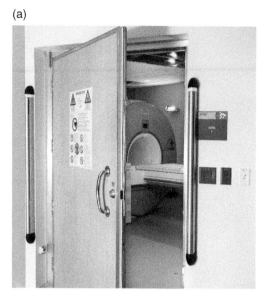

(b)

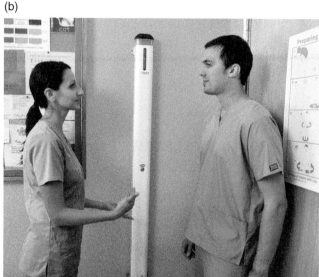

Figure 12.7   Ferromagnetic detection systems: (a) Ferroguard Assure mounted by the magnet room entrance; (b) screening system for ambulant patient inspection. Source: Metrasens Ltd. (www.metrasens.com/mri-safety). Used with permission.

Changing rooms and lockers

The changing of patients into gowns or scrubs has become a standard means of ensuring that no loose ferromagnetic items can be brought into the room. Lockers can be provided for patients' personal effects: cell phones, purses, wallets, watches, and loose jewellery.

Fire extinguishers

MR safe fire extinguishers, appropriately labeled, should be available in Zone III. These should use carbon dioxide rather than water as the extinguishing agent. The safety pin may be ferromagnetic and should be removed before entering Zone IV. In the event of a serious fire requiring fully equipped fire-fighters to enter Zone IV, the magnet should be quenched.

Fire exits

The provision of sufficient fire exits will depend upon local fire regulations. This may entail there being more than one possible door into the MR suite. Any additional fire doors should enable exit only, not entrance.

Resus equipment

Emergency resuscitation equipment should be accessible. This would not be used in Zone IV, and must be appropriately labeled.

MRI PROJECT MANAGEMENT

As MRI safety begins with design, it is imperative that the project group overseeing the procurement and installation of the system includes professionals with the appropriate range of skills. These may include hospital managers, radiologists, lead MR technologists, MRSO, MRMD, MRSE, medical physicists, hospital estates engineers, MR manufacturer engineers, project managers, anaesthetic staff, electrical and building contractors, architect, and RF shield contractors.

The following is a suitable design process (Figure 12.8.).

1. The project begins with a statement of the clinical need, or business case, detailing the range and number of patients and referrals. This informs the choice of *technical specifications*.
2. The technical specifications may be a statement of required functionality or performance and/or a detailed technical questionnaire addressed to prospective suppliers.
3. An *Operational Policy* outlines the proposed day-to-day functioning of the unit. For example, how ambulant and trolley patients are handled, where patient screening, anesthesia, recovery, etc. takes place. The "patient's journey" is an important consideration [14].
4. The Operational Policy informs the architect on the design features required. Room *data sheets* specify the features and services (e.g. electrical supply, medical gases, data ports, plumbing, etc) required in each room.
5. Prospective MR manufacturers may provide detailed technical drawings and information regarding placement of the magnet, power, water, ventilation, floor loading requirements, and fringe field containment. Magnetic shielding may be specified.
6. Following the award of purchase, the project group oversees the installation process.
7. Testing and commissioning include the testing of the RF shield, magnet shimming, manufacturer's test procedures, customer *acceptance testing* [15,16]. This should include a fringe field survey and an inspection of the safety features.
8. The manufacturer's applications specialist will provide training to the MR staff and assist with the customization of MR scanning protocols.

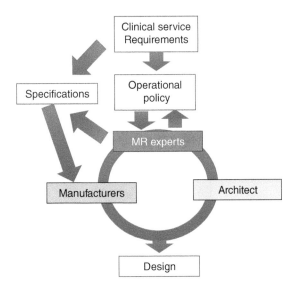

Figure 12.8   MRI suite design process.

SPECIALIST SYSTEMS

Specialist systems include mobile MR, extremity or open scanners, interventional systems, MR-positron emission tomography (PET) scanners or MR-linear accelerator (Linac) systems. These have particular safety requirements.

Mobile MRI systems

MRI systems mounted in a truck or trailer may be moved from site to site, to provide access to MRI for populations remote from a major healthcare facility. The safety requirements are similar to static systems. However, due to the constrained space available, the 0.5 mT region may extend into the control room and extra care is needed regarding projectiles. Additionally, the remoteness from main hospital facilities may restrict the ability to deal with medical emergencies. Consequently, mobile systems are best suited for ambulant, outpatient referrals. A fringe field survey should confirm that the 0.5mT contour is contained within the vehicle, and if not, suitable signage and barriers should be erected on site. The magnet will be transported between sites in a cold state. This will increase the risk of quench or explosion in the event of a road traffic accident. Consideration must be given to local regulations regarding the transportation of dangerous goods.

Interventional MRI systems

Interventional MRI systems include:

- The combined use of conventional MR with X-ray angiography, using a common patient table system transferrable between an X-ray room and an MR room (the Myabi solution)
- The use of a mobile fluoroscopy system within the MR environment
- The MR system suspended on rails, movable into the operating theatre or room.

In each case, the key safety aspect is the control of ferromagnetic surgical instruments and equipment, particularly where large teams on non-MR staff are involved [17].

Extremity and open MRI systems

Orthopedic clinics may have dedicated extremity MRI systems. These are generally low field (< 0.4 T) using permanent or resistive electromagnets. The latter have the advantage of their field being turned off when not in use. The fringe fields of these magnets lie close to the magnet and hence the controlled access area (Zone IV) may be locally defined around the magnet.

Open systems, employing a vertical field, may have B_0 up to 1 T. The safety requirements are similar to conventional closed-bore systems; however, the fringe field and fringe field spatial gradient maps may be dissimilar. Refer to the manufacturer's Compatibility Data [9] (Chapter 11).

PET-MRI and MR-linac

The combination of MRI with radiation equipment adds a further layer of complexity to safety [18]. In MR-PET this involves the administration of radio-active materials producing high energy (511 keV) gamma rays. Additional radiation shielding, signage, and radiation laboratory design features are required. These will be subject to local ionizing radiation regulations.

With an MR-linac, a linear accelerator is incorporated in the MR to enable dynamic, real-time external beam radiation therapy to be administered (Figure 12.9a). Additional adherence to local

(a)
(b)

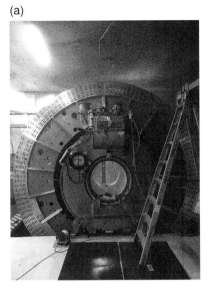
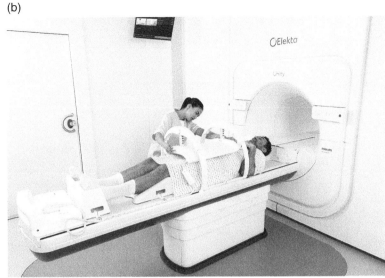

Figure 12.9 MRI-Linac: (a) MRI-linac gantry surrounding the MRI scanner during installation at the Townsville Hospital, QLD, Australia; (b) patient set-up. Note the door from the magnet room into the linac machine room. Source: Elekta Ltd. Used with permission.

radiation safety regulations will also be required [19]. Depending upon the radiation bunker design, access to the linac machine room, required for servicing and QC of the collimator, may be via the magnet room (Figure 12.9b).

A key aspect of both MR-PET and MR-linac operation is the training of nuclear medicine and oncology staff unfamiliar with MRI safety, and the training of MR staff unfamiliar with radiation safety [20]. The ACR guidance on MR safe practices has recently been updated to include consideration of such systems [21].

CONCLUSIONS

The design and layout of the MR suite is paramount to its safe operation. By including appropriately qualified healthcare, engineering, and professional experts at the earliest stage of a new scanner project, mistakes and design flaws can be avoided. The fundamental principle of design should be the ACR four Zones scheme. As with radiation safety, the MRI suite design should be signed off by the MRSO and MRSE. MRI safety begins with suite design. For further information on design and installation issues consult your MR manufacturer's installation guides and the Further reading and resources at the end of this chapter.

Revision questions

1. Regarding ferromagnetic detection systems. They
   A. ensure no ferromagnetic items can be brought into the scanner room
   B. replace the need for intrusive questioning
   C. can act as final confirmatory check, provided they are situated in an environment where there is no moving metal

D. can act as final confirmatory check, provided they are situated in an environment where there is no moving ferromagnetic material
E. do not work.

2. During a quench
   A. the cryogens rapidly boil off and are vented to the atmosphere
   B. the magnet heats up
   C. the magnetic field collapses
   D. there is a loud noise
   E. all of the above.

3. Which of the follow are not essential safety features of an MRI scanner:
   A. Quench button
   B. Ferromagnetic detection system
   C. Patient intercom
   D. Patient alarm
   E. Emergency couch release.

4. An MRI unit lacks a Zone 2. Which of the following are true?
   A. It is operating illegally
   B. It is unsafe
   C. Additional control measures may be required to ensure safety of staff, visitors and patients
   D. It will be shut down
   E. It does not comply with accepted safety guidance.

5. Which of the following should be on an MR project group?
   A. MR safety officer
   B. MR safety expert
   C. Lead MR technologist/radiographer
   D. Architect
   E. All of the above.

6. The MR controlled access area or Zone IV is usually defined by:
   A. The extent of the 0.5 mT contour
   B. The extent of the 0.5 G contour
   C. The extent of the 3 mT contour
   D. The extent of the 0.5 T m^{-1} contour
   E. The extent of the 200 mT contour.

References

1. American Association of Physicists in Medicine (1986). *Site planning for magnetic resonance imaging systems.* AAPM Report 20. New York: AAPM.
2. Medical Devices Directorate (1993). *Guidelines for Magnetic Resonance Diagnostic Equipment in Clinical Use – with Particular Reference to Safety.* London: MDD.
3. Kanal, E., Borgstede, J.P., Barkovich, A.J. et al. (2002). American College of Radiology white paper on MR safety. *American Journal of Roentgenology* 178:1335–1347.
4. Royal Australian and New Zealand College of Radiologists (2017). *MRI safety guidelines version 2.0.* Sydney: RANZCR. Available from https://www.ranzcr.com/college/document-library/ranzcr-mri-safety-guidelines (accessed 21 June 2019).
5. Australasian Health Facilities Alliance (2016). *Australasian Health Facility Guidelines: AHFG B.0440.* Sydney: AHFA. Available from https://www.healthfacilityguidelines.com.au/part/part-b-health-facility-briefing-and-planning-0 (accessed 25 May 2019).
6. Department of Veterans Affairs (2008). *MRI Design Guide.* Washington DC: DVA.
7. European Society of Radiology (ESR) and the European Federation of Radiographer Societies (2019). Patient safety in medical imaging: a joint paper of the European Society of Radiology (ESR) and the European Federation of Radiographer Societies (EFRS). *Radiography* 25: e26–e38.

8. Medicines and Healthcare products Regulatory Agency (2015). *Safety Guidelines for Magnetic Resonance Imaging Equipment in Clinical Use. MHRA DB2007.* London: MHRA.

9. International Electrotechnical Commission (2015). *IEC 60601-2-33 Medical Electrical Equipment - Part 2–33: Particular Requirements for the Basic Safety and Essential Performance of Magnetic Resonance Equipment for Medical Diagnosis, Edn 3.3.* Geneva: IEC.

10. Krestin, G.P., Leijh, P.C.J., Stubbs, P. et al. (2008). *Using MRI Safely: Practical Rules for Employees.* The Hague: Government of the Netherlands. Available at http://docs.minszw.nl/pdf/92/2008/92_2008_1_22102.pdf. (Accessed 25 May 2019)

11. Directive 2013/35/EU of the European Parliament and of the Council of 26 June 2013 on the minimum health and safety requirements regarding the exposure of workers to the risks arising from physical agents (electromagnetic fields) (20th individual Directive within the meaning of Article 16(1) of Directive 89/391/EEC) and repealing Directive 2004/40/EC. *Official Journal of the European Union* L 179/1.

12. *Statutory Instrument 1999 No. 2001. The Pressure Equipment Regulations 1999.* London; Her Majesty's Stationary Office. Available from http://www.opsi.gov.uk/si/si1999/19992001.htm (accessed 25 May 2019).

13. Keene, M. (2014). Using ferromagnetic systems in the MRI environment. In: *MRI bioeffects, safety, and patient management* (Ed. F.D. Shellock and J.V. Crues III) pp. 299–327. Los Angeles, CA: Biomedical Research Publishing Group.

14. NHS Estates (2001). *Facilities for Diagnostic Imaging and Interventional Radiology HBN 6.* Norwich: Her Majesty's Stationery Office.

15. McRobbie, D.W. and Quest, R.A. (2002). Effectiveness and relevance of MR acceptance testing: results of an eight-year audit. *British Journal of Radiology* 75:523–531.

16. American Association of Physicists in Medicine (2010). *Acceptance testing and quality assurance procedures for magnetic resonance imaging facilities.* AAPM Report no. 100. New York: AAPM.

17. White, M.J., Thornton, J.S., Hawkes, D.J. et al. (2015). Design, operation, and safety of single-room interventional MRI suites: practical experience from two centers. *Journal of Magnetic Resonance Imaging* 41:34–43.

18. Brix, G., Nekolla, E.A., Nosske, D. et al. (2009). Risks and safety aspects related to PET/MR examinations. *European Journal of Nuclear Medicine* 36 Suppl 1(S1):S131–8.

19. Rai, R., Kumar, S., Vikneswary, B. et al. (2017). The integration of MRI in radiation therapy: collaboration of radiographers and radiation therapists. *Journal of Medical Radiation Sciences* 64:61–68.

20. O'Meara, C., Burns, S., Menezes, L. et al. (2013) Implementing a magnetic resonance (MR) safety training programme for nuclear medicine technologists – Initial UK experience. *Journal of Nuclear Medicine* 54 (supplement 2):2647–2647.

21. ACR Committee on MR Safety (2019). ACR Guidance Document on MR Safe Practices: Updates and Critical Information 2019. *Journal of Magnetic Resonance Imaging* https://doi.org/10.1002/jmri.26880.

Further reading and resources

ACR Committee on MR Safety (2019). ACR Guidance Document on MR Safe Practices: Updates and Critical Information 2019. *Journal of Magnetic Resonance Imaging* https://doi.org/10.1002/jmri.26880.

Department of Veterans Affairs (2008). *MRI Design Guide.* Washington DC:DVA.

Joint Commission (2017). *Planning, Design, and Construction of Health Care Facilities, Revised Third Edition Revised.* Oak Brook, Illinois: Joint Commission Resources. Available from https://camrt-bpg.ca/patient-safety/mri-safety/mri-facility-design-rtmr/ (accessed 25 May 2019).

Kanal, E., Barkovich, A.J., Bell, C.M. et al. (2013). ACR Guidance Document on MR Safe Practices: 2013, American College of Radiology Expert panel on MR Safety. *Journal of Magnetic Resonance Imaging* 37:501–530.

NHS Estates (1997). *Magnetic Resonance Imaging: Health Guidance Notes.* London: The Stationery Office Books (Agencies).

13

But what about us? Occupational exposure

INTRODUCTION

So far, we have considered the safety of our patients and other staff, from biological and physical hazards arising from MRI. It is now time to think about ourselves! As MR workers what is our exposure to EM fields, what are the implications of this, and how is our exposure regulated?

In the normal course of your duties as an MR technologist/radiographer you will encounter the following exposures:

- The static field spatial gradient dB/dz of the B_0 fringe field
- A fraction of B_0 close to the bore entrance, whilst positioning a patient
- Acoustic noise in the magnet room during scanning – see Chapter 6.

Even if you remain in the room during scanning your exposure to time-varying magnetic fields from the gradients and RF will be negligible unless you are very close to or partially within the bore.

This chapter outlines the nature and range of occupational (worker) exposures and limits encountered in MRI. The biological consequences of static field exposure were reviewed in Chapter 3.

OCCUPATIONAL EXPOSURE LIMITS

The nature of occupational exposure limits differs from those applied to patients and the public. A patient is deemed to gain health benefit from their medical exposure (assuming an appropriate risk–benefit ratio). Patient limits are set by the IEC operating modes [1] rather than by regulation or law. With ionizing radiation there are *legal* limits for workers, e.g. 20 mSv (milli-sieverts) per year. There are few legally-enforceable limits to exposure from electromagnetic fields that relate to MRI, but there are guidelines, recommendations, and advisory limits, some of which may have quasi-legal status, i.e. they could be referenced in safety at work regulations or used as evidence in legal cases. EMF exposure limits are commonly arranged in a two-tier system relating to the *induced fields* directly responsible for acute physiological effects, and *incident fields* generated by the EM source.

Essentials of MRI Safety, First Edition. Donald W. McRobbie.
© 2020 John Wiley & Sons Ltd. Published 2020 by John Wiley & Sons Ltd.

Basic restrictions

"Basic Restrictions" (BR), "Exposure Limit Values" (ELV), "Exposure Reference Values" (ERV), or "Dosimetric Reference Levels" (DRL) relate to the induced field in tissue. They are based upon the minimum threshold for a biologically significant field quantity to elicit an *acute* physiological event. For example, the induced electric field E is used to characterize the onset of peripheral nerve stimulation (PNS). EMF occupational limits do not usually consider long term effects, such as potential cancer induction. If there is no demonstrable harm, we cannot set an exposure level based upon its avoidance. Nevertheless, it is impossible to exclude some as yet unforeseen detrimental effect. For this reason, the *Precautionary Principle*, a risk management policy applied in circumstances where there is scientific uncertainty, is often invoked. In practice, each limit is set below the threshold for *any* detectable effect whether harmful or not, possibly including a safety factor or margin.

Reference levels

Basic Restrictions are frequently specified in quantities which cannot be readily measured, e.g. induced current density or local SAR. "Reference Levels" (RL), "Action Levels" (AL), or "Exposure Reference Levels" (ERL) are provided as an alternative *measurable* quantity of the incident fields, usually magnetic flux density. In any given situation, if compliance with the RL is demonstrated, then compliance with the Basic Restriction is assumed. If the RL is exceeded however, establishing compliance with BR requires full determination of the induced fields by EM modeling [2–4].

NATIONAL AND INTERNATIONAL LIMITS

National and international guidance on limits include the International Commission for Non-Ionizing Radiation Protection [5–8], the Institute of Electrical and Electronic Engineers [9], the European Union [10], the Australian Radiation Protection and Nuclear Safety Agency [11]. IEC 60601-2-33 [1] provides occupational exposure limits specifically for the MR industry. Although the ICNIRP limits (endorsed by the World Health Organization) are widely used, occupational and public limits for RF exposure may differ significantly between countries [12]. Check which limits apply in your part of the world.

Static field

The most commonly cited static field limits are those recommended by ICNIRP [5] (Table 13.1). The ICNIRP limit is 2 T to the head and truck. However, in so-called "controlled situations" this can be increased to 8 T. MRI is considered to be a controlled system, bringing it into harmony with IEC60601-2-33. The public limit is 0.4 T (400 mT), but for persons with cardiac pacemakers this is reduced to 0.5 mT in line with MRI practice.

Separate limits exist for movement within the static field [8]. The Basic Restrictions are shown in Table 13.2 and Figure 13.1. The Reference Levels are shown in Table 13.3. ΔB represents a step change in B occurring over a three second interval; B_{pk-pk} is the peak-to-peak value of a time-varying magnetic field. In some ways, staff will be self-regulating, as they learn how to

Table 13.1   Static field occupational exposure limits [1,5].

Standard	Uncontrolled		Controlled	Public
	Head and trunk (T)	Limbs (T)	Head and trunk (T)	Any part (T)
ICNIRP	2	8	8	0.4
IEC (MRI only)		8	8	NA

Table 13.2   ICNIRP Basic Restrictions for movement within the static magnetic field [8].

Frequency (Hz)	Uncontrolled			Controlled
	ΔB^1 (T)	$B_{pk\text{-}pk}{}^2$ (T)	Induced E^3 (V m^{-1})	Induced E^4 (V m^{-1})
0	2	–	–	–
0–1	–	2	–	–
0–0.66	–	–	1.1	1.1
0.66–1	–	–	0.7 / f	1.1

f in Hz.
Critical effects are stated to be:
[1] "Vertigo due to motion in B-field"; [2] "Vertigo due to time-varying B-field"; [3] "PNS effects due to movement in the B-field or time-varying B-field"; [4] "Phosphenes due to movement in the B-field or time-varying B-field."

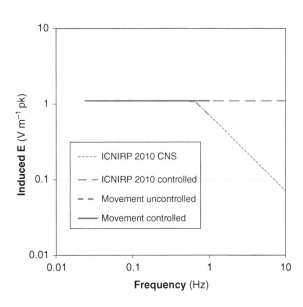

Figure 13.1   ICNIRP Basic Restrictions for movement within the static magnetic field (red lines). Blue lines indicate the Basic Restriction above 1 Hz [8].

Table 13.3   ICNIRP Reference Levels for movement within the static magnetic field [8].

Frequency (Hz)	Uncontrolled[1]	Controlled[2]
	$(dB/dt)_{pk}$ (T s^{-1})	
0–0.66	2.7	2.7
0.66–1	1.8 / f	2.7

f in Hz.
Critical effects are stated to be:
[1] "Phosphenes due to movement in the B field or time-varying B field"; [2] "Phosphenes due to movement in the B field or time-varying B field".

avoid acute effects by modifying their movements.[1] The IEC limit of 8 T only applies to MR workers; workers in other fields should observe the ICNIRP or other relevant national limits.

Time-varying magnetic fields: 1–100 kHz

Basic Restrictions for exposure to time-varying magnetic fields are shown in Figure 13.2. We can observe a discrepancy of almost two orders of magnitude- so some of them must be wrong! The Reference Levels [7] (Table 13.4) are most easily presented on a graph (Figure 13.3). The IEC limit is simply "to avoid PNS", represented by the green line in the figures.

The IEC limit is much less conservative than the other ones. This is because the IEC limit is based upon measured and well characterized studies of PNS in volunteers, whereas other limits rely upon various diverse observations, not all relevant to MRI, and upon extrapolations from theoretical considerations. The ICNIRP limits are anchored by the minimum observed threshold for visual phosphenes, considered by ICNIRP to be the most sensitive acute sensory effect. In actuality, when expressed in terms of ΔB, PNS has the lowest threshold [13]. The IEC limit only applies to MR personnel.

Time-varying magnetic fields: RF

The ICNIRP guideline limits cover the entire RF range from 100 kHz to 300 GHz [6]. Relevant ICNIRP and IEC limits up to 300 MHz are shown in Tables 13.5 and 13.6. Be aware of specific country variations, e.g. ARPANSA limits in Australia. A commonly used metric for RF limitation is the power density (W m^{-2}). This is applicable to plane wave exposures, e.g. from broadcasting, mobile telephony or WiFi, and is not relevant to MRI exposures.

EMF exposure limitation in the European Union

A particular situation exists within the European Union. Directive 2004/40/EC [14] sought to protect workers from "harmful" acute effects from EMF by setting ELVs and Action Values based upon ICNIRP 1998 guidelines [15]. The European MR community considered the limits to be prejudicial to certain aspects of clinical and research MRI: particularly interventional or intra-operative MRI, MRI with anesthesiology, any scan requiring a patient escort to be present in the room, and other scenarios [16,17]. A period of political lobbying spearheaded by the Alliance for MRI (see https://www.myesr.org/article/514, accessed 2 June 2019), and numerous studies of occupational exposure led to Directive 2008/46/EC [18] which postponed the adoption of the 2004

---

[1] PNS and phosphenes are unlikely to be caused by movement through dB/dz in MRI.

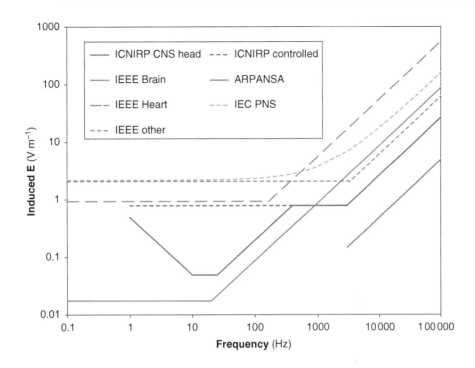

Figure 13.2   Basic Restrictions 0.1 Hz to 100 kHz: ICNIRP [7], IEEE [9], ARPANSA [11], IEC [1] PNS threshold. Values are RMS except IEC PNS (peak). IEEE values are for persons permitted in a restricted environment. ARPANSA limits are expressed as current density, converted to V m⁻¹ assuming tissue conductivity of 0.2 S m⁻¹.

Table 13.4   ICNIRP limits for time-varying magnetic fields from 1 Hz–100 kHz [7]. Note these are RMS values.

Frequency (Hz)	Basic Restriction (V m⁻¹ RMS)		Frequency (Hz)	Reference Level (T RMS)
	CNS tissues in the head	All tissues- head and body		
1–10	$0.5/f$	0.8	1–8	$0.2/f^2$
10–25	0.05	0.8	8–25	$2.5 \times 10^{-2}/f$
25–400	$2 \times 10^{-3}/f$	0.8	25–300	1×10^{-3}
400–3000	0.8	0.8	300–3000	$0.3/f$
3000–1 00 000	$2.7 \times 10^{-4}\ f$	$2.7 \times 10^{-4}\ f$	3000–1 00 000	1×10^{-4}

f in Hz.

Directive pending the publication of new (the current) ICNIRP limits. Directive 2013/35/EC replaces the earlier one, with new Exposure Limit Values and high and low Action Levels (AL) [10]. These are based upon the avoidance of "health effects" such as tissue heating or neuro-muscular stimulation (high AL), and "sensory effects" (Low AL). The ALs for 1 Hz to 10 MHz are shown in Table 13.7. The ELVs are identical to the ICNIRP Basic Restrictions, although expressed as peak rather than RMS values. There are also static field ALs: 0.5 mT to avoid pacemaker malfunction and 3 mT to avoid projectiles. The ALs for RF exposures (10– 400 MHz) are identical to the ICNIRP Reference Levels.

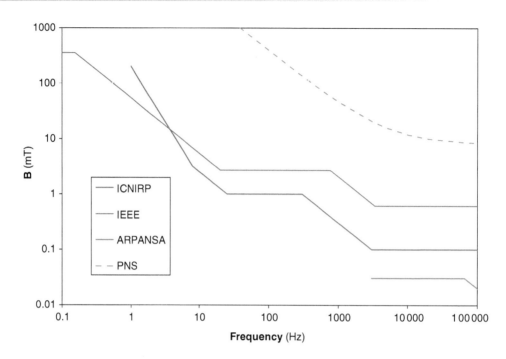

Figure 13.3   Reference Levels 0.1 Hz to 100 kHz: ICNIRP [7], IEEE [9], and ARPANSA [11]. Values are RMS except PNS (peak). The PNS threshold is derived from [13].

Table 13.5   ICNIRP Basic Restrictions RF [6].

Standard	SAR (W kg⁻¹)			
	Frequency	Whole body	Localized (head and trunk)	Localized (limbs)
ICNIRP	10 MHz–10 GHz	0.4	10	20
IEC 60601-2-33	All MRI	4	20	40

Table 13.6   ICNIRP Reference Levels RF [6].

	Frequency	E (V m⁻¹)	H (A m⁻¹)	B (μT)	Power density (W m⁻²)
ICNIRP	10–400 MHz	61	0.16	0.2	10

Crucially there is a derogation from the limits for MRI: ELVs *may* be exceeded for exposures related to the installation, testing, use, development, maintenance of, or research related to MRI for patients in the health sector, subject to the following conditions:

- A *risk assessment*² has shown that ELVs are exceeded
- All technical and organizational measures (of exposure limitation) are applied.

---

² Risk assessment is a term with a legal meaning under EU and UK Health and Safety at Work legislation and Directives.

Table 13.7   Action Levels from EU Directive 2013/35/EC [10].

Frequency	B (μT RMS)		
	Low ALs (sensory effects)	High ALs (health effects)	ALs for localized exposure to limbs
1–8 Hz	$2 \times 10^5/f^2$		
8–25 Hz	$2.5 \times 10^4/f$	$3.0 \times 10^5/f$	$9.0 \times 10^5/f$
25–300 Hz	1.0×10^3		
300 Hz–3 kHz	$3.0 \times 10^5/f$		
3 kHz–10 MHz	1.0×10^2	1.0×10^2	3.0×10^2

f in Hz.

- Circumstances justify exceeding the ELV
- The characteristics of the workplace, equipment or practices have been taken into account
- The employer demonstrates that workers are still protected against adverse health effects and against safety risks.

This means that the limits do not strictly apply to MRI, but the remaining obligations of the Directive do: risk assessments, implementation of action plans, training, and health surveillance.

The Directive also directs member states to provide non-binding practical guidance [19,20]. UK legislation [21] directs the employer to keep exposures "as low as reasonably practicable" (ALARP) wherever an ELV is exceeded. The ALARP principle is usually applied to the limitation of ionizing radiation to provide protection from stochastic or cancer-inducing effects which may arise from even a small exposure. In MRI, however, we are dealing with short term effects with known thresholds. The Directive remains unaffected by the UK's departure from the EU [22]. The Directive establishes the *minimum* health and safety requirements; member states may legislate for more stringent standards if they so choose. MR practitioners in the other 27 European Union states should refer to their own country's implementation of the Directive.

SURVEYS OF OCCUPATIONAL EXPOSURE LEVELS

Concerns about the implications of the EU Directives led to significant work measuring occupational exposure levels, particularly with regard to the static field and movement within the static field [23–30].

Static field exposure

Peak B

Figure 13.4 shows measurements of field exposures of over 164 shifts on 11 scanners from 0.6–4 T [23–24]. The average peak exposure is around 40% of B_0. One of the largest studies was conducted in the Netherlands [25] involving 271 MR workers over 419 shifts in varying occupations (Figure 13.5).

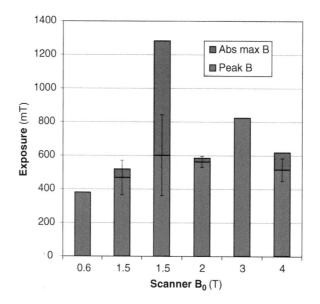

Figure 13.4   Peak occupational B field exposures. Data from [23,24]. The absolute maximum values measured is shown red bars. Blue bars denote the mean.

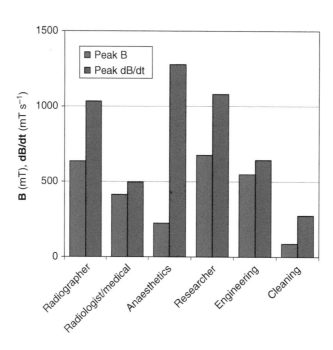

Figure 13.5   Peak B and dB/dt exposures by occupation. Data from [25].

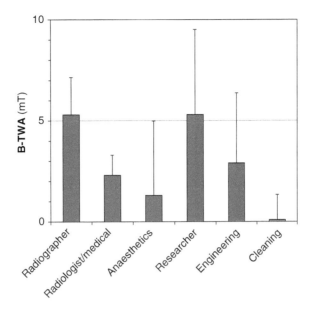

Figure 13.6   Time-weighted average (over a shift) B-field exposure by occupation. Data from [25].

Time-weighted average B

The time-weighted average (TWA) B is also used as a metric for occupational exposure, although its health or biological significance is unclear. Figure 13.6 shows the mean TWA over shift duration by occupation [25]. Unsurprisingly radiographers and researchers showed the highest exposures, but only of the order of 5 mT in agreement earlier data [23–24].

Example 13.1   TWA exposure

An MR tech scans 10 patients in one 7.5 hour shift, spending 45 s positioning each patient in a fringe field of 0.4 T. What is his/her cumulative and time-weighted average exposure?

Cummulative exposure $= 0.4 \times 10 \times 0.75 = 3\,T - min.$

Time – weighted average exposure over the shift is $B_{TWA} = \dfrac{3}{7.5 \times 60} = 6.7 \times 10^{-3} = 6.7\,mT.$

The 24 hour TWA exposure is $B_{TWA,24} = \dfrac{3}{24 \times 60} = 2.1 \times 10^{-3} = 2.1\,mT$

Peak dB/dt from movement within the fringe field

The above studies showed peak dB/dt exposures from moving within the fringe field (spatial gradient) of around 1–2 T s⁻¹. Figure 13.5 shows measurements of maximum dB/dt from movement by professional group [25].

Example 13.2   Movement through dB/dz

How quickly does an MR staff member have to move through a 2 T m⁻¹ fringe field spatial gradient in a 1 second period in order to exceed an ICNIRP Reference Level?

A 1 s movement is equivalent to a frequency of 1 Hz. Apply the Controlled limit of 2.7 T s⁻¹:

$$\frac{dB}{dt} = \frac{dB}{dz} \cdot \frac{dz}{dt} < 2.7$$

Velocity $= \dfrac{dz}{dt}$ *so the velocity required to exceed the limit is*

$$v > \frac{2.7}{2} = 1.35\,m\,s^{-1}.$$

This is similar to an average walking speed of 4.9 km hr⁻¹ (3 mph). Moral of the story? Don't run near scanners!

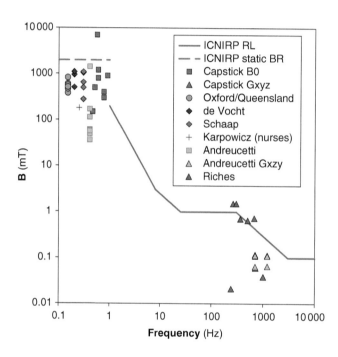

Figure 13.7   Occupational field exposures (peak values) versus frequency relative to the ICNIRP Reference Levels (RMS values). Data from [23-30].

Time-varying B from the imaging gradients

Figure 13.7 shows a collation of published occupational exposures from both B₀ and the gradients plotted alongside the ICNIRP Reference Levels. These encompassed a range of real-life activities (interventional procedures, biopsy, general anesthesia monitoring, cardiac stress testing, tactile fMRI, manual contrast injection, EEG adjustment, emergency evacuation, and in-bore cleaning) and clinical pulse sequences. The majority of exposures are significantly below the action level [26,27]. Two activities which were shown to exceed the Reference Levels: an interventional procedure within the bore of a 1 T open MR system, and the research EEG adjustment at 7 T, were investigated further using EM modeling and were shown to comply with the Basic Restrictions [27].

Time-varying B$_1$

The RF B$_1$ field in air (but not in the patient's body) attenuates rapidly outside the transmit coil. Measurements of the RF exposure outside the bore for 1.5 and 3 T scanners gave a maximum time-averaged RMS E$_1$ of less than 48 V m^{-1} and an H$_1$ of less than 0.36 A m^{-1} [27], within the ICNIRP Reference Levels (Table 13.6). RF exposures to persons, other than the patient, in the proximity of the scanner, are not considered to be of concern.

SURVEY INSTRUMENTATION

Exposure to the static field is the most critical element for monitoring MRI occupational exposure. The monitoring device should be sensitive to the magnetic field in three orthogonal axes, from which the magnitude of B may be calculated:

$$|B| = \sqrt{B_x^2 + B_y^2 + B_z^2} \tag{13.1}$$

Suitable devices may use the Hall effect [31] or induction coils and accelerometers with integrating circuitry [24]. This latter method has sufficient temporal resolution to measure dB/dt from motion within the B$_0$ spatial gradient. Devices used to monitor occupational exposure require calibration and correction for any drift. An alternative approach is to visually record or monitor staff movement and calculate exposures by reference to a detailed fringe field plot [27, 32]. The range of instruments suitable for measuring electric and magnetic fields from the imaging gradients and RF transmission is reviewed in [33].

INCIDENCE OF BIO-EFFECTS AMONG MAGNET FACILITY AND MR WORKERS

The evidence for biological effects of static magnetic fields was reviewed in Chapter 3. A few studies have specifically concentrated on looking for effects amongst MRI and magnet factory workers as a consequence of their work activities. Slight dizziness, slight or mild headache, and eye strain occurred during 4% of the measured shifts from 104 MR workers in the UK [34]. Vertigo incidences amongst MR workers at 1.5, 3, and 7 T were 3.5%, 7.6%, and 22.6% with nausea incidences of 1.2, 1.5 and 3.2% [35]. The occurrence of some acute effects confirms the validity and importance of occupational exposure limits.

Minor changes in hearing threshold amongst MRI factory workers who have undergone up to 60 scans as volunteers has been reported [36]. See Figure 6.8.

CONCLUSIONS

So, should you worry about your exposure to electromagnetic fields?

Probably not. Peak exposures to the static field are around 40% of B$_0$, with a time-averaged exposure of around 5 mT. Exposures to dB/dt from the imaging gradients and RF transmission field are negligible. At higher field strengths (3 T and above) short term sensory effects are well documented. Those associated with vertigo are the most likely to affect task performance. Sensory effects can be minimized by moving slowly and by avoiding the highest field and spatial gradient regions. In other words: don't run near magnets, and don't stick your head into the bore (or if you really must, do so slowly)!

Revision questions

1. You position a patient for an MRI scan, then leave the magnet room to initiate the acquisition. Which of the following contributed to your occupational exposure?
   A. The static magnetic field
   B. The static field spatial gradient
   C. The imaging gradients dB/dt
   D. The RF B_1 field
   E. Acoustic noise.

2. Which of the following are occupational limits for exposure to electromagnetic fields *not* designed to provide protection from?
   A. Excessive tissue heating
   B. Short term acute sensory effects
   C. Long term health effects
   D. Peripheral nerve stimulation
   E. Cancer induction.

3. Which of the following are legally binding?
   A. ICNIRP occupational exposure limits
   B. IEC 60601-2-33 occupational exposure limits
   C. European Union Directive 2013/35/EC
   D. ARPANSA occupational exposure limits for electromagnetic fields
   E. The Institute of Electrical and Electronic Engineers (IEEE) standards.

4. Which of the following quantities is *not* used as a Basic Restriction in occupational exposure limits to electromagnetic fields?
   A. Static field B (T)
   B. dB/dt (T s^{-1})
   C. Induced electric field (V m^{-1})
   D. Power density (W m^{-2})
   E. Specific absorption rate (W kg^{-1}).

5. The mean time-weighted average (TWA) static magnetic field exposure (B) for an MR technologist/radiographer is around:
   A. 0.5 mT
   B. 5 mT
   C. 10 mT
   D. 200 mT
   E. 400 mT.

6. Within the European Union which of the following is true:
   A. MRI does not need to comply with Directive 2013/35/EC on electromagnetic fields
   B. Occupational exposures from MRI must comply with the Action Levels but not the Exposure Limit Values
   C. MRI must comply with all Action Levels and Exposure Limit Values
   D. MRI does not need to comply with the Exposure Limit Values but must follow the remainder of the Directive
   E. In the UK the Directive will not apply after Brexit.

References

1. International Electrotechnical Commission (1995). *Medical Electrical Equipment – Part 2–33: Particular Requirements for the Safety of Magnetic Resonance Equipment for Medical Diagnosis.* IEC 60601-2-33 3.3 edn. Geneva: IEC.

2. Li, Y., Hand, J.W., Wills, T. et al. (2007). Numerically simulated induced electric field and current density within a human model located close to a z-gradient coil. *Journal of Magnetic Resonance Imaging* 26:1286–1295.

3. Liu, F., Zhao, H., Crozier, S. (2003). Calculation of electric fields induced by body and head motion in high-field MRI. *Journal of Magnetic Resonance Imaging* 161:99–107.

4. Crozier, S., Wang, H., Trakic, A. et al. (2007). Exposure of workers to pulsed gradients in MRI. *Journal of Magnetic Resonance Imaging* 26:1236–1254.

5. International Commission on Non-Ionizing Radiation Protection (2009). Guidelines on limits to exposure from static magnetic field. *Health Physics* 96:504–514.

6. International Commission on Non-Ionizing Radiation Protection (2009). ICNIRP statement on the "Guidelines for limiting exposure to time-varying electric, magnetic, and electromagnetic fields (up to 300 GHz)". *Health Physics* 93:257–258.

7. International Commission on Non-Ionizing Radiation Protection (2010). ICNIRP guidelines for limiting exposure to time-varying electric, magnetic, and electromagnetic fields (up to 100 kHz). *Health Physics* 99:818–836.

8. International Commission on Non-Ionizing Radiation Protection (2014). ICNIRP guidelines for limiting exposure to electric fields induced by movement of the human body in a static magnetic field and by time-varying magnetic fields below 1Hz. *Health Physics* 106:418–425.

9. Institute of Electrical and Electronics Engineers (2019). *IEEE Standard for Safety Levels with Respect to Human Exposure to Radio Frequency Electromagnetic Fields. 0 Hz to 300 GHz, C95.1-2019*. New York, USA: IEEE.

10. Directive 2013/35/EC of the European Parliament and of the Council (2013). *Official Journal of the Union*, L 179/1.

11. Australian Radiation Protection and Nuclear Safety Agency (2002). *RPS-3 Maximum Exposure levels to Radiofrequency Fields 3 kHz–300 GHz*. Yallambie, Vic: ARPANSA.

12. Madjar, H.M. (2016). Human radio frequency exposure limits: An update of reference levels in Europe, USA, Canada, China, Japan and Korea. *IEEE International Symposium on Electromagnetic Compatibility* 2016:467–473.

13. McRobbie, D.W. (2012). Occupational exposure in MRI. *British Journal of Radiology* 85:293–312.

14. Directive 2004/40/EC of the European Parliament and of the Council (2004). *Official Journal of the Union*, L 159.

15. International Commission on Non-Ionizing Radiation Protection (1998). Guidelines for limiting exposure to time-varying electric, magnetic, and electromagnetic fields (up to 300 GHz). *Health Physics* 74:494–522.

16. Keevil, S.F, Gedroyc, W., Gowland, P. et al. (2005). Electromagnetic field exposure limitation and the future of MRI. Commentary. *British Journal of Radiology* 78:973–975.

17. Young, I., McRobbie, D., Keevil, S. et al. (2006). Unintended consequences of an unwarrantedly cautious approach to safety. *British Journal of Hospital Medicine* 67:174–175.

18. Directive 2008/46/EC of the European Parliament and of the Council (2008). *Official Journal of the Union*, L 114/88.

19. European Commission (2015). *Non-binding guide to good practice for implementing Directive 2013/35/EU Electromagnetic Fields*. Luxembourg: Publications Office of the European Union.

20. Health and Safety Executive (2016). *Electromagnetic fields at work. A guide to the control of electromagnetic fields at Work Regulations 2016*. London: HSE. Available from: http://www.hse.gov.uk/pubns/priced/hsg281.pdf. [Accessed 4 June 2019].

21. The Control of Electromagnetic Fields at Work Regulations (2016). SI 2016/588. London: The Stationery Office.

22. Keevil, S.F. and Lomas, D.J. (2017). The Control of Electromagnetic Fields at Work Regulations 2016 and medical MRI. *British Journal of Radiology* 90:1070.

23. Bradley, J.K., Nyekiova, M., Price, D.L. et al. (2007). Occupational exposure to static and time-varying gradient magnetic fields in MR units. *Journal of Magnetic Resonance Imaging* 26:1204–1209.

24. Fuentes, M.A., Trakic, A., Wilson, S.J. et al. (2008). Analysis and measurements of magnetic field exposures for healthcare workers in selected MR environments. *IEEE Transactions in Biomedical Engineering* 55:1355–1364.

25. Schaap, K., Christopher-de Vries, Y., Crozier, S. et al. (2014). Exposure to static and time-varying magnetic fields from working in the static magnetic stray fields of MRI scanners: A comprehensive survey in the Netherlands. *Annals of Occupational Hygiene* 5:1094–1110.

26. McRobbie, D.W. (2013). Occupational Exposures During MRI. In: *Magnetic Resonance Procedures: Health Effects and Safety* (Ed. F. G. Shellock and J.V. Crues, III) pp. 624–647. Los Angeles CA: Biomedical Research Publishing Group.

27. Capstick, M., McRobbie, D., Hand, J., et al (2008). *An investigation into occupational exposure to electromagnetic fields for personnel working with and around medical magnetic resonance imaging equipment. Report on Project VT/2007/017 of the European Commission Employment, Social Affairs and Equal Opportunities DG*. Available from www.myesr.org/html/img/pool/VT2007017FinalReportv04. pdf [Accessed 4 June 2019].

28. Riches, S.F., Charles-Edwards, G.D., Shafford, J.C. et al. (2007). Measurements of occupational exposure to switched gradient and spatially varying magnetic fields in areas adjacent to 1.5T clinical MRI systems. *Journal of Magnetic Resonance Imaging* 26:1346–1352.

29. Andreuccetti, D., Contessa, G.M., Falsaperla, R. et al (2013). Weighted-peak assessment of occupational exposure due to MRI gradient fields and movements in a nonhomogeneous static magnetic field. *Medical Physics* 40 https://doi.org/10.1118/1.4771933.

30. Karpowicz, J. and Gryz, K. (2013). The pattern of exposure to static magnetic field of nurses involved in activities related to contrast administration into patients diagnosed in 1.5 T MRI scanners. *Electromagnetic Biology and Medicine* 32:182–191.

31. Cavagnetto, F., Prati, P., Ariola, V. et al. (1993). A personal dosimeter prototype for static magnetic fields. *Health Physics* 65:172–177.

32. Hartwig, V., Vanello, N., Giovannetti, G. et al. (2011). A novel tool for estimation of magnetic resonance occupational exposure to spatially varying magnetic fields. *MAGMA* 24:323–330.

33. Reeves, J. (2010). Measurement techniques and technology. In: *Guidance on the measurement and use of EMF and EMC, IPEM Report 98*. York: Institute of Physics and Engineering in Medicine. p28–44.

34. De Vocht, F., Batistatou, E., Mölter, A. et al. (2015). Transient health symptoms of MRI staff working with 1.5 and 3.0 Tesla scanners in the UK. *European Radiology* 25:2718–2726.

35. Schaap, K., Christopher-DeVries, Y., Mason, C.K. et al. (2014). Occupational exposure of healthcare and research staff to static magnetic stray fields from 1.5–7 tesla MRI scanners is associated with reporting of transient symptoms. *Occupational & Environmental Medicine* 71:423–439.

36. Bongers, S., Slottje, P., and Kromhout, H. (2017). Hearing loss associated with repeated MRI acquisition procedure-related acoustic noise exposure: an occupational cohort study. *Occupational and Environmental Medicine* 74:776–784.

Further reading and resources

European Commission (2015). *Non-binding guide to good practice for implementing Directive 2013/35/EU Electromagnetic Fields*. Luxembourg: Publications Office of the European Union.

McRobbie, D.W. (2012). Occupational exposure in MRI. *British Journal of Radiology* 85:293–312.

14

Organization and management

INTRODUCTION

This last topic is not the least. It is essential for MRI safety and binds all the earlier material together, consolidating theoretical knowledge into practice through policy, procedure, and organizational culture. This chapter is for everyone, but particularly for those entrusted with the management of health and safety within their institution. We will examine the overall organization and governance of MR safety, duty-holder roles, policy documentation and implementation, relevant standards and guidelines, accreditation, and training. A key component is patient and staff safety screening.

ROLES IN MR SAFETY

In 2016 a consensus document produced by a number of leading professional bodies[1] recommended the roles of *MR Medical Director* (MRMD), *MR Safety Officer* (MRSO), and *MR Safety Expert* (MRSE) [1]. Whilst similar roles had been in existence in Europe and the UK for decades before [2], the consensus document established a uniform model that could be adopted worldwide. This model has been endorsed widely by professional bodies the USA, Europe, and Australasia [3-5]. A similar document covers the situation of human scanning in a research environment [6]. These three roles act together with clear lines of responsibility and function between them (Figure 14.1).

MR Medical Director – MRMD

The MRMD has overarching responsibility for MR safety, either in person or via delegation to another appropriately licensed and/or qualified individual. This covers patients, staff, and visitors. The MRMD is a suitably registered or licensed medically qualified person. Access to the MRMD, their delegate, or a responsible radiologist should be available at all times when scanners are operating.

---

[1] International Society for Magnetic Resonance in Medicine, Section for MR Technologists, European Federation of Organisations for Medical Physics, European Federation of Radiographer Societies, European Society of Radiology, European Society of Magnetic Resonance in Medicine and Biology.

Essentials of MRI Safety, First Edition. Donald W. McRobbie.
© 2020 John Wiley & Sons Ltd. Published 2020 by John Wiley & Sons Ltd.

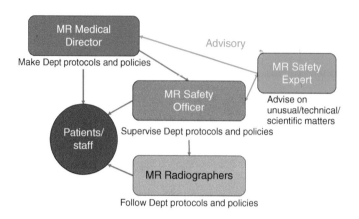

Figure 14.1 The inter-relationship between roles in a MR safety framework.

The MRMD ensures the overall safety governance of the MR operation, including the appointment of an appropriately qualified and skilled MRSO for each scanner, and a MRSE. The MRMD ensures that policies and procedures are current and appropriate for the range of patients, imaging procedures, and equipment within their remit. A key role is to ensure that safety related incidents are properly investigated, analyzed, and reported, with records kept. The MRMD ensures that appropriate risk assessments are carried out and that quality assurance (QA) programs are implemented.

MR Safety Officer – MRSO

The MRSO has the key role for the day-to-day safe operation of the MRI unit, requiring ready accessibility and availability to MRI system operators at all times when the MRI facility is active. The MRSO supervises safety practice "on the ground" by:

- Ensuring that proper policies and procedures for MR safety are enforced
- Developing, documenting, and implementing safe working procedures for the MR environment in conjunction with the MRMD
- Ensuring that adequate written safety procedures, work instructions, emergency procedures, and operating instructions are issued to all MR staff
- Ensuring that measures for minimizing risks to health arising from the use of equipment and from associated exposures are implemented and monitored
- Managing hazards posed by the MR equipment, and monitoring related protection measures
- Ensuring that all heads of departments and senior medical staff members who are responsible for personnel who will be involved with the MR system are informed of the formal procedures for training and authorization
- Ensuring the provision of regular MR safety training and keeping training records for staff
- Providing safety advice regarding the selection, procurement, and installation of MR-related equipment in consultation with the MRSE as required
- Providing safety advice on the modification of MR protocols in consultation with the MRSE as required
- Ensuring that there is a clear policy for the purchasing, testing, and marking of all equipment to be used in the MR environment.

This is a big job with wide-ranging responsibility. The employer should provide the MRSO with sufficient resources of time, access to training, and professional development in order to fulfil their duties. The employer should also ensure that the MRSO holds a sufficiently senior post (and is properly remunerated for their efforts!) The MRSO discharges these duties under the authority of, and reporting to, the MRMD; the MRSO is the MRMD's eyes and ears in the MR department. The MRSO maintains regular contact with the MRSE and all other stakeholders including safety committees. The most appropriate person to be appointed as MRSO is a senior MR radiographer or technologist, registered as required by national professional standards or legislation.

MR Safety Expert – MRSE

Formerly known as the MR Safety Adviser [2], the MRSE is a person with a deep technical knowledge of the MR equipment, physics and biophysics of electromagnetism, including interactions with medical devices. The MRSE provides high-level advice on the engineering, scientific, and administrative aspects of the safe use of MR equipment, and may be called upon to:

- Advise on the development or evaluation of a MR safety framework
- Advise on the development of local rules and procedures
- Provide safety and image quality advice regarding the modification of MR protocols
- Provide safety advice on non-routine MR procedures, including dealing with unfamiliar implants or scanning scenarios, e.g., assessing the risks from off-label scanning
- Advise on the choice of MR safety and QA programmes.

The MRSE has a key role in the selection, procurement, and installation of the MR system and related equipment with regard to safety. Project managers and architect must liaise with the MRSE prior to and during the planning of a new installation. The MRSE also advises on acceptance testing of the equipment before its first use on clinical or research subjects.

The most suitable person to fulfil the role of MRSE is a MR-trained medical physicist, or engineer, registered or licensed by the appropriate national body. As a provider of independent MR safety advice, their ongoing professional development is crucial to their effectiveness in the role, and employers must facilitate and resource this. The MRSE may be remote from the MR unit, providing their advice from another organization on a service level agreement basis.

In the UK this role has been in existence since the early days of MRI and is currently summarized as [7]:

> The MR SAFETY EXPERT should be in a position to adequately advise on the necessary engineering, scientific and administrative aspects of the safe clinical use of the MR devices including site planning, development of a safety framework, advising on monitoring the effectiveness of local safety procedures, procurement, adverse incident investigation and advising on specific patient examinations. Their knowledge of MR physics should enable them to advise on the risks associated with individual procedures and on methods to mitigate these risks.

The UK's Institute of Physics and Engineering in Medicine [8] and the European Federation of Organisations for Medical Physics [9] have issued policy statements on the role of the medical physicist in MR safety. These include summaries of the required knowledge base. A deep understanding of all the material in this book, including the appendices, is required.

MR Responsible Person

The United Kingdom's organizational approach to MR safety was developed from the early 1990s. This designates a "MR Responsible Person" [2,7]. This may be the clinical director, head of the department, a clinical scientist, medical physicist, or MR superintendent (lead) radiographer.

323

Their managerial role in MRI safety role mirrors the administrative activities of the MRMD. The Responsible Person should not be the MRSE. In many instances, the Responsible Person will be a consultant radiologist (equivalent to the MRMD) with the MRSO role fulfilled by the MR superintendent radiographer.

MYTHBUSTER:

The organizational or managerial aspects of the MR safety framework are not the same in all countries.

The wider organization

It is ineffective for the MR safety framework to exist or operate only within the MR or radiology department. There need to be avenues for formal engagement with the wider medical/hospital community to communicate information on risks, training, incidents, and compliance with occupational health laws.

Local committees

A MR safety representative (MRMD, MRSO, or MRSE) should sit on appropriate departmental or hospital committees. These may include the Radiation Safety, Clinical Governance, Risk Management, Health and Safety, and Research Ethics (IRB) committees. MR safety management also requires access to nursing, infection control, fire, security, anesthetics, and clinical emergency response teams. In larger organizations it may be advisable to have a dedicated MR Safety Committee. It is important that senior clinicians and managers are involved in such committees so that policy decisions and directives can be effectively implemented with due authority.

Fire department

The MRSO should liaise with the local fire department and in-house fire safety officers to ensure that in the event of fire in MRI, the firefighters are aware of MRI safety issues:

- Ferromagnetic projectile risk
- The need to quench should firefighting equipment be brought into Zone IV
- The location of the quench buttons
- The helium exhaust system
- Health risks arising from cold helium gas
- An appreciation of the cryostat as a pressure vessel with a risk of explosion.

POLICY AND SAFETY DOCUMENTATION

Each MR department should have a written MR safety policy and/or a set of MR safety procedures or local rules. These should be written by the MRSO and MRMD with input from the MRSE and other stakeholders: e.g. security, infection control, anesthetics, work health and safety, as appropriate. There should be a formal process for review and authorization by the appropriate committees, heads of department, and managers. The documentation must be readily available to all staff who may work in the MR environment. The MRSO will ensure that all such staff have read and understood their specific instructions and responsibilities.

Exercise 14.1   MR Safety Policy.

Before you start writing your MR safety policy consider:
   What is it for?
   Who is it for?
   Who should write the policy?
   What are your sources of information/authority?
   Who are the stakeholders?
   Who will ratify/review the policy?
   How will you distribute the policy?
   What subjects will be covered?
   The answers to these questions may serve as a template for your policy document – so write them down!

Policy content

Sections of the documentation may be derived from an appropriate national standard or guideline, but should be customized to your local practice. These may include (this list is not exclusive):

- Identity, contact details, and description of the roles of the MRMD, MRSO, and MRSE
- A brief description of the equipment and associated hazards
- Explanation of the four Zones, with a map and fringe field diagrams
- Security and access:
  - list of staff authorized for access
- Patient and staff screening
- Dealing with implants, including specialized work instruction for specific devices, e.g. MR conditional pacemakers and neuro-stimulators
- Fringe field spatial gradient information
- Requirement for hearing protection
- Pregnancy:
  - patient
  - staff
- Administration of contrast agents
- Emergency procedures:
  - fire
  - projectile incident
  - quench, including who can authorize and under which circumstances
  - resuscitation
  - contrast reaction
- Training and staff induction:
  - definition and identification of categories of MR safety trained staff
  - records of training
- Record keeping
  - patient exposures including GBCA administration
  - incidents
- Research requirements (if any)
- Incident investigation and reporting
- General anesthesia and sedation
- Infection control and cleaning
- Occupational exposure and field limits
- References to national and international standards and guidance.

The documentation should be subject to review at regular pre-defined intervals (e.g. every one or two years) or whenever significant changes in practice occur.

CHECKLIST AND SCREENING

A key aspect of practical MRI safety is the process of patient and staff screening. Referrers and administrative staff must also be aware of key issues that may impact patient safety or scanning preparation, such as the presence of implanted medical devices. Referral and booking systems need a method to alert key MRI staff at the earliest opportunity.

Safety checklist

On arrival at the MR unit, the patient is required to complete the local MR safety checklist, being guided where necessary. Ideally this takes place in Zone II. An example of a highly detailed checklist is provided on www.mrisafety.com [10] and this can be customized to suit local practice. Figure 14.2 gives an example of a shorter, simpler checklist [11]. The checklist must comply with any local regulations, standards or requirements for communication with the patient. For example, there may be a specified minimum typeface font size or a requirement for its availability in different languages.

When designing a checklist, it is good practice to place the most critical questions first: for example, "do you or have you ever had a heart pacemaker?" using the most simple and clear language. The staff conducting the screening should be suitably knowledgeable and trained (Level II in ACR nomenclature) and be prepared to sign-off the form. It is a legal document and must be stored in keeping with the requirements for patient records. A clear procedure should exist for when an implant or other potential contraindication or complication is indicated. In every case, the form must contain all the appropriate responses with additional "full stop" verbal confirmation prior to the patient entering the magnet room (Zone IV) [12].

Patient preparation

Patients are instructed to remove all loose metal objects, watches, jewellery, body-piercings (if possible), hairpins and clasps, and magnetic sensitive objects (credit cards, travel cards for bus or metro, etc.) These can be stored in a locker. Medical patches that contain metal foil backing should be removed. It is generally considered good practice to have patients change into scrubs or hospital gowns to ensure no dangerous objects remain on their person, and because some clothing may contain metal fibers that can affect the RF or cause burns [12]. In many countries there are particular requirements for patient privacy and dignity, e.g. segregation of the sexes, to be incorporated into the workflow, the patient's journey, and the structural facilities.

Some sites deploy ferromagnetic detection systems (see Chapter 12, page 299) as an adjunct deterrent against the introduction of unsafe objects into the MR environment. These are capable of detecting fields as low as 0.5 nT (10^{-9} T) and, at their highest sensitivity, have been shown to be capable of detecting ferromagnetic material in implanted devices [13] (Figure 14.3). However many sites operate safely without their use. Ferromagnetic detection devices do not replace the need for robust and thorough screening procedures and need to be adequately incorporated into the physical infrastructure in order to be fully effective.

BAMRR MRI SAFETY QUESTIONNAIRE

Name.. Date of Birth...

Address..

Height... Weight..

	YES	NO	DETAILS
Have you ever had an MRI scan before?			
Do you, or have you ever had, a cardiac pacemaker or implantable cardioverter defibrillator (ICD)?			
Have you ever had any surgery to your heart?			
Have you ever had any brain surgery or surgery to your eyes or ears			
Do you have a hydrocephalus shunt? If Yes, Is it a programmable shunt?'			
Do you have any type of electronic, mechanical or magnetic implant or device?			
Have you ever had any surgery involving the use of pins, clips, Plates, screws or stents?			
Have you ever had an endoscopy procedure involving swallowing a capsule "Pillcam"			
Have you ever had any accidents where metal may have entered any part of your body, especially your eyes? Eg shrapnel.			
Are you wearing any form of drug delivery patch eg Nicotine replacement or pain relief?			
Do you have any tattoos or body piercings of any type?			

FOR CONTRAST EXAMINATIONS
   1.   Do you have any allergies
   2. Are your kidneys working well			

FEMALES ONLY
   1.   Are you or could you be pregnant?
   2.   Are you breastfeeding
   3. Do you have a contraceptive coil (IUD)			

Before entering the scan room you will need to remove any loose metal objects such as coins, keys, watch, jewellery and hairclips.

You may be asked to remove any makeup.

You may be asked to change into metal free clothing especially if you are wearing sportswear with metal threads.

PATIENT SIGNATURE	AUTHORISED STAFF SIGNATURE	DATE

Figure 14.2 Example patient questionnaire. Advisory document only. Reproduced with permission of the British Association of MR Radiographers (BAMRR).

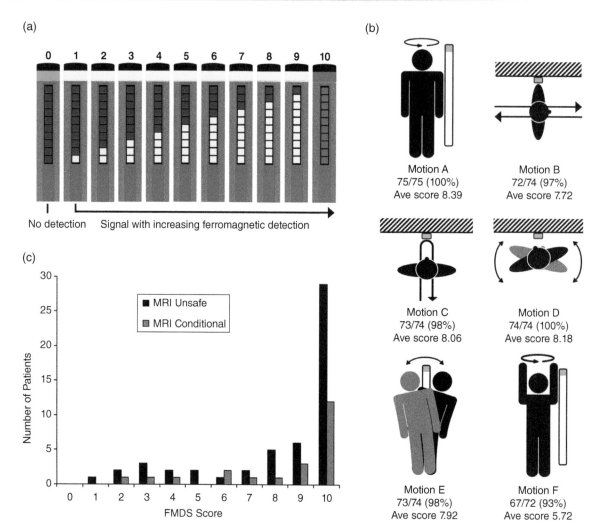

Figure 14.3 Detection of cardiac implants by a Metrasens ferromagnetic detection system: (a) Device indicator; (b): patient screening motions; (c) detection of implanted cardiac devices. Source: [13]. Reproduced with permission of Wiley.

INCIDENTS

A robust system for investigating adverse incidents is required. This is greatly facilitated if there is a "no blame" culture. Where an institutional culture of intimidation exists (this is not as uncommon as you might wish), there may be tendency to under-report, covering up accidents and near-miss events. This undermines the MR safety framework. The purpose of the investigation is to discover the root causes and to learn from the episode, not to assign blame. Local policy, national standards, and regulations determine the actions required following an incident or near-miss.

All incidents should be reported to and investigated by the MRSO and MRMD, with the assistance of the MRSE. Local reporting systems should be used with an initial report logged as soon as practicable. Records of incidents and their investigations should be maintained, with a summary reported to the appropriate hospital committees. An incident resulting in an injury or equipment damage may be reportable to the relevant national authorities such as the FDA's Manufacturer and User facility Device Experience (MAUDE) database (https://www.accessdata.fda.gov/scripts/cdrh/cfdocs/cfMAUDE/search.CFM, accessed 19 June 2019), the Medicines and Healthcare products Regulatory Agency (MHRA) in the UK, the Therapeutic Goods Administration (TGA) in Australia, MedSafe in New Zealand, or the National System for Incident Reporting (NSIR) in Canada. In federated countries, local state or province requirements may also apply. Be aware of the reporting requirements that apply in your country of practice.

EMERGENCIES

Local MR policies and procedures should include written instructions for dealing with emergencies: both medical and physical. Those outlined here are not exclusive.

Cardiac arrest

A patient suffering a cardiac arrest within the scanner or Zone IV and requiring the use of resuscitation equipment (external defibrillator) should be removed urgently from Zone IV to a place where resuscitation may be initiated. One staff member removes the patient – using the emergency manual couch release if required, whilst another calls for help and secures the Zone IV entrance. Solo operation of MR scanners is not best practice.

Projectile incident

In the event of a ferromagnetic projectile becoming attached to the MR magnet, a quench is only required in the case of serious or life-threatening injury to a person. For an incident without injury, for example as in Figure 14.4, the MR manufacturer can be contacted and the field "ramped down" without quenching the magnet for safe removal of the object. Following re-establishment of the magnetic field QC procedures should confirm the scanner's performance. In the case of impalement, trapping or serious injury to a person, the magnet may need to be quenched. Local policy must detail when to quench, and who is authorized to initiate one.

Fire

A minor fire occurring within Zone IV can be tackled by appropriately trained persons using MR safe or conditional fire extinguishers. The nozzle and safety pin of such may be ferromagnetic so hold on tight, and watch where you throw the pin! If ferromagnetic firefighting equipment (breathing apparatus, axes, etc.) is required in Zone IV, the magnet must be quenched prior to entry. Liaison with the local fire service at the earliest opportunity is a key task for the MRSO.

Quench

In any quench incident, whether operator-initiated or spontaneous, all persons must evacuate Zone IV immediately, closing the door behind them. Quenching and helium hazards were considered in Chapter 12. It is important to know the circumstances when a quench should be initiated and

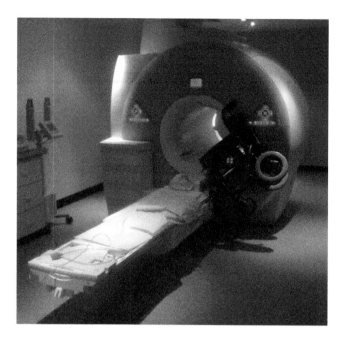

330

Figure 14.4   An incident involving a ferromagnetic object, but without injury. A magnet quench is not required, but ramping down the field enables the object to be detached.

who has the authority so to do. A quench will result in significant downtime and cost, and carries a risk of damaging the magnet. It is a last resort response to a serious emergency situation.

TRAINING

MRI safety training has two main components: the academic training required by your profession in order to practice or be licenced to practice, and local MRI specific safety training provided by your department. The ACR [3] and MHRA [7] documents specify levels of training required for different staff groups.

ACR staff categories

- **Level 1 MR Personnel**: have minimal MR safety education to ensure their own safety as they work in Zone III. They may enter Zone IV and supervise non-MR personnel in Zone III (but not Zone IV)
- **Level 2 MR Personnel**: are identified by the MRMD and have more extensive training and education in MR safety issues, including issues related to RF heating or burns and PNS from gradient dB/dt
- **Non-MR Personnel**: anyone else, including MR staff who have not attended the designated MR training within the previous 12 months. They must be supervised by a Level 2 person when in Zones III and IV and satisfy safety screening requirements.

The MRMD is responsible for approving the training, ensuring its implementation, and for the designation of MR Personnel.

Table 14.1   Summary of training requirements for categories of staff. Adapted from [7].

Staff Category	Training Requirements
A, B, C, and D	Awareness of the location of the MR Environment and its hazards.
A, B, and C	Understanding of the significance of the MR Controlled Area, MR Environment, and MR Projectile Zone. Fully conversant with: • the projectile effect; • effect of magnetic field on implant and prostheses; • effect of magnetic fields upon personal effects such as credit cards and watches. Understanding of safety aspects relating to the main static field and associated equipment.
A and B	Understanding of safety aspects relating to: • electrical safety of the equipment; • RF fields and associated equipment; • gradient magnetic fields and associated equipment. Understanding of local regulations and procedures for the MR equipment and its location. Understanding of emergency procedures arising from causes other than equipment failure. Understanding of the consequences and effects of a magnet quench. Full awareness of the recommendations on exposure to MR. Having full instruction in, and understanding of the consequences of, the correct selection, fitting, and use of ear protection.
A	Having full training and instruction from the MR manufacturer in the use of the equipment, its hazards, and actions to take in an emergency. Full awareness of the relevant contents of the MRI instructions for use.

331

MHRA staff training requirements

The MHRA guidelines identify four categories of staff in relation to MRI:

- **Category A**: the MR Operator (whether radiographer/technologist, engineer, or physicist)
- **Category B**: a person other than a MR Operator who may be present *during* scanning, e.g., radiologist, anesthetist, nurse, etc.
- **Category C**: a staff member who enters the MR Environment when scanning is *not* taking place, e.g., maintenance staff, cleaners (if magnet room cleaning is not performed by the MR staff)
- **Category D**: all other staff who may be in the MR Controlled Area (equivalent to Zone III) but not the MR Environment (equivalent to Zone IV).

The guidance offers a detailed schedule of training and education requirements for each category as summarized in Table 14.1.

ACCREDITATION AND CERTIFICATION

Departmental

Accreditation or certification is a key element for the provision of health services by organizations, or the for the professional conduct of healthcare workers. Accreditation of a hospital or department may be a condition for their receiving of government rebates, funding for services, or being allowed to operate. Accreditation may be voluntary, as in the USA's Joint Commission [14] or statutory, as in the inspections of the Care Quality Commission in the UK (www.cqc.org.uk accessed 22 July 2019).

Practitioners

For the individual practitioner there may be differing requirements for basic, undergraduate, or postgraduate education, and for statutory registration as a healthcare professional. These vary by country: an entitlement to practice as a MR technologist in one country may not entitle you to work in the same role in another without further training or professional assessment.

Radiographers and MR technologists

In New Zealand a postgraduate diploma in MRI is a prerequisite to working as a MR technologist and is additional to registration with the Medical Radiation Technologists Board (MRTB). In Canada registration with the Canadian Association of Medical Radiation Technologists (CAMRT) in the discipline of MRI is required, along with other province-specific requirements [15]. In Australia MR radiographers are registered as Medical Radiation Practitioners. The Australian Society of Medical Imaging and Radiation Therapy (ASMIRT) operates a non-mandatory accreditation system with two-part training: Level 1 covering MR theory, safety, and practice is examined; Level II requires three years clinical experience [16]. Professional capabilities specific to MRI (and other medical imaging disciplines) are set by the Medical Radiation Practice Board [17] under the auspices of Australian Health Practitioner Regulation Agency (AHPRA). In the UK all MR radiographers and medical physicists must be registered with the Health and Care Professions Council (HCPC) possessing appropriate undergraduate or postgraduate degrees. The HCPC defines mandatory professional practice standards for radiographers [18]. For those working in MRI these include knowledge of and competence in MRI safety.

The US situation is more fragmented; different requirements apply in individual states. The American Society of Radiologic Technologists (ASRT) provides training and standards of professional practice in radiography (including MRI), but registration is not compulsory in all states. Some states have specific licensing of MR technologists. Others do not require radiographic qualifications to perform MRI scans. Partly to address this issue, the American Board of Magnetic Resonance Safety (ABMRS) offers certification as MRMD, MRSO, or MRSE by examination. Whilst this certification may be useful, it is important for individuals to recognize legal limits to, or requirements for, their scope of practice in their country of employment. Possession (or otherwise) of ABMRS certification is not prerequisite for acting in the role of MRMD, MRSO, or MRSE. These roles or their equivalent predate the formation of the ABMRS. The appointment of individuals to these roles is a matter for the employer and local or national professional requirements.

MYTHBUSTER:

It is not necessary to have certification from the American Board of MR Safety in order to function as a MRMD, MRSO, or MRSE.

Radiologists, physicians

In most countries radiologists receive basic theoretical and practical on-the-job training in MRI. The scope and extent of MRI-safety specific training may be small, insufficient to equip them adequately to assess the risks inherent in, for example, introducing particular implants into the

MR environment. It is particularly important for the MRMD to have a solid training in MR safety, although this is seldom mandated by radiology colleges.

Medical Physicists

The level of MRI and MR safety training for medical physicists also varies by country. In the UK the Institute of Physics and Engineering in Medicine has published guidelines on the role of the medical physicist in MR safety [8], and the national training scheme for medical physicists includes detailed MRI and non-ionizing radiation safety modules.

STANDARDS AND GUIDANCE

Most of the relevant standards have appeared elsewhere in this book. Here we summarize those that apply mainly in the Anglophone regions: North America, the UK, and Australasia. You should be conversant with the contents of the standards that apply in your country of residence. Standards provide authoritative guidance on safe practice of MR scanning.

Other sources of authority include peer-reviewed journal articles. A MRMD, MRSO, or MRSE should have access to the relevant journals, and be adept at carrying out literature searches. A common source of information is through social media. You should exercise caution regarding advice given, for example, on Facebook, from someone you do not know or whose professional credentials you cannot verify or who is not subject to the same standards of professional conduct that apply in your country. Be aware that offering clinical or related advice about specific patients or devices may be beyond the scope of practice of those offering such advice. The internet does not respect country boundaries. The advice on offer may violate national professional standards or regulations in your region. Never disclose identifiable patient information on the internet.

The following national and international guidance and standards *can* be trusted. All web addresses accessed 15 August 2019.

American College of Radiology

ACR guidance document on MR safe practices [3]

Link: https://www.acr.org/Clinical-Resources/Radiology-Safety/MR-Safety
   Status: US-based professional guidance.
   Summary: addresses numerous MR safety-related topics including:

- Translational and rotational forces on ferromagnetic materials
- Induced voltage, auditory considerations and thermal issues
- Qualifications and training
- Site access restrictions
- Pregnancy-related issues
- Guidelines on claustrophobia, anxiety, sedation, analgesia, and anesthesia
- Safety of MR scanning of device patients
- MR siting considerations- the four zones
- Emergency preparedness planning.

Updated guidance was published in 2019 [12]. This included advice on specialist and high field systems, and further explanation of B_0 spatial gradients.

333

American Society for Testing and Materials

F2503-13 Standard Practice for Marking Medical Devices and Other Items for Safety in the Magnetic Resonance Environment [19]

Link: https://www.fda.gov/downloads/medicaldevices/deviceregulationandguidance/guidance documents/ucm107708.pdf
Status: Applies internationally as IEC 62570:2014.
Summary: specifies the permanent marking of items, which are used in the MR environment, by means of terms and icons (shown in Figure 11.1) and definitions for MR Safe, MR Conditional, and MR Unsafe (see Chapter 11).

ASTM standards relating to the testing and labeling of devices and implants were considered in Chapter 9.

Australian Radiation Protection and Nuclear Safety Agency

Safety guidelines for magnetic resonance diagnostic facilities RHS 34

Link: https://www.arpansa.gov.au/regulation-and-licensing/regulatory-publications/radiation-health-series
Status: Australian guidance, withdrawn, replaced by "Trusted International Standard" *Medical Magnetic Resonance (MR) Procedures: Protection of Patients* [20].
Summary: See ICNIRP guidelines below.

Food and Drug Administration

FDA Criteria for Significant Risk Investigations of Magnetic Resonance Devices [21]

Link: https://www.fda.gov/media/71385/download
Status: Non-binding recommendations for the USA.
Summary: Sets guideline exposure levels indicating significant risk to adults, children and neonates. Exceeding these levels requires specific FDA approval. Levels are:

- 8 T, with 4 T for younger neonates
- Whole-body SAR not exceeding 4 W kg^{-1} averaged over 15 minutes
- Head SAR not exceeding 3.2 W kg^{-1} averaged over 10 minutes
- Avoidance of discomfort or painful PNS from gradient dB/dt
- Acoustic noise level not exceeding 140 dB(Z) unweighted or 99 dB(A)RMS (A-weighting).

FDA Establishing Safety and Compatibility of Passive Implants in the Magnetic Resonance (MR) Environment, Guidance for Industry and Food and Drug Administration Staff [22]

Link: https://www.fda.gov/downloads/MedicalDevices/DeviceRegulationandGuidance/Guidance Documents/ucm107708.pdf?source=govdelivery&utm_medium=email&utm_source=govdelivery
Status: US-based guidance focused on passive implants that function without electronic power.
Summary: addresses the testing and labeling of passive implants for safety and compatibility in the MR environment. ASTM testing methodologies and standards are referenced. Active implants or devices that are not implants are not considered.

Health Protection Agency

Protection of patients and volunteers undergoing MRI procedures [23]

Link: https://www.gov.uk/government/uploads/system/uploads/attachment_data/file/329364/Protection_of_patients_and_volunteers_undergoing_MRI_procedures.pdf

Status: current UK guidance on bio-effects and exposure limits for MR patients and research volunteers.

Summary: Similar to ICNIRP guidance.

International Commission on Non-Ionizing Radiation Protection

Medical magnetic resonance (MR) procedures: protection of patients [20]

Link: http://www.icnirp.org/cms/upload/publications/ICNIRPMR2004.pdf

Status: voluntary guidance intended for use by international or national medical device regulatory authorities, MR users and health professionals, and MR equipment manufacturers. This document replaces ARPANSA RHS 34 in Australia.

Summary: contains a detailed review of biological effects of static, time-varying gradient and RF magnetic fields, acoustic noise, and special cases arising from disease or medication, childhood and pregnancy. Contraindications, precautions, and safety considerations for patients are given. A section covers research scanning and use of the 2nd Level (Experimental Mode) plus practical guidance on operational and magnet safety issues.

An amendment increases the normal mode static field limit to 4 T, the first level to 8 T and second level to greater than 8 T [24].

International Electrotechnical Commission

IEC 60601-2-33 Medical Electrical Equipment - Part 2-33: Particular Requirements for the Basic Safety and Essential Performance of Magnetic Resonance Equipment for Medical Diagnosis [25]

Link: https://webstore.iec.ch/publication/22705

Status: Current. All MR equipment manufacturers comply with its requirements. Costs CHF 450.

Summary: this is a highly technical document published in English and French. It is not for general reading, but the MRSE should have access to a copy. Contents include:

- Modes of operation: Normal, First Level, Second Level
- Safety instructions
- Standardized methodologies for the measurement scanner safety-related field parameters:
  - B_0 fringe field
  - dB/dz spatial gradient
  - gradient dB/dt
  - SAR
  - B_{1+}RMS.
- The requirement for *compatibility data* specifies field measurements that must be made available to customers, required to assess implant conditions and occupational exposures
- Exposure limits for patients and workers (Table 14.2)

Table 14.2 IEC patient exposure limits for each Operating Mode [25].

Mode	Static field (T)	Median threshold for peripheral nerve stimulation (PNS) (%)	Core temperature rise (° C)	SAR (W kg⁻¹)	
				Head	Whole Body
Normal	3	80	0.5	3.2	2.0
First Level Controlled	8	100	1	3.2	4.0
Second Level Controlled	>8	120	2	>3.2	>4.0

- Signage specifications
- The fixed parameter option FPO:b via standard TS10974 [26] regarding active implant safety in the MR environment.

International Organization for Standardization

ISO/TS 10974:2018. Assessment of the Safety of Magnetic Resonance Imaging for Patients with an Active Implantable Medical Device [26]

Link: https://www.iso.org/standard/46462.html

Status: Industry standard for active implant manufacturers.

Summary: Outlines the design specifications and testing methodology to establish and determine MR compatibility of active implants for hydrogen scanning at 1.5T in closed-bore systems.

Medicines and Healthcare products Regulatory Agency

Safety Guidelines for Magnetic Resonance Imaging Equipment in Clinical Use [7]

Link: https://www.gov.uk/government/publications/safety-guidelines-for-magnetic-resonance-imaging-equipment-in-clinical-use

Status: Current UK Government guidance published by the Department of Health. Non-binding, standard practice.

Summary: A highly practical and comprehensive publication covering most aspects of MR safety including installation and cryogen handling. It contains references to UK legislation, but this does not negate the value of the guidance.

National Electrical Manufacturer's Association

Link: https://standards.globalspec.com/std/10149021/nema-ms-12

Status: Industry standard for MR manufacturers.

Summary: industry consensus methodologies on measuring MRI system performance. Whilst they deal primarily with image quality, Standards MS 4, 8 and 10 are relevant for patient safety:

NEMA MS 4 - *Acoustic Noise Measurement Procedure for Diagnostic Magnetic Resonance Imaging Devices* [27]

NEMA MS 8 - *Characterization of the Specific Absorption Rate (SAR) for Magnetic Resonance Imaging Systems* [28]

NEMA MS 10 - *Determination of Local Specific Absorption Rate (SAR) in Diagnostic Magnetic Resonance Imaging Systems* [29].

Royal Australian and New Zealand College of Radiologists

MRI safety guidelines version 2.0 [5]

Link: https://www.ranzcr.com/college/document-library/ranzcr-mri-safety-guidelines

Status: Current guidance from the Faculty of Clinical Radiology in Australasia. Best practice, non-binding.

Summary: Covers the practical, organizational and training aspects of MR safety in the clinical setting. Recommends the roles of MRMD, MRSO, and MRSE. Exposure limits are consistent with the current IEC standard [25]. Procedural guidance is provided regarding passive and active implants. Guidance on the use of gadolinium-based contrast agents has been updated by a separate statement: https://www.ranzcr.com/whats-on/news-media/171-ranzcr-statement-on-gadolinium-retention (accessed 8 March 2019).

EXPOSURE LIMITS

Whilst various jurisdictions and international organizations may specify exposure limits for patients [20-25], the standard which underpins what your scanner actually does is likely to be IEC 60601-2-33 [25]. The IEC patient (and staff) exposure limits are summarized in Table 14.2. (See Chapters 3–5 for the complete set of limits). The RF exposure limit is given in terms of core body temperature rise rather than SAR, because the hazard is thermal (see Chapter 5). As the in-vivo measurement of core body temperature is not feasible, SAR is used as a surrogate limiting parameter. Full SAR limits were shown in Table 5.6.

CONCLUSIONS: THE LAST WORD

Not only is this the conclusion of this chapter, it is also the conclusion of *Essentials of MRI Safety*. A strong organizational framework is essential for ensuring the safety of patients, staff, and visitors. This entails the three roles: MRMD, MRSO, MRSE; written safety policies and documentation, robust screening procedures, regular training, record-keeping, accreditation, professional development, adherence to guidelines, standards, and exposure limits, and where applicable, national or local regulations.

As a final statement, let us quote from the popular textbook *MRI from Picture to Proton* [30]:

"With hundreds of millions of people having been scanned over the last four decades, it seems unlikely that some unthought-of detrimental effect from the field exposures should appear now...

Ultimately the everyday dangers arise from the magnetic attractive and twisting forces and from implant heating or malfunction. Unfortunately accidents are usually caused by people, not machines.

MRI is only as safe as you are in your practice."

Figure 14.4 serves as a suitable visual reminder. Go and do no harm.

Revision questions

1. Which of the following is/are not recognized MR safety roles:
   A. MR Safety Officer
   B. MR Responsible Person
   C. MR Medical Officer
   D. MR Medical Director
   E. MR Safety Expert.
2. Which of the following should be addressed in a MRI safety policy:
   A. Definition of the four zones as specified by the ACR
   B. Procedure of dealing with implants
   C. Site security
   D. Infection control
   E. All of the above.
3. Your MRI scanner console offers the choice to select First Level Mode at patient registration, before any scans have taken place. What should you do?
   A. Carry on regardless- the scanner knows best
   B. Change the patient weight so that Normal Mode is selected
   C. Deselect First Level mode and start in the Normal Mode
   D. Abort the examination
   E. Obtain informed consent from the patient and carry on.
4. In which of the following situations should you press the quench button?
   A. A steel oxygen tank was brought into the scan room and has flown across the room and stuck to the magnet, trapping a staff member's chest and causing serious injury
   B. There is a fire alarm and call to evacuate the building
   C. A cleaner has entered the room with a large floor polisher which is now stuck to the magnet. No one is hurt, but he can't pull the machine away from the magnet
   D. All of the above
   E. None of the above.
5. Under the ACR designation of categories of MR personnel, a Level 1 person:
   A. May work and supervise other staff in all Zones
   B. May only work in Zones I, II and III
   C. Must know how to control SAR and dB/dt
   D. Must have passed the ABMRS exam
   E. May enter Zone IV and supervise non-MR personnel in Zone III.
6. If a patient undergoes a cardiac arrest whilst in the scanner requiring resuscitation equipment
   A. They should be resuscitated on the scanner couch immediately to avoid risk of death
   B. The magnet should be quenched to allow resuscitation in Zone IV
   C. Only MR trained staff should bring the resuscitation equipment into Zone IV
   D. They should be removed from Zone IV prior to resuscitation
   E. The system electrical power can be turned off to allow resuscitation equipment to be used in the magnet room.

References

1. Calamante, F., Ittermann, B, Kanal, E. et al. (2016). The Inter-Society Working Group on MR Safety: Recommended responsibilities for management of MR safety. *Journal of Magnetic Resonance Imaging* 44:1067–1069.
2. Medical Devices Directorate (1993). *Guidelines for Magnetic Resonance Diagnostic Equipment in Clinical Use – with Particular Reference to Safety.* London: MDD.
3. Kanal, E., Barkovich, A.J., Bell, C.M. et al. (2013). ACR guidance document on MR safe practices: 2013. *Journal of Magnetic Resonance Imaging* 37:501–530.

4. European Society of Radiology and the European Federation of Radiographer Societies (2019). Patient safety in medical imaging. *Radiography* 25: e26–e38.

5. Royal Australian and New Zealand College of Radiologists (2017). *MRI safety guidelines version 2.0*. Sydney: RANZCR.

6. Calamante, F., Faulkner, W., Ittermann, B. et al. (2015). Recommended minimum requirements for performing MRI in human subjects in a research setting. *Journal of Magnetic Resonance Imaging* 41:899–902.

7. Medicines and Healthcare products Regulatory Agency (2015). *Safety Guidelines for Magnetic Resonance Imaging Equipment in Clinical Use.' MHRA DB2007*. London: MHRA.

8. Institute of Physics and Engineering in Medicine (2017). Policy statement: Scientific safety advice to magnetic resonance imaging units that undertake human imaging. York, UK: IPEM. http://www.ipem.ac.uk/Publications/IPEMStatementsandNotices.aspx (accessed 4 August 2019).

9. Hand, J., Bosmans, H., Caruana, C. et al. (2013). The European Federation of Organisations for Medical Physics Policy Statement No 14: The role of the Medical Physicist in the management of safety within the magnetic resonance imaging environment: EFOMP recommendations. *Physics in Medicine and Biology* 29:122–125.

10. www.mrisafety.com (accessed 4 August 2019).

11. www.bamrr.org (accessed 4 August 2019).

12. ACR Committee on MR Safety (2019). ACR Guidance Document on MR Safe Practices: Updates and Critical Information 2019. *Journal of Magnetic Resonance Imaging* https://doi.org/10.1002/jmri.26880.

13. Watson, R.E., Walsh, S.M., Felmlee, J.P. et al. (2019). Augmenting MRI safety screening processes: reliable identification of cardiac implantable electronic devices by a ferromagnetic detector system. *Journal of Magnetic Resonance Imaging* 49:e297–e299.

14. Joint Commission (2015). *Standard EC.02.01.01 Environment of Care*. Oakbrook Terrace, IL: Joint Commission. https://www.jointcommission.org/assets/1/18/AHC_DiagImagingRpt_MK_20150806.pdf (accessed 19/06/2019).

15. Smith, K. (2014). MRI standards and safety guidelines in Canada. In: *MRI bioeffects, safety, and patient management* (Ed. F.D. Shellock FD and J.V. Crues JV III) pp 678–693. Los Angeles, CA: Biomedical Research Publishing Group.

16. Brown, G. (2014). MRI standards and safety guidelines in Australia. In: *MRI bioeffects, safety, and patient management* (Ed. F.D. Shellock FD and J.V. Crues JV III) pp 694–712. Los Angeles, CA: Biomedical Research Publishing Group.

17. Medical Radiation Practice Board (2019). *Professional capabilities for medical radiation practitioners*. Melbourne, Vic: Australian Health Practitioner Regulation Agency. https://www.medicalradiationpracticeboard.gov.au/Registration/Professional-Capabilities.aspx (accessed 7 January 2020).

18. Health and Care Professions Council. *The standards of proficiency for radiographers*. London: HCPC. https://www.hcpc-uk.org/standards/standards-of-proficiency/radiographers/ (accessed 21 June 2019)

19. ASTM International F2503-13 (2013). *Standard Practice for Marking Medical Devices and Other Items for Safety in the Magnetic Resonance Environment*. West Conshohocken, PA: ASTM International.

20. International Commission on Non-Ionizing Radiation Protection (2004). ICNIRP statement on medical magnetic resonance (MR) procedures: protection of patient. *Health Physics* 87:197–216.

21. Food and Drug Administration (2014). *Criteria for significant risk investigations of magnetic resonance diagnostic devices*. Rockville, MD: Center for Devices and Radiological Health, FDA.

22. Food and Drug Administration (2014). *Establishing Safety and Compatibility of Passive Implants in the Magnetic Resonance (MR) Environment, Guidance for Industry and Food and Drug Administration Staff*. Rockville, MD: Center for Devices and Radiological Health, FDA. https://www.fda.gov/regulatory-information/search-fda-guidance-documents/establishing-safety-and-compatibility-passive-implants-magnetic-resonance-mr-environment (accessed 4 August 2019).

23. Health Protection Agency (2008): Protection of patients and volunteers undergoing MRI procedures. *Documents of the Health Protection Agency*. RCE-7 Didcot: HPA.

24. International Commission on Non-Ionizing Radiation Protection (2009). Amendment to ICNIRP statement on medical magnetic resonance procedures: protection of patients. *Health Physics* 97:259–261.

25. International Electrotechnical Commission (2015). *IEC 60601-2-33 Medical Electrical Equipment - Part 2-33: Particular Requirements for the Basic Safety and Essential Performance of Magnetic Resonance Equipment for Medical Diagnosis, Edn 3.2*. Geneva: IEC.

26. International Organization for Standardization (2018). *ISO/TS 10974 Assessment of the Safety of Magnetic Resonance Imaging for Patients with an Active Implantable Medical Device*. Geneva: ISO.

339

27. NEMA (2010). MS 4 - *Acoustic Noise Measurement Procedure for Diagnostic Magnetic Resonance Imaging Devices*. Rosslyn, VA: National Electrical Manufacturers Association

28. NEMA (2016). MS 8 - *Characterization of the Specific Absorption Rate (SAR) for Magnetic Resonance Imaging Systems*. Rosslyn, VA: National Electrical Manufacturers Association.

29. NEMA (2010). MS 10 - *Determination of Local Specific Absorption Rate (SAR) in Diagnostic Magnetic Resonance Imaging Systems*. Rosslyn, VA: National Electrical Manufacturers Association.

30. McRobbie, D., Moore, E., Graves, M. et al. (2017). *MRI from picture to proton (3rd Edition)* pp 356. Cambridge, UK: Cambridge University Press.

Further reading and resources

ACR Committee on MR Safety (2019). ACR Guidance Document on MR Safe Practices: Updates and Critical Information 2019. *Journal of Magnetic Resonance Imaging*. https://doi.org/10.1002/jmri.26880.

American Board of MR Safety. www.abmrs.org (accessed 15 August 2019).

European Society of Radiology (ESR) and the European Federation of Radiographer Societies (EFRS). (2019). Patient safety in medical imaging. *Radiography* 25: e26–e38.

European Society for Magnetic Resonance in Medicine and Biology. www.esmrmb.org (accessed 21 June 2019).

European Society of Radiology www.myesr.org (accessed 15 August 2019).

International Society for Magnetic Resonance in Medicine *safety resources*. https://www.ismrm.org/mr-safety-links/ (accessed 15 August 2019).

Kanal, E., Barkovich, A.J., Bell, C.M. et al. (2013). ACR Guidance Document on MR Safe Practices: 2013, American College of Radiology Expert panel on MR Safety. *Journal of Magnetic Resonance Imaging* 37:501–530.

MHRA (2015). *Safety Guidelines for Magnetic Resonance Imaging Equipment in Clinical Use. MHRA DB2007*. London: Medicines and Healthcare products Regulatory Agency.

Society and College of Radiographers (2019). *Safety of magnetic resonance imaging*. London: SCOR. Available from https://www.sor.org/learning/document-library/safety-magnetic-resonance-imaging-2 (accessed 15 August 2019).

Appendix 1

One hundred equations you need to know

This appendix is intended as compulsory reading for those wishing to act as a MRSE. The results derived here are used without proof elsewhere in this book. In this appendix the scalar or "dot" product is denoted "•", and the vector or "cross" product is denoted "×". Vectors are denoted in bold typeface. A brief description of vector calculus is presented in Appendix 2.

MAXWELL'S EQUATIONS

The fundamental laws of magnetism are summarized by Maxwell's four equations expressed in two equivalent forms, differential and integral:

Differential		Integral	
Gauss's Law			
$\nabla \cdot \mathbf{E} = \dfrac{Q_V}{\varepsilon_0}$	(A1.1a)	$\int_s \mathbf{E} \cdot \mathbf{dS} = \dfrac{Q_t}{\varepsilon_0}$	(A1.1b)
Gauss's Law for magnetism			
$\nabla \cdot \mathbf{B} = 0$	(A1.2a)	$\int_s \mathbf{B} \cdot \mathbf{dS} = 0$	(A1.2b)
Faraday's Law			
$\nabla \times \mathbf{E} = -\dfrac{d\mathbf{B}}{dt}$	(A1.3a)	$\oint \mathbf{E.dl} = -\dfrac{d}{dt}\int_s \mathbf{B} \cdot \mathbf{dS} = \mu_0 I_t$	(A1.3b)
Ampere's Law			
$\nabla \times \mathbf{B} - \dfrac{1}{c^2}\dfrac{d\mathbf{E}}{dt} = \mu_0 \mathbf{J}_m$	(A1.4a)	$\oint \mathbf{B} \cdot \mathbf{dl} = \mu_0 \int_s \left[\mathbf{J}_m + \varepsilon_0 \dfrac{d\mathbf{E}}{dt} \right] .\mathbf{dS}$	(A1.4b)

Essentials of MRI Safety, First Edition. Donald W. McRobbie.
© 2020 John Wiley & Sons Ltd. Published 2020 by John Wiley & Sons Ltd.

where the following definitions apply:

Q_v total volume charge
Q_t total surface charge
ε_0 permittivity of free space
c   speed of light
J_m displacement current.

A conceptual description of these laws is given in Chapter 2 illustrated in Figures 2.1–2.4.

MAGNETIC FIELD INDUCTION

B from a long straight conductor

The field from a current I flowing through a long straight conductor is:

$$B_\theta = \frac{\mu_0 I}{2\pi r} \tag{A1.5}$$

The magnetic field has circular field lines with directionality according to a right-hand rule (Figure 2.5). There are no radial or z-components of field for an infinitely long wire.

B from a single loop conductor

The field on the z-axis from a circular loop of radius a is directed along the z-direction:

$$B_z = \frac{\mu_0 I a^2}{2\left(z^2 + a^2\right)^{3/2}} \tag{A1.6}$$

At the center of the loop z = 0 and

$$B_z = \frac{\mu_0 I}{2a} \tag{A1.7}$$

At long distances the loop can be considered as a magnetic dipole of area A having a magnetic dipole moment **m** with magnitude:

$$m = IA \tag{A1.8}$$

B at distance r from a dipole has components B_r and B_θ (in spherical polar coordinates: r, θ, φ)

$$B_r = \frac{\mu_0}{4\pi} \frac{2m}{r^3} \cos\theta; \qquad B_\theta = \frac{\mu_0}{4\pi} \frac{m}{r^3} \sin\theta; \qquad B_\varnothing = 0 \tag{A1.9}$$

On axis θ = 0, r = z and the z component is

$$B_z = \frac{\mu_0}{4\pi} \frac{2m}{z^3} \tag{A1.10}$$

The field gradient on the z axis with $\theta = 0$ from a dipole is

$$\frac{dB_z}{dz} = -\frac{\mu_0}{2\pi}\frac{3m}{z^4} \qquad (A1.11)$$

showing an inverse 4th power dependence upon distance z from the dipole.

B from a solenoidal coil

The field generated at the center of a solenoid of length l with windings of density N turns per meter is

$$B_z = \frac{\mu_0}{2}\int_{-l/2}^{l/2}\frac{INr^2}{2\left(z^2 + r^2\right)^{3/2}}\,dz \qquad (A1.12)$$

$$= \mu_0 NI\sin\theta \qquad (A1.13)$$

θ is the angle measured from the vertical at iso-center to the end of the solenoid (Figure 2.7). For long solenoids $\theta \rightarrow 90°$ $(\pi/2)$ and the field is

$$B_z = \mu_0 NI \qquad (A1.14)$$

The magnetic field strength or intensity, H, in A m^{-1} is

$$H_z = NI \qquad (A1.15)$$

B_z along the axis of a solenoid of length 2d is

$$B_z = \frac{\mu_0 IN}{2d}\left(\cos\theta_1 + \cos\theta_2\right) \qquad (A1.16)$$

where θ_1 and θ_2 are the angles subtended from position z to either end of the coil:

$$\theta_1 = \frac{d-z}{\sqrt{\left[r^2 + \left(d-z\right)^2\right]}}; \qquad (A1.17a)$$

$$\theta_2 = \frac{d+z}{\sqrt{\left[r^2 + \left(d+z\right)^2\right]}} \qquad (A1.17b)$$

B from a multi-layer solenoid

B at the iso-center of a multi-layer solenoid of inner radius r_1 and outer radius r_2 and length l is

$$B = \frac{\mu_0 NIl}{2}\ln\left\{\frac{\alpha + \left(\alpha^2 + \beta^2\right)^{1/2}}{1 + \left(1 + \beta^2\right)^{1/2}}\right\}; \quad \alpha = \frac{r_2}{r_1}; \quad \beta = \frac{l}{2r_1} \qquad (A1.18)$$

The Biot-Savart Law

A generalized method of computing the magnetic field from an arbitrary coil geometry is given by:

$$\mathbf{B} = \frac{\mu_0}{4\pi} I \oint \frac{d\mathbf{l} \times \mathbf{r}}{r^2}$$ (A1.19)

$d\mathbf{l}$ is an incremental vector along the coil path and $\mathbf{r}$ is the 3-dimensional spatial vector (x,y,z). Figure 2.6 shows the attenuation in distance of the B_z from various coil geometries.

MRI gradient coils

The gradient fields are

$$G_x = \frac{dB_z}{dx}$$ (A1.20a)

$$G_y = \frac{dB_z}{dy}$$ (A1.20b)

$$G_z = \frac{dB_z}{dz}$$ (A1.20c)

and the total field during imaging is

$$B_z(x, y, z) = B_0 + xG_x + yG_y + zG_z$$ (A1.21)

However, B_z cannot exist in isolation as it does not satisfy Maxwell's equation A1.2b. Concomitant fields [1] in the x and y directions must exist such that

$$\mathbf{B}(x, y, z) = ax\,G_z\hat{\imath} + byG_z\hat{\jmath} + zG_z\hat{k}$$ (A1.22)

$\hat{\imath}, \hat{\jmath}, \hat{k}$ are unit vectors with magnitude equal to 1, pointing along the x, y and z directions. For a Maxwell pair coil a = b = –0.5.

For the x and y gradients, Ampere's law (equation A1.4) at low frequency and in the absence of displacement current, $\nabla \times \mathbf{B} = 0$, requires that there is an additional z-component, e.g. for G_x and G_y

$$\mathbf{B}(x,z) = z\,G_x\hat{\imath} + xG_x\hat{k}; \qquad \mathbf{B}(y,z) = z\,G_y\hat{\imath} + yG_y\hat{k}$$ (A1.23)

From an imaging point of view, these additional terms can usually be neglected as only the z-component is relevant, but for patient exposure, the field patterns will be different in direction and amplitude. The amplitude of the x-gradient field is:

$$|B| = G_x\sqrt{x^2 + z^2}$$ (A1.24)

The gradient field has zero z-dependence only in the plane of the iso-center.

MAGNETIC MATERIALS

In an external field, the magnetization **M** of a material is

$$\mathbf{M} = \chi \mathbf{H} \tag{A1.25}$$

χ is the material's magnetic susceptibility. In an isotropic medium χ is independent of orientation or position.

The nett B in the medium is

$$\mathbf{B} = \mu_0 \left(\mathbf{H} + \mathbf{M} \right) \tag{A1.26}$$

If the material is linear and isotropic then

$$\mathbf{B} = \mu_0 \left(1 + \chi \right) \mathbf{H} \tag{A1.27}$$

The relative permeability μ_r is

$$\mu_r = 1 + \chi \tag{A1.28}$$

and

$$\mathbf{B} = \mu_0 \mu_r \mathbf{H} \tag{A1.29}$$

Demagnetizing field and factors

Figure 2.13 illustrates how the magnetization within the object produces virtual north and south poles which sustain a demagnetizing field $\mathbf{H}_d$ opposed to **B** and **M**. The apparent susceptibility χ_{app} underestimates the true value:

$$\chi_{app} = \frac{\chi}{1 + d} \tag{A1.30}$$

where d is the shape or demagnetizing factor. For simple shapes (ellipsoids of rotation, cuboids and cylinders) there are three demagnetizing factors: d_1 along the principal axis, d_2 and d_3 along the minor axes with a sum equal to 1. Some representative values are shown in Table A1.1. and plotted in Figure 2.14.

For cylinders of arbitrary length to diameter ratio, n, the following gives approximately correct values [2]:

$$d_1 = \left(\frac{4n}{\sqrt{\pi}} + 1 \right)^{-1} \text{ and } d_2 = d_3 = \frac{1 - d_1}{2} \tag{A1.31}$$

FORCES AND TORQUE

Forces on circuits

The force on a conductor a carrying current I_a from the B-field of another conductor is

$$\mathbf{F} = I_a \oint d\mathbf{l}_a \times \mathbf{B} \tag{A1.32}$$

Table A1.1 Demagnetizing factors for various geometries. d_1 is for the principal axis. Values from [2,3].

Shape	Length/diameter ratio	d_1	d_2	d_3
Flat sheet	0	1.00	0.00	0.00
Sphere	1	0.333	0.333	0.333
Cylinder	0.1	0.797	0.102	0.102
	0.5	0.475	0.263	0.263
	1	0.312	0.344	0.344
	2	0.182	0.409	0.409
	5	0.080	0.460	0.460
	10	0.042	0.479	0.479
	∞	0.00	0.500	0.500

Force between two long parallel conductors

The magnitude of the force between two parallel long conductors of length d, separated by a is

$$F = \frac{\mu_0 I_1 I_2}{2\pi a}\, d \qquad\qquad (A1.33)$$

If I_1 and I_2 flow in the same direction the force is attractive, if they follow in opposite directions the force will be repulsive.

Force on a straight conductor in a B-field

The force on a current-carrying conductor of length d in a magnetic field is:

$$F = IdB\sin\theta \qquad\qquad (A1.34)$$

Energy and force: non-ferromagnetic materials

The magnetic force can be calculated from the magnetic energy U. If the object is initially un-magnetized the energy acquired by introducing it into the field is:

$$U = \frac{1}{2}\mathbf{m}\cdot\mathbf{B_0} = \frac{1}{2}MVB_0\cos\theta \qquad\qquad (A1.35)$$

where $\mathbf{m}$ (=$\mathbf{M}V$) is the magnetic moment. For diamagnetic and paramagnetic materials where $|\chi|$ is very small, we can neglect demagnetizing factors. The magnetic force is given by the spatial derivative of U. The z-component is

$$F_z = \frac{1}{2}\frac{d}{dz}MVB_0 = \frac{1}{2}\frac{d}{dz}\frac{\chi}{\mu_0}VB_0{}^2 \qquad\qquad (A1.36)$$

The magnetic force on a paramagnetic object is therefore

$$F = \frac{\chi}{\mu_0} V B_0 \frac{dB}{dz} \tag{A1.37}$$

For a diamagnetic material the force is negative.

Forces on ferromagnetic objects

In this section we derive the force applied to a cylinder or ellipsoid with equal minor axes [4]. The H-field in a magnetizable object in an external field H_0 is

$$\mathbf{H} = \mathbf{H_0} - \mathbf{d}\,\mathbf{M} \tag{A1.38}$$

with demagnetizing factor $\mathbf{d}$. As $M = \chi H$

$$\mathbf{H} = \mathbf{H_0} - d\chi \mathbf{H} \tag{A1.39}$$

so

$$\mathbf{H} = \mathbf{H_0}\, \frac{1}{1 + d\chi} \tag{A1.40}$$

From equation A1.27

$$\mathbf{B} = \mu_0 \mathbf{H_0}\, \frac{1 + \chi}{1 + d\chi} \tag{A1.41}$$

$$\mathbf{M} = \frac{1}{\mu_0}\mathbf{B_0}\, \frac{\chi}{1 + d\chi} \tag{A1.42}$$

If demagnetizing factor $d = 0$ this gives Equations A1.25 and A1.27.
In a cylinder of length l, radius r the axial and radial magnetizations are (Figure A1.1)

$$M_1 = H \frac{\chi}{1 + d_1\chi}; \quad M_2 = H \frac{\chi}{1 + d_2\chi} \tag{A1.43}$$

If the long axis of the cylinder makes an angle θ with the external B_z we have:

$$H_1 = H \cos\theta; \quad H_2 = H \sin\theta \tag{A1.44}$$

and

$$M_1 = \frac{1}{\mu_0} B_0 \frac{\chi}{1 + d_1\chi} \cos\theta; \quad M_2 = \frac{1}{\mu_0} B_0 \frac{\chi}{1 + d_2\chi} \sin\theta \tag{A1.45}$$

M_z is the sum of $M_1\cos\theta$ and $M_2\sin\theta$:

$$M_z = \frac{\chi}{\mu_0} B_0 \left[\frac{\cos^2\theta}{1 + d_1\chi} + \frac{\sin^2\theta}{1 + d_2\chi} \right] \tag{A1.46}$$

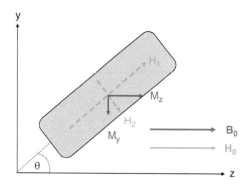

Figure A1.1 Magnetization of a ferromagnetic object in an external B_0.

and

$$M_y = \frac{\chi^2}{\mu_0} B_0 \left[\frac{d_2 - d_1}{(1 + d_1 \chi)(1 + d_2 \chi)} \right] \cos\theta \sin\theta \qquad (A1.47)$$

M_z simplifies to equation A1.25 for $\chi \ll 1$, whilst a sphere will have zero y (or x) magnetization.

A general form for the magnetic force from equations A1.36 and A1.46 is

$$F_z = \frac{\chi}{\mu_0} V B_0 \frac{dB_0}{dz} \left[\frac{\cos^2\theta}{1 + d_1\chi} + \frac{\sin^2\theta}{1 + d_2\chi} \right] \qquad (A1.48)$$

Strongly ferromagnetic (unsaturated) materials ($\chi \gg 1$)

If $\chi \gg 1$, the force on an ellipsoid or cylinder at angle θ to B_0 is

$$F_z = \frac{1}{\mu_0} V B_0 \frac{dB}{dz} \left(\frac{\cos^2\theta}{d_1} + \frac{\sin^2\theta}{d_2} \right) \qquad (A1.49)$$

The force does not depend upon magnetic susceptibility as long as $\chi \gg 1$.

Weakly ferromagnetic materials ($\chi \ll 1$)

If χ is small ($\ll 1$) as for "weakly ferromagnetic" materials such as 316 series stainless steel then $(1 + d\chi) \approx 1$ and Equation A1.48 reduces to Equation A1.37. Notably, the shape dependence disappears and the force depends upon susceptibility again.

Soft saturated ferromagnetic material

For a saturated metal the magnetization is at a maximum M_{sat} and $\chi \to 0$ as the external H (or B) increases. In terms of the "saturation field" B_{sat} [1]

---

[1] It is magnetization which saturates rather than flux density. However B is more familiar so B_{sat} is used here and elsewhere.

$$F_z \approx \frac{1}{\mu_0} V B_{sat} \frac{dB}{dz}$$ (A1.50)

Permanent magnet

For a permanent magnet we are not reliant on the external B_0 to magnetize the object, so the factor ½ in equation A1.35 is dropped. The force is given by the spatial derivative of the total energy but **m** is the remanent magnetization of the material:

$$F_z = \frac{dU}{dz} = \frac{d}{dz}(\mathbf{m} \cdot \mathbf{B}) = \frac{V}{\mu_0} B_{rem} \cos\theta \frac{dB}{dz}$$ (A1.51)

Torque

A non-spherical object with its principal axis unaligned with B_0 will experience torque acting to align the object along z (Figure 2.21). Torque, **T**, is

$$\mathbf{T} = \mathbf{m} \times \mathbf{B}_0$$ (A1.52)

349

For B_0 along the z-axis

$$\mathbf{T} = \begin{vmatrix} \hat{\mathbf{i}} & \hat{\mathbf{j}} & \hat{\mathbf{k}} \\ m_x & m_y & m_z \\ 0 & 0 & B_0 \end{vmatrix} = m_y B_0 \hat{\mathbf{i}} - m_x B_0 \hat{\mathbf{j}}$$ (A1.53)

To calculate **T** consider the effect of the demagnetizing fields along each axis of the object, then deduce M_x and M_y terms. Due to rotational symmetry we need only calculate M_y [4].

From equations A1.47 and A1.53 the general form for torque is

$$\mathbf{T} = \frac{\chi^2}{\mu_0} B_0{}^2 V \left[\frac{d_2 - d_1}{(1 + d_1\chi)(1 + d_2\chi)} \right] \cos\theta \sin\theta$$ (A1.54)

Torque on diamagnetic and paramagnetic objects

From Equation A1.54 and using the trigonometric identity $\sin 2\theta = 2\sin\theta\cos\theta$, if $|\chi| \ll 1$ the magnitude of torque on a cylindrical or symmetric ellipsoid is

$$\mathbf{T} = \frac{1}{2\mu_0} \chi^2 V B_0^2 (d_2 - d_1) \sin 2\theta$$ (A1.55)

The maximum torque is exerted at 45° (Figure 2.22a). The maximum torque for an elongated object is

$$T_{elong} \propto \frac{1}{4\mu_0} \chi^2 V B_0^2$$ (A1.56a)

For a flat sheet object:

$$T_{sheet} \propto \frac{1}{2\mu_0} \chi^2 V B_0^2 \qquad\qquad (A1.56b)$$

These expressions also hold for "weakly" ferromagnetic objects up to values of around $\chi < 0.1$.

Torque on soft unsaturated ferromagnetic objects

The torque on a soft ferromagnetic material with $\chi \gg 1$ is

$$T = \frac{1}{2\mu_0} V B_0^2 \frac{(d_2 - d_1)}{d_1 d_2} \sin 2\theta \qquad\qquad (A1.57)$$

This is independent of susceptibility.

Torque on saturated ferromagnetic objects

When the metal is saturated the torque depends upon the square of its saturation magnetization and becomes independent of B_0. As χ is the ratio of M/H and $B_0 = \mu_0 H$, from Equation A1.54 the torque on a saturated object becomes [5]

$$T_{max,sat} = \frac{\mu_0}{2} V M_{sat}^2 (d_2 - d_1) \sin 2\theta \qquad\qquad (A1.58)$$

or, in terms of B_{sat} the maximum torque is

$$T_{max,sat} \approx \frac{1}{2\mu_0} V B_{sat}^2 (d_2 - d_1) \qquad\qquad (A1.59)$$

FORCES ON MOVING CHARGES

Maxwell's equations inform us that moving charges are subject to an additional force, the Lorentz force; also that charge moving within an external magnetic field will produce an electric field by the *hydrodynamic* or *Hall effect*.

Lorentz force

The Lorentz force on a charge Q possessing velocity **v** (Figure 2.25a) is given as

$$\mathbf{F} = Q(\mathbf{E} + \mathbf{v} \times \mathbf{B}) \qquad\qquad (A1.60)$$

We can ignore the electric field term. The magnitude of the force is

$$F = QvB \sin\theta \qquad\qquad (A1.61)$$

The direction of action is determined by Fleming's left-hand rule (Figure 2.25b).

Magneto-hydrodynamic effect

The magneto-hydrodynamic effect is the generation of an electric field $\mathbf{E}_i$ by the flow of charge within an external magnetic field (Figure 2.26). This is analogous to the Hall effect observed in semiconductors:

$$E_i = vB \sin\theta \tag{A1.62}$$

In terms of voltage or electrical potential, V, where

$$V = E\,d \tag{A1.63}$$

and d is the distance between charged surfaces (as in a capacitor), we have an induced voltage

$$V_i = dvB \sin\theta \tag{A1.64}$$

This is the source of the ECG artefact in MRI.

LAWS OF INDUCTION

Maxwell's third equation or Faraday's law, equation A1.3 states that an electric field will be induced by a time-varying magnetic field with an electric field strength equal to the rate of change of *magnetic flux* Φ

$$\Phi = \int_s \mathbf{B} \cdot \mathbf{dS} \tag{A1.65}$$

measured in webers (Wb). For a uniform B, Φ is the product of area A and B, so that

$$\oint \mathbf{E.dl} = -A\frac{dB}{dt} \tag{A1.66}$$

Induced fields from dB/dt

If we consider a wire loop within a uniform time-varying B-field we have [6]

$$2\pi rE = -\pi r^2 \frac{dB}{dt} \tag{A1.67}$$

The magnitude of the induced E-field is

$$|E| = \frac{r}{2}\frac{dB}{dt} \tag{A1.68}$$

The direction of E follows a left-hand rule, as the magnetic field produced by the induced current in the wire will oppose the rate of change of flux that induced the current (Figure 2.3).

In a uniform volume conductor with conductivity σ current density $\mathbf{J}$ is given by

$$\mathbf{J} = \sigma\mathbf{E} \tag{A1.69}$$

Its magnitude is

$$J = \sigma \frac{r}{2} \frac{dB}{dt}$$

(A1.70)

Induction in an elliptical cross section

The maximum E and J for an elliptical cross-section are [7]

$$E = \frac{a^2 b}{a^2 + b^2} \frac{dB}{dt}$$

(A1.71)

$$J = \frac{a^2 b}{a^2 + b^2} \sigma \frac{dB}{dt}$$

(A1.72)

where a is the semi-major axis and b the semi-minor axis (Figure 4.3).

Induction from magnetic field gradients

A simplified **E** solution for a cylinder of radius r_0 has been stated as [8]

$$E_x = \frac{xy}{2} \frac{dG_x}{dt} + \frac{r_0^2 - x^2 + y^2}{4} \frac{dG_y}{dt} + \frac{xz}{2} \frac{dG_z}{dt}$$

(A1.73)

$$E_y = \frac{-xy}{2} \frac{dG_y}{dt} - \frac{r_0^2 - x^2 + y^2}{4} \frac{dG_x}{dt} - \frac{xz}{2} \frac{dG_z}{dt}$$

(A1.74)

$$E_z = -yz \frac{dG_x}{dt} + xy \frac{dG_z}{dt}$$

(A1.75)

Human anatomy, with irregular shapes and differing tissue conductivities, will exhibit much more complex behavior, with E-field lines and current loops altered by tissue boundaries and electrostatic charges induced on these boundaries according to Gauss's Law.

RF INDUCTION FROM THE RADIOFREQUENCY FIELD

Absorbed power density is given by:

$$P_V = \mathbf{J} \cdot \mathbf{E} = \sigma E^2$$

(A1.76)

Specific absorption rate (SAR) is defined as the power deposited in tissue per unit mass:

$$SAR = 0.5 \frac{\sigma}{\rho} E^2$$

(A1.77)

ρ is tissue density. In the simplest case of a uniform sphere of radius r, the maximum SAR from a rectangular constant amplitude B_1 pulse repeated N times per TR period can be calculated from equation A1.68

$$SAR_{max} = \frac{\sigma\pi^2 r^2 f^2 B_1^2 D}{2\rho}$$ (A1.78)

where D is the duty cycle.

Average SAR in a uniform sphere

The equivalent resistance R_m of a sphere of uniform conductivity σ is [9]

$$R_m = \frac{2}{15}\pi\sigma\omega^2 \left(\frac{B_1}{I}\right)^2 r^5$$ (A1.79)

The average power deposited (from $P = 0.5I^2R$) is

$$P = \frac{1}{15}\pi\sigma\omega^2 B_1^2 r^5 D$$ (A1.80)

The average SAR is

$$SAR_{ave} = P/\rho\frac{4}{3}\pi r^3 = \frac{1}{20\rho}\sigma\omega^2 B_1^2 r^2 D$$ (A1.81)

For a sphere, the average SAR is 0.4 of the peak SAR. In terms of flip angle α, for a rectangular B_1 pulse of duration t_p is:

$$SAR_{ave} = \frac{1}{5\rho\gamma^2}\sigma\pi^2 f^2 \alpha^2 r^2 \left(\frac{N}{t_p TR}\right)$$ (A1.82)

Average SAR in a uniform cylinder

A general approach to calculating R_m uses the magnetic vector potential [10]. For a uniform cylinder within a transverse B_1:

$$R_m = \frac{1}{8}\pi\sigma\omega^2 \left(\frac{B_1}{I}\right)^2 r^4 d\Gamma\left(\frac{d}{r}\right)$$ (A1.83)

$\Gamma(d/r)$ is a geometric function. For an approximation to the human torso with d = 4r, $\Gamma\approx1.3$ and the average SAR is

$$SAR_{ave} \cong \frac{1}{6\rho}\sigma\omega^2 B_1^2 r^2 D$$ (A1.84)

Skin depth

The "skin effect" is caused by induced eddy currents within a conductor resulting in a relationship between current and depth x:

$$I(x) = I_{surface} e^{-\frac{x}{\delta}} \tag{A1.85}$$

The skin depth δ is

$$\delta = \sqrt{\frac{1}{\pi f \sigma \mu_0 \mu_r}} \tag{A1.86}$$

where f is frequency. In MRI it is only significant for B_1. At 128 MHz the skin depth in muscle is around 53 mm; in titanium it is 0.028 mm.

SAR AND TISSUE HEATING

The relationship between SAR and heating is non-linear, heterogeneous and heavily influenced by the thermal properties of tissue and cooling from perfusion and conduction.

Perfusion cooling

A simple model for bulk heat transport and temperature T in tissue is [11]

$$C_t \frac{dT}{dt} = -g_b C_b (T - T_b) + SAR \tag{A1.87}$$

where C_t and C_b are the specific heat capacities for tissue and blood (J kg^{-1} °C^{-1}), g_b is the bulk blood flow (kg s^{-1} kg^{-1}), and T_b is blood temperature. At t = 0 the tissue temperature equals the blood temperature. For the steady state dT/dt = 0 so the final equilibrium temperature rise is

$$\Delta T_f = \frac{SAR}{C_b g_b} \tag{A1.88}$$

The solution to equation A1.87 is

$$\Delta T = \Delta T_f \left(1 - e^{-t/\tau}\right) \tag{A1.89}$$

where the time constant is

$$\tau = \frac{C_t}{C_b g_b} \tag{A1.90}$$

It terms of blood flow F_b in ml min^{-1} kg^{-1}, using C_b = 3617 J kg^{-1} °C^{-1}, Equations A1.88 and A1.90 become:

$$\Delta T_f = 15.8 \frac{SAR}{F_b} \qquad\qquad\text{(A1.91)}$$

$$\tau = 15.8 \frac{C_t}{F_b} \qquad\qquad\text{(A1.92)}$$

Convection cooling

Convection cooling by a fluid or air is similar to perfusion cooling (Equation A1.87):

$$C\frac{dT}{dt} = -\frac{hA}{\rho V}(T - T_\infty) + SAR \qquad\qquad\text{(A1.93)}$$

where T_∞ is the background fluid temperature, A is the cooling surface area, and h is the heat transfer coefficient (W m^{-2} °C^{-1}). This implies exponential behavior similar to Equation A1.89 with a time constant

$$\tau = \frac{\rho VC}{hA} \qquad\qquad\text{(A1.94)}$$

355

and an equilibrium temperature rise

$$\Delta T_f = \frac{\tau\, SAR}{C} \qquad\qquad\text{(A1.95)}$$

In the absence of fluid flow, h can be calculated from the thermal conductivity

$$h = \frac{\kappa}{L} \qquad\qquad\text{(A1.96)}$$

L is the ratio of volume to surface area or the "characteristic length" of the cooling object. For a sphere of radius r_0, $L = r_0/3$; for a cylinder $L = r_0/2$.

Conduction cooling

The effect of cooling by thermal conduction can be obtained from the thermal conduction equation:

$$\frac{d^2T}{dr^2} + 2r\frac{dT}{dr} + \frac{\rho}{K}SAR = 0 \qquad\qquad\text{(A1.97)}$$

where ρ is tissue density and κ is its thermal conductivity (W m^{-1} °C^{-1}). This gives a temperature rise at distance r from the maximum temperature (at r = 0) [11] of

$$\Delta T = \frac{\rho r^2}{6\kappa} SAR \qquad \text{(A1.98)}$$

This allows us to estimate the heating in a non-perfused spherical region of tissue.

Radiative cooling

The cooling of a body of surface area A by radiative processes is given by Stefan's Law:

$$P = \frac{dU}{dt} = e\,A\,s\left(T_1^{\,4} - T_0^{\,4}\right) \qquad \text{(A1.99)}$$

T_1 and T_0 are the hotter and cooler temperatures (in kelvin), e is the emissivity (values 0-1) and the Stefan–Boltzmann constant s = 5.67×10^{-8} W m^{-2} K^{-4}. Power P is the rate of change of thermal energy U. Radiative cooling can be incorporated into a simple transient heating model:

$$\frac{dU}{dt} = 4\,e\,A\,s\,T_0^{\,3}\Delta T \qquad \text{(A1.100)}$$

where the temperature is given in kelvin. The multiplier of the temperature difference then has the same units as heat transfer coefficient h and can be incorporated into Equation A1.93.

References

1. Norris, D.G. and Hutchison, J.M.S. (1990). Concomitant magnetic field gradients and their effects on imaging at low magnetic field strengths. *Magnetic Resonance Imaging* 8:33–37.
2. Sato, M. and Ishii, Y. (1989). Simple and approximate expressions of demagnetizing factors of uniformly magnetized rectangular rod and cylinder. *Journal of Applied Physics* 66:983–985.
3. Osborne, J.A. (1945). Demagnetizing factors of the general ellipsoid. *Physical Review* 67:351–357.
4. Schenck, J.F. (2000). Safety of strong static magnetic fields. *Journal of Magnetic Resonance Imaging* 12:2–19.
5. Abbot, J.J., Ergeneman, O., Kummer, M.P. et al. (2007). Modeling magnetic torque and force for controlled manipulation of soft-magnetic bodies. *IEEE Transactions on Robotics* 23:1247–1252.
6. Budinger, T.F. (1979). Thresholds for physiological effects due to RF and magnetic fields used in NMR imaging. *IEEE Transactions on Nuclear Science* NS-26:2821–2825.
7. McRobbie, D.W. (1987). Relationship between changing B and induced electric and physiological effects. In: *Safety Assessment of NMR Imaging* (ed. K. Schmidt), Stuttgart: Georg Thieme Verlag, pp.64–70.
8. Turk, E.A., Kopanoglu, E., Guney, S. et al. (2012). A simple expression for the gradient induced potential on active implants during MRI. *IEEE Transactions on Biomedical Engineering* 59:2845–2851.
9. Hoult, D.I and Lauterbur, P.C. (1979). The sensitivity of the zeugmatographic experiment involving human samples. *Journal of Magnetic Resonance* 34:71–85.
10. Harpen, M.D. (1989). Eddy current distributions in cylindrical sample: effect on equivalent sample resistance. *Physics in Medicine and Biology* 34:1229–1238.
11. Athey, T.W. (1989). A model of the temperature rise in the head due to magnetic resonance imaging procedures. *Magnetic Resonance in Medicine* 9:177–184.

Appendix 2
Maths toolkit

COORDINATE SYSTEMS

Cartesian coordinates

The Cartesian coordinate system is the usual orthogonal "real world" system comprising axes x, y and z (Figure A2.1a). The axes are depicted in the right-handed orientation with +x coming out of the page, y is left-right, and z vertical.

The unit vectors for x, y, z are $\hat{\mathbf{i}}, \hat{\mathbf{j}}, \hat{\mathbf{k}}$.
The incremental elements are dx, dy, dz.
The incremental volume dV = dx dy dz

Cylindrical polar coordinates

Cylindrical polar coordinates are convenient for situations with cylindrical symmetry, e.g. solenoidal coils. The coordinates are r, θ, z where r is the radial distance in the x–y plane, orthogonal to the z-axis (Figure A2.1b). In Cartesian coordinates:

$$r = \sqrt{x^2 + y^2}; \qquad \tan\theta = \frac{y}{x}; \qquad z = z \qquad \text{(A2.1)}$$

and

$$x = r\cos\theta; \qquad y = r\sin\theta; \qquad z = z \qquad \text{(A2.2)}$$

The unit vectors are $\hat{\mathbf{r}}, \hat{\boldsymbol{\theta}}, \hat{\mathbf{k}}$
 The incremental elements are dr, rdθ, dz so that

$$\mathbf{dr} = dr\,\hat{\mathbf{r}} + rd\theta\,\hat{\boldsymbol{\theta}} + dz\,\hat{\mathbf{k}} \qquad \text{(A2.3)}$$

Essentials of MRI Safety, First Edition. Donald W. McRobbie.
© 2020 John Wiley & Sons Ltd. Published 2020 by John Wiley & Sons Ltd.

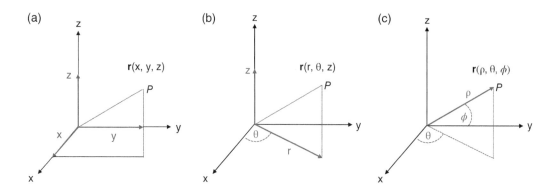

Figure A2.1   Coordinate systems showing the positional vector **r** and its components to a point *P*: (a) Cartesian; (b) cylindrical polar; (c) spherical polar.

The incremental volume is

$$dV = r\,dr\,d\theta\,dz \qquad \text{(A2.4)}$$

Spherical polar coordinates

Spherical polar coordinates are convenient for situations with spherical symmetry. The coordinates are ρ, θ, ϕ where ρ is the radial distance from the origin to a point of interest *P*, θ is the angle from the x–y plane as for cylindrical coordinates and ϕ is the angle from the x–y plane to *P* (Figure A2.1c). In terms of Cartesian coordinates:

$$x = \rho\sin\phi\,\cos\theta; \quad y = \rho\sin\phi\,\sin\theta; \quad z = \rho\cos\phi \qquad \text{(A2.5)}$$

In terms of cylindrical coordinates:

$$r = \rho\sin\phi; \qquad \theta = \theta; \quad z = \rho\cos\phi \qquad \text{(A2.6)}$$

The unit vectors are $\hat{\rho}, \hat{\theta}, \hat{\phi}$
   The incremental elements are $d\rho$, $\rho d\theta$, $\rho\sin\theta\,d\phi$ so that

$$\mathbf{dr} = d\rho\,\hat{\rho} + \rho d\theta\,\hat{\theta} + \rho\sin\theta\,d\phi\,\hat{\phi} \qquad \text{(A2.7)}$$

The incremental volume is

$$dV = \rho^2\sin\theta\,d\rho\,d\theta\,d\phi \qquad \text{(A2.8)}$$

VECTOR ALGEBRA

Vectors, denoted by bold typeface have scalar components in the each of the directions defined by the coordinate system. For example, the position vector, **r**, in Cartesian coordinates is

$$\mathbf{r} = x\hat{\mathbf{i}} + y\hat{\mathbf{j}} + z\hat{\mathbf{k}} \qquad \text{(A2.9)}$$

The magnitude of **r**, denoted r is

$$r = |\mathbf{r}| = \sqrt{x^2 + y^2 + z^2} \qquad \text{(A2.10)}$$

Vectors, e.g., the magnetic flux density **B** have components B_x, B_y and B_z:

$$\mathbf{B} = B_x\hat{\mathbf{i}} + B_y\hat{\mathbf{j}} + B_z\hat{\mathbf{k}} \qquad \text{(A2.11)}$$

with a magnitude B:

$$B = |\mathbf{B}| = \sqrt{B_x^2 + B_y^2 + B_z^2} \qquad \text{(A2.12)}$$

Vector addition (and subtraction) is achieved by adding the respective components together:

$$\mathbf{A} + \mathbf{B} = \left(A_x + B_x\right)\hat{\mathbf{i}} + \left(A_y + B_y\right)\hat{\mathbf{j}} + \left(A_z + B_z\right)\hat{\mathbf{k}} \qquad \text{(A2.13)}$$

The scalar product, denoted "•" between vectors **A** and **B** at an angle θ to each other is

$$\mathbf{A} \cdot \mathbf{B} = AB\cos\theta \qquad \text{(A2.14)}$$

In terms of components

$$\mathbf{A} \cdot \mathbf{B} = \left(A_xB_x\right) + \left(A_yB_y\right) + \left(A_zB_z\right) \qquad \text{(A2.15)}$$

A and B are the magnitudes of **A** and **B**. The scalar product is commutative and distributive:

$$\mathbf{A} \cdot \mathbf{B} = \mathbf{B} \cdot \mathbf{A} \qquad \text{(A2.16)}$$

$$\mathbf{A} \cdot \left(\mathbf{B} + \mathbf{C}\right) = \mathbf{A} \cdot \mathbf{B} + \mathbf{B} \cdot \mathbf{C} \qquad \text{(A2.17)}$$

The vector product or *cross product*, denoted "×" between vectors **A** and **B** at an angle θ to each other is

$$\mathbf{A} \times \mathbf{B} = \begin{bmatrix} \hat{\mathbf{i}} & \hat{\mathbf{j}} & \hat{\mathbf{k}} \\ A_x & A_y & A_z \\ B_x & B_y & B_z \end{bmatrix}$$

$$= \left(A_yB_z - A_zB_y\right)\hat{\mathbf{i}} + \left(A_zB_x - A_xB_z\right)\hat{\mathbf{j}} + \left(A_xB_y - A_yB_x\right)\hat{\mathbf{k}} \qquad \text{(A2.18)}$$

Its magnitude is

$$|\mathbf{A} \times \mathbf{B}| = AB\sin\theta \qquad \text{(A2.19)}$$

The direction of the resultant vector is perpendicular to the plane containing the two initial vectors. The cross product is distributive but not commutative:

$$\mathbf{A} \times \mathbf{B} = -\mathbf{B} \times \mathbf{A} \qquad \text{(A2.20)}$$

VECTOR CALCULUS

Maxwell's equations utilize vector calculus. The following simply defines each operator. Consult a mathematics or electromagnetic physics textbook for a full discussion of the various theorems and identities.

The derivative

The derivative of a function f(x) with respect to x, denoted $\dfrac{df(x)}{dx}$ or f'(x) is the gradient of f measured over an infinitesimal increment Δx:

$$\frac{df(x)}{dx} = \lim_{\Delta x \to 0} \frac{f(x + \Delta x) - f(x)}{\Delta x} \tag{A2.21}$$

If f(x) is linear, then its derivative is a constant. For example, in MRI, the gradients are:

$$G_x = \frac{dB_z}{dx}; \qquad G_y = \frac{dB_z}{dy}; \qquad G_y = \frac{dB_z}{dz} \tag{A2.22}$$

The derivative of a constant is zero.

The time derivative of a vector **B** is

$$\frac{d\mathbf{B}}{dt} = \frac{dB_x}{dt}\hat{\mathbf{i}} + \frac{dB_y}{dt}\hat{\mathbf{j}} + \frac{dB_z}{dt}\hat{\mathbf{k}} \tag{A2.23}$$

The divergence and curl of a vector

The *divergence* of a vector is a scalar defined as

$$\nabla \cdot \mathbf{B} = \frac{dB_x}{dx} + \frac{dB_y}{dy} + \frac{dB_z}{dz} \tag{A2.24}$$

The *curl* of a vector is defined as

$$\nabla \times \mathbf{E} = \begin{bmatrix} \hat{\mathbf{i}} & \hat{\mathbf{j}} & \hat{\mathbf{k}} \\ \dfrac{d}{dx} & \dfrac{d}{dy} & \dfrac{d}{dz} \\ E_x & E_y & E_z \end{bmatrix} \tag{A2.25}$$

which expands as

$$\nabla \times \mathbf{E} = \left(\frac{dE_z}{dy} - \frac{dE_y}{dz}\right)\hat{\mathbf{i}} + \left(\frac{dE_x}{dz} - \frac{dE_z}{dx}\right)\hat{\mathbf{j}} + \left(\frac{dE_y}{dx} - \frac{dE_x}{dy}\right)\hat{\mathbf{k}} \tag{A2.26}$$

Vector integration

The integral of f(x) is equal to the area under the curve (Figure A2.2):

$$A = \int_{x_1}^{x_2} f(x)\, dx \tag{A2.27}$$

Integrals can be visualized by dividing the curve of f(x) into thin strips of thickness Δx and adding the areas of each of these strips together.

$$A = \sum_{x_1}^{x_2} f(x)\, \Delta x \tag{A2.28}$$

As $\Delta x \rightarrow 0$ the summation Equation A2.28 becomes the integral Equation A2.27. Integration is evaluated over limits x_1 and x_2. Often the limits are 0, ∞ (infinity) or $-\infty$ (minus infinity). For example, the integral

$$\int_0^2 x\, dx = \left[\frac{x^2}{2}\right]_0^2 = \frac{2^2}{2} - \frac{0^2}{2} = 2$$

In electromagnetic theory there are line integrals where the incremental component is **dl** or **dr**. Faraday induction utilizes a contour integral, evaluated around a loop or closed path:

$$\oint \mathbf{E} \cdot \mathbf{dl} = -\frac{d\Phi}{dt} \tag{A2.29}$$

Φ is the magnetic flux. Φ is given by a surface integral with two integrations, e.g. for dx and dy:

$$\Phi = \iint_S \mathbf{B} \cdot \mathbf{dS} \tag{A2.30}$$

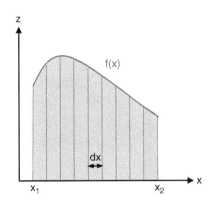

Figure A2.2   Integration and summation of a function f(x) with respect to x. The integral is the area of the shaded region.

For example, the magnetic flux from a uniform B normal to a surface of area A is

$$\Phi = \iint_S B_z \, dx \, dy = B_z A \tag{A2.31}$$

Volume integrals have three integrations with respect to each of the elemental increments dx, dy and dz or polar equivalents.

$$\iiint_V f(x,y,z) \, dx \, dy \, dz = \iiint_V f(r,\theta,z) r \, dr \, d\theta \, dz = \iiint_V f(\rho,\theta,\phi) \rho^2 \sin\theta \, d\rho \, d\theta \, d\phi \tag{A2.32}$$

For example, the volume of a sphere of radius a, using spherical coordinates is:

$$V = \int\int\int_{0,0,0}^{a,\pi,2\pi} dV = \int\int\int_{0,0,0}^{a,\pi,2\pi} \rho^2 \sin\theta \, d\rho \, d\theta \, d\phi$$

$$= \int_0^a \rho^2 \, d\rho \int_0^\pi \sin\theta \, d\theta \int_0^{2\pi} d\phi$$

$$= \left[\frac{1}{3}\rho^3\right]_0^a \left[-\cos\theta\right]_0^\pi \left[\phi\right]_0^{2\pi}$$

$$= \frac{1}{3}a^3 \left[1-(-1)\right] 2\pi = \frac{4}{3}\pi a^3$$

Appendix 3
Symbols and constants

Symbol	Definition	Unit	Value
α	flip angle	°	
$\not\gamma$	H^1 gyromagnetic ratio	MHz T^{-1}	42.58
γ	H^1 gyromagnetic ratio	radian s^{-1} T^{-1}	2.68×10^8
Γ	geometric factor for equivalent resistance		
δ	skin depth	m, μm	
ε_0	permittivity of free space	farads m^{-1}, F m^{-1}	8.85×10^{-12}
ε_r	relative permittivity		
η	coefficient of friction		
K	thermal conductivity	W m^{-1} $°C^{-1}$	
λ	wavelength	m	
μ_0	permeability of free space	henrys m^{-1}, H m^{-1}	$4\pi \times 10^{-7}$
μ_r	relative permeability		
ρ	density	kg m^{-3}	
σ	conductivity	siemens m^{-1}, S m^{-1}	
τ	time constant	s	
T	torque	newton-meter, N m	
Φ	magnetic flux	webers, Wb	
χ	magnetic susceptibility		
χ_{app}	apparent magnetic susceptibility		
ω	angular frequency = $2\pi f$	radian s^{-1}	
A	area	m^2	
a	radius, semi-major axis (ellipse)	m	

Essentials of MRI Safety, First Edition. Donald W. McRobbie.
© 2020 John Wiley & Sons Ltd. Published 2020 by John Wiley & Sons Ltd.

Symbol	Definition	Unit	Value
B	magnetic flux density	tesla, T	
B_0	MRI magnetic flux density	tesla, T	
B_1	RF magnetic field amplitude	μT	
B_{1+}	rotating RF magnetic field amplitude	μT	
b	radius, semi-minor axis (ellipse)	m	
C	specific heat capacity	$J\ kg^{-1}\ {}^\circ C^{-1}$	
c	velocity of light	$m\ s^{-1}$	3×10^8
C_A	concentration of contrast agent	$mmol\ kg^{-1}$	
Ch	chronaxie (strength-duration curve)	ms	
D	duty cycle		
d	diameter, length	m	
$d_{1,2,3}$	demagnetizing factor		
E	electric field	$volts\ m^{-1}$, $V\ m^{-1}$	
e	emissivity		
F	force	newton, N	
f	frequency	hertz, Hz	
f_0	Larmor/resonant frequency	MHz	
F_b	blood perfusion rate	$mL\ min^{-1}\ kg^{-1}$	
g	acceleration due to gravity	$m\ s^{-2}$	9.8
g_b	bulk blood flow	$kg\ s^{-1}\ kg^{-1}$	
$G_{SS,FE,PE}$	gradient amplitude (functional)	$mT\ m^{-1}$	
$G_{x,y,z}$	gradient amplitude (physical)	$mT\ m^{-1}$	
H	magnetic field strength or intensity	$A\ m^{-1}$	
H(f)	acoustic transfer function		
h	heat transfer coefficient	$W\ m^{-1}\ {}^\circ C^{-1}$	
I	current	ampere, A	
J	current density	$A\ m^{-2}$	
k	Boltzmann constant	$J\ K^{-1}$	1.38×10^{-23}
K_{cond}	conditional stability constant	log_{10}	
K_{therm}	thermodynamic stability constant	log_{10}	
L	characteristic length (thermal)	m	
L_{eq}	equivalent sound pressure level (SPL)	decibel, dB	
$L_{eq,d}$	daily equivalent SPL	decibel, dB	
L_{pk}	peak acoustic noise, Z-weighting	dB(Z)	
M	magnetization	$A\ m^{-1}$	

Symbol	Definition	Unit	Value
m	magnetic moment	A m^2	
m	mass	kg	
M_0	macroscopic magnetization (MRI)	A m^{-1}	
M_{xy}	transverse magnetization (MRI)		
M_z	longitudinal magnetization (MRI)		
N	number of turns per meter		
n	ratio of length to diameter of a cylinder		
N_A	Avogadro number, molecules per mole		6.022×10^{23}
P	power	watt, W	
p	pressure	pascal, Pa	
P_V	power density	W m^{-3}	
q	charge of an electron	C	1.602×10^{-19}
Q	electric charge	coulomb, C	
r	linear distance	m	
R	electrical resistance	ohm, Ω	
Rh	rheobase (strength-duration curve)	V m^{-1}, T s^{-1}	
R_m	equivalent resistance (tissue)	Ω	
r_1, r_2	relaxivity	L mmol^{-1} s^{-1}	
s	Stefan–Boltzmann constant	W m^{-2} K^{-4}	5.67×10^{-8}
S_0	reference sound intensity	pW m^{-2}	1
S_i	sound intensity	W m^{-2}	
t	time	second, s	
T	temperature	° kelvin (K) or celsius (C)	
T_1	longitudinal relaxation time	s	
T_2	transverse relaxation time	s	
T_c	critical temperature (superconductor)	kelvin, K	
TE	echo time	s	
TI	inversion time	s	
t_p	pulse duration	ms, µs	
TR	pulse sequence repetition time	s	
U	energy	joule, J	
v	velocity	m s^{-1}	
V	voltage (potential difference)	volt, V	
V	volume	m^3 or litre, L	
x, y, z	position	m	

Answers to revision questions

Chapter 1
1–C; 2–B; 3–E; 4–B; 5–D; 6–C, E

Chapter 2
1–A; 2–E; 3–D; 4–C, E; 5–C; 6–C; 7–C, D; 8–D; 9–E; 10–A

Chapter 3
1–C; 2–B; 3–E; 4–B; 5–D, E; 6–D.

Chapter 4
1–D; 2–B; 3–A; 4–C,D,E; 5–C; 6–A.

Chapter 5
1–T; 2–A; 3–B; 4–D; 5–E; 6–C or D; 7–E; 8–D.

Chapter 6
1–E; 2–D; 3–E; 4–D; 5–A; 6–B.

Chapter 7
1–E; 2– A, D; 3–A, B; 4–C, E.

Chapter 8
1–C; 2–B; 3–D; 4–C; 5–D; 6–E.

Chapter 9
1–E; 2–B; 3–B; 4–A; 5–D; 6–C; 7–B; 8–C; 9–D; 10–D; 11–B; 12–E.

Chapter 10
1–A; 2–E; 3–E; 4–B; 5–A, B, D; 6–B; 7–E; 8–C; 9–D; 10–D.

Chapter 11
1–E; 2–E; 3–C; 4–D; 5–B; 6–B; 7–D; 8–D.

Essentials of MRI Safety, First Edition. Donald W. McRobbie.
© 2020 John Wiley & Sons Ltd. Published 2020 by John Wiley & Sons Ltd.

Chapter 12
1–D; 2–E; 3–B; 4–C, E; 5–E; 6–A.

Chapter 13
1–A, B; 2–C, E; 3–C; 4–D; 5–B; 6–D.

Chapter 14
1–C; 2–E; 3–C; 4–A; 5–E; 6–D.

Index

Page numbers in **bold** indicate tables or boxes; page numbers in *italic* indicate figures

Essentials of MRI Safety, First Edition. Donald W. McRobbie.
© 2020 John Wiley & Sons Ltd. Published 2020 by John Wiley & Sons Ltd.

371